FACULTY
OF COLOR
IN THE
HEALTH
PROFESSIONS

DENA HASSOUNEH

Foreword by Charles R. Thomas Jr., MD

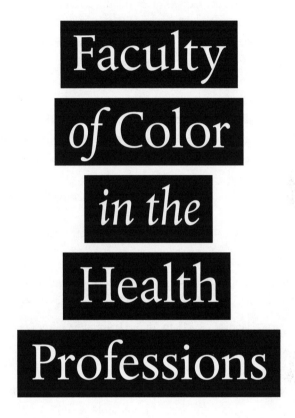

Faculty of Color in the Health Professions

STORIES OF SURVIVAL AND SUCCESS

Dartmouth College Press | Hanover, New Hampshire

Dartmouth College Press

An imprint of University Press of New England

www.upne.com

© 2018 Trustees of Dartmouth College

All rights reserved

Manufactured in the United States of America

Designed by Mindy Basinger Hill

Typeset in Albertina MT Pro

For permission to reproduce any of the material in this book,
contact Permissions, University Press of New England, One Court Street,
Suite 250, Lebanon NH 03766; or visit www.upne.com

Library of Congress Cataloging-in-Publication Data

NAMES: Hassouneh, Dena, author. | Thomas, Charles R., Jr.,
1957– writer of foreword.

TITLE: Faculty of color in the health professions: stories of survival and success /
Dena Hassouneh; foreword by Charles R. Thomas Jr., MD.

DESCRIPTION: Hanover, New Hampshire: Dartmouth College Press, [2017] |
Includes bibliographical references and index.

IDENTIFIERS: LCCN 2017007510 (print) | LCCN 2017009296 (ebook) |
ISBN 9781512601213 (cloth: alk. paper) | ISBN 9781512601220 (pbk.: alk. paper) |
ISBN 9781512601237 (epub, mobi, & pdf)

SUBJECTS: | MESH: Faculty, Medical—psychology | Prejudice |
Minority Groups—psychology | Attitude of Health Personnel |
Cultural Diversity | Leadership | United States

CLASSIFICATION: LCC R727 (print) | LCC R727 (ebook) | NLM W 19 AA1 |
DDC 610.73/706—dc23

LC record available at https://lccn.loc.gov/2017007510

5   4   3   2   1

The idea

that some lives

matter less

is the root of all

that is wrong

with the world.

Paul Farmer

CONTENTS

FOREWORD

Charles R. Thomas Jr., MD

Every faculty member of color, at one time or another, must try to reconcile experiences of racism with dominant cultural claims of equal opportunity, professionalism, and merit while serving in the academy. A key to surviving challenges and learning how to exploit opportunities in academic medicine and other health professions is to have a framework to navigate the terrain. To that end, *Faculty of Color in the Health Professions: Stories of Survival and Success*, by Dena Hassouneh, fills an important void by helping readers understand the experiences of faculty of color in US academic health centers and other health professions schools. This text was developed as a career development toolkit. I am very privileged to write this foreword to a long-overdue resource.

Over the past three decades I and my colleagues have learned to harness adaptive strategies to combat the bias that may shape how larger medical and health-care environments see us. To survive has taken a lot of emotional energy and no doubt has taken some vital years of my life. I suspect that if I had had access to the information that Dr. Hassouneh so eloquently articulates here, my road would have been less hazardous. For example, nearly every single academic physician from the African American diaspora with whom I have developed a deep professional and personal trust has shared an example of when he or she was in danger of being terminated from school, postgraduate training, and/or a faculty position. To be honest, these routine experiences of marginalization, invalidation, invisibility, and of course microaggressions happen to us throughout our educational and professional lives, beginning in elementary school and going on through attainment of senior leadership roles; they are synonymous with DWB (driving while black). Quite frankly, such experiences are an unnecessary and harmful rite of passage.

It is a tremendous burden knowing our human imperfections have the potential to reduce or eliminate opportunities for those who will come behind us. I feel this challenge on a regular basis and in response have practiced a form of de facto race-conscious professionalism throughout my career. Race-conscious professionalism is the process blacks confront when attempting to "navigate the competing demands of professionalism, racial obligations, and personal integrity" (1) p.914. Hassouneh's "Diversity and Equity Climate Stages Rubric" is novel and presents a concrete framework that institutional leaders and faculty can use throughout the ranks and in leadership. Furthermore, this book describes a myriad of coping strategies that come alive in participants' narratives, including one of my favorite methods, "strategic disengagement," a health (mental and physical) and career *survival* tool.

The most important aspect of *Faculty of Color in the Health Professions* is the solution-based message that is communicated to the reader. Such a message can extend far beyond academic medicine and other health professions, as our country has arrived at an important historical moment eerily similar to that in early 1930s Germany, when large numbers of people supported an explicitly xenophobic political platform. As I write this, xenophobia in political discourse has reached a fevered pitch in the United States. A substantial number of Americans support limiting the civil liberties of Muslims and banning this group from the country altogether in the context of an international refugee crisis. Walling off the Mexican border and questioning the qualifications of a supreme court justice on the basis of ethnicity is now part of the public sphere. Moreover, images of police dressed in military combat gear fighting citizens in cities across America have become commonplace as people have risen in outrage to protest the continued slaughter of black men. Although many have grieved over the murder of black boys at the hands of police, too many others rationalize these tragedies. Politically charged xenophobia toward diverse populations in the West ironically appears to be heightening as the sun sets on the Obama administration.

As such, I believe that this text is required reading for every chair of a faculty search committee, dean, department chair, research institute or center director, and diversity consultant, as well as faculty who want to broaden their perspective and develop a more sophisticated toolbox in this domain. The narratives and consistent themes described in this book, along with mandatory implicit bias training, will contribute to making *all* leaders in academic medicine and other health professions (current and future) more capable of addressing diversity and equity in health professions academe.

ACKNOWLEDGMENTS

I am deeply grateful for the contributions my friends and colleagues, Drs. Ann Beckett and Kristin Lutz, made to the study presented in this book. Ann and I began working together on studies of racism in nursing education sixteen years ago. She is a talented interviewer and a committed friend. Kristin, a grounded theory expert, joined our team for this study and lent valuable methodological expertise. I am indebted to Kristin for taking time out of her busy schedule to read and edit drafts of the chapters. She also went out of her way to send me information such as articles and data that proved useful in writing the book.

I would also like to express gratitude to my mentors, Drs. Christine Tanner and Judith Baggs, for their help and support. Dr. Tanner has had a profound influence on my career and as my Macy mentor provided me with guidance about how to secure a contract for this book. Dr. Baggs was generous with her time, reading and editing nearly every chapter in the book and offering encouragement along the way. I would also like to acknowledge the contributions of PhD students at Oregon Health & Science University, who assisted me with the analysis of data at various points.

Thank-you, Dr. Phyllis Deutsch, for being a wonderful editor and for your encouragement and support during what has been an arduous process.

I was fortunate to receive generous funding support from the Josiah Macy Jr. Foundation, which gave me precious time and funding to work on this project. I would also like to recognize the financial support of Sigma Theta Tau International, the Oregon Health & Science University Foundation, and the Oregon Health & Science University School of Nursing. Finally, I would like to express my profound gratitude to the participants for their willingness to share their stories, making this book possible.

Some quotations in this book were published previously. We received permission to reprint this text as follows:

Hassouneh, D., Akeroyd, J., Lutz, K., Beckett, A. Exclusion and control: patterns aimed at limiting the influence of faculty of color. *JNE*. 2012;51(6)314–325. Reprinted with permission from SLACK Incorporated.

Hassouneh, D. & Lutz, K. (2013). Faculty of color having influence in schools of nursing. *Nursing Outlook, 61,* 153–163. Reprinted with permission from Elsevier. http://www .nursingoutlook.org/article/S0029–6554(12)00290–4/abstract

Lutz, K.F., Hassouneh, D., Akeroyd, J., & Beckett, A. Balancing survival and resistance: experiences of faculty of color in predominantly Euro-American schools of nursing. *Journal of Diversity in Higher Education,* 6, 127–146. Published in 2013 by APA and reprinted with permission.

FACULTY
OF COLOR
IN THE
HEALTH
PROFESSIONS

Introduction

Revolution is not a one-time event.

Audre Lorde (2) p.140

More than ten years ago the Sullivan Commission on Diversity in the Health Care Workforce found that access to a health career was "largely separate and unequal" (3) p.iv. Despite this warning, underrepresentation of people of color in the health professions continues to be severe. This lack of racial and ethnic diversity has crippled the nation's ability to address the disproportionately high rates of morbidity and mortality affecting communities of color.

Significantly increasing the number and influence of faculty of color has the potential to unlock radical change in health care. Because of their life experiences, faculty of color are more likely than whites to understand the needs of patients, students, and communities of color and are therefore as a whole better able to improve educational and health outcomes for these groups. Greater understanding of the experiences of people of color is also important for the education of white students (4). Without strong and thriving faculty of color, equity and excellence in education and health care cannot be achieved. Yet health professions academe must change for faculty of color to thrive in greater numbers.

Opportunities in American life have been cumulatively shaped by the social construction of race and ethnicity since colonization. In the words of Garrison-Wade and colleagues, it is important "to remember that the lack of diversity in higher education is not some random accident" (5) p.108. The endemic nature of racism has created and continues to maintain structural, institutional, and interpersonal inequities in health professions education. In this book you will find ways to create policies, practices, and climates that promote the satisfaction and success of faculty of color and lead to a long-term shift toward social justice and equity in health professions education. This book presents findings from a national study of the experiences of faculty of color and makes recommendations for change. As you read participants' stories, I invite you to enter a space of understanding and make a personal commitment to eliminating inequities in health professions education, which in turn will transform health care. The stories offer detailed accounts of participants' experiences of racism and the strategies they used to cope with exclusion and control to achieve success. The stories also offer a rich description of participants' contributions to the health professions through their passionate dedication to students, patients, and communities.

Although conceptualizations of diversity and equity should not be used to define or limit perceptions of faculty of color, a book focused on their satisfaction and success in the context of social inequities requires an examination of these terms. *Diversity* has gained ground over unpopular equity frameworks in higher education by emphasizing the value of diverse workers as a marketable commodity (4, 6–9). Diversity is broadly defined and includes everyone. The goal of inclusion is to support differences in the workforce to enable all employees to fully contribute to the institution. This broad approach is less threatening to whites than *equity*, which focuses on correcting the historical disadvantages experienced by members of specific groups (10). With equity there is an expectation that health professions education should work equally well for all groups and result in equal outcomes. Thus, equity allows for differences in individual treatment if it helps groups achieve parity and close racial and ethnic gaps caused by systemic racism. Diversity and equity scholars have expressed concern that preference for the word *diversity* signals institutional indifference to change and may even be used to fortify rather than challenge social privilege (9). As you read this book, I urge you to think about the social and historical contexts that shaped participants' stories and the need to embrace equity to achieve a racially and ethnically diverse faculty and leadership in health professions education.

Little has been written about health professions education from the perspective of faculty of color. I explored the following questions through their lenses:

Why do so few faculty of color, in proportion to their representation in health professions schools, attain the rank of full professor and serve in academic leadership roles?

Why are health professions schools unable to recruit and retain a critical mass of faculty of color?

What factors are important for supporting faculty of color in health professions education?

What strategies can faculty of color use to be successful despite barriers?

How can we create an equitable structure and climate in health professions education and build avenues for success that benefit all faculty?

An Overview of Health Professions Education

Whites are overrepresented among health professions faculty, researchers, and clinicians compared to other groups, particularly in leadership (11–16). Blacks, Latino/as, and Native Americans are underrepresented minorities (URMs) across the health professions (17). Asians are overrepresented in all the professions but are underrepresented in nursing faculty (18); Native Hawaiian and Pacific Islanders are underrepresented in some areas but not others (18–20). Some authors have cited underrepresentation of US-born faculty of color as an unrecognized problem, suggesting the need to consider representation at the granular level (21, 22). These inequities have limited our ability to effectively provide education and health care to people of color in this country. Increasing the number and influence of faculty of color in health professions education advances equity while improving excellence in education, practice, and research (23). Recognizing the importance of racial and ethnic diversity for health professions education and the nation's health, some organizations such as the American Association of Medical Colleges (AAMC) and National League for Nursing (NLN) have called for an increase in the proportion of faculty of color in colleges and universities (24, 25).

The United States has approximately 272,261 health professions faculty in 2,043 nursing, 145 medical, 33 osteopathic, 135 pharmacy, and 66 dental schools (19, 20, 26–33). Each of these professions has its own culture as well as departments and specialties that operate as subcultures.

Academic health professions institutions have a common hierarchical structure. Higher academic rank and administrative leadership roles have greater institutional power, but faculty of color are underrepresented in these positions (16, 34, 35). Education, research, and practice are the missions of most institutions, and achievements in both teaching and research are usually necessary to achieve tenure. Hence, an investment of time to conduct research is important for faculty success in promotion and tenure. There are large numbers of non-tenure-track clinical faculty in the health professions; scholarship expectations for this group are different than for tenure-track faculty but can still be substantial. Institutional support is crucial to the success of faculty who want to launch a research program. This support often includes funding for graduate research assistants, research and laboratory equipment and materials, office space and support, computers and software, and starting a project or lab. How much an institution will invest in faculty research time and materials is often individually negotiated with administration, making it a potential source of inequity among faculty.

Teaching and mentoring students takes a great deal of time. For the purpose of simplicity, throughout this book the word *student* refers to a learner at any level, whether an undergraduate, a graduate, or a postgraduate trainee, unless otherwise specified in a specific context. Students often feel more comfortable with faculty from similar backgrounds and seek them out for classes or mentorship. When faculty of color are few, as is the case with URMs, these student relationships, though fulfilling, can lead to overload. Despite this reality, study findings and the higher education literature generally indicate that faculty of color do not receive additional workload credit to compensate them for this contribution, which means they have less time to meet other goals. Further, although institutions use the rhetoric of diversity, they tend not to reward diversity- and equity-related teaching, research, service, and practice (36). Therefore, faculty of color, who are heavily overrepresented among those engaged in diversity and equity work, are disadvantaged as scholars. There are also other covert barriers to faculty of color's getting promotion and tenure that are not widely acknowledged. I describe some of these covert barriers in this book.

Contributions of Faculty of Color That Are Crucial to the Nation's Health

Persistent and embarrassing health inequities in the United States have put health professions education in the spotlight. Thirty-one years ago the *Report of the Secretary's Task Force on Black & Minority Health*, or the Heckler Report (37), called for action to eliminate health inequities. Several landmark reports have followed, documenting racial and ethnic inequities in health and health-care delivery and recommending that health professions education make changes to increase the racial and ethnic diversity of the health-care workforce (3, 38, 39). Increasing the number and influence of faculty of color in the health professions must happen to achieve this goal.

In an increasingly diverse US society, differences in perspectives between whites and people of color must be bridged to achieve the effective delivery of care. A pronounced and therefore easy to recognize example of differences in perspective between racial groups is evident in white and black Americans' perceptions of the criminal justice system. A 2013 survey of racial equity found that seven in ten black respondents and about one-third of whites believe blacks are treated less fairly in their dealings with the police (40). Other fairness questions on the survey also revealed large racial differences, reflecting the different life experiences of whites and blacks with the criminal justice system. There are also differences between the experiences of whites and blacks in many other areas of life, as is the case with other racial and ethnic groups. Some of these differences are stark, and others are subtle. Because human experience and health are intricately interconnected, understanding and addressing diverse life stories is an essential part of effective health-care delivery (41). The diverse perspectives faculty of color bring to health care add strength to the professions, but it is the responsibility of all faculty, regardless of race or ethnic background, to make these human connections.

The contributions of faculty of color to health professions education, which benefit all groups, are extensive and far-reaching. Although work on diversity and equity is not the sole purview of faculty of color, and their contributions extend well beyond this focus, the literature reflects their strong influence on teaching cultural humility and professionalism (42); minority student recruitment, mentoring, and retention (4, 43, 44); and clinical practice and research with minority and medically underserved communities (45–47). The findings of the study reported here are consistent with this literature. Moreover, the unique perspectives of participants prompted many to investigate research questions based on their communities' needs and concerns, even though these lines of inquiry are often devalued in higher education, making it more difficult to obtain research funding and publish scholarly work (48–54). The hegemonic influence of empiricism in science fields has been identified as detrimental to the faculty pipeline because scholars of color are more likely to choose fields such as the humanities or education, which are more supportive of the use of social justice lenses in research (4, 55). Yet it was because of their understanding and connection with communities of color that participants' research was powerful.

Efforts to Increase Faculty of Color
in the Health Professions

Efforts to increase the number of faculty of color in the health professions include pipeline programs, recruitment and retention plans, debiasing interventions, and faculty development and mentoring programs (56–65). The need to increase the racial and ethnic diversity of the health-care workforce and thereby promote the nation's health has been cited by the Institute of Medicine and other organizations as the reason why health professions education should devote time and resources to such programs (39). Although it is clear the nation's educational and health inequities cannot be corrected without faculty of color, and findings from this study provide further support for the urgent need to increase the number and influence of racially and ethnically diverse faculty, it is important to recognize the rights of people of color to equal representation in the health professions as the primary justification for diversity and equity efforts. By virtue of their humanity, people of color have a right to enjoy equitable power, access, opportunities, treatment, impacts, and outcomes in the health professions and in health professions education (66, 67). Working to achieve this racial justice is essential for health professions education to move forward to a more socially just and equitable future.

The State of Diversity in Health Professions Education

Current representation of faculty of color is inconsistent with numerous and long-standing calls for increased racial and ethnic diversity in the health professions, such as those issued by the Institute of Medicine (39), health professions educational organizations (24, 68–70), and colleges and universities. The most recent data available on representation of students and faculty of color in nursing, medicine, pharmacy, and dentistry relative to the general population are provided in tables 1 and 2.

A review of trends in the representation of faculty of color in health professions education reveals a disturbing lack of progress among URMs. The American Association of Colleges of Nursing (AACN) reported an increase in all URM faculty combined between 2006 and 2015 of 4.4 percent (18). Considering that the annual growth rate of the US Latino/a population alone from 2005 to 2010 was 3.4 percent, a 4.4 percent increase over nine years in combined URM nursing faculty does not reflect real progress (78). Moreover, the AAMC reported that from 2007 to 2011 the percentage of black, Native American, Mexican American, Puerto Rican, Cuban, and multiple Hispanic faculty remained exactly the same. Asian, Native Hawaiian and other Pacific Islander, multiple races, and other Hispanic categories decreased during that period (79). Pharmacy faculty have

TABLE 1. Enrollment of Racial and Ethnic Minorities in Health Professions Schools Relative to US Higher Education and the General Population

ENROLLMENT IN US INSTITUTIONS	BLACK (PERCENT)	LATINO/A (PERCENT)	NATIVE AMERICAN/ ALASKA NATIVE (PERCENT)	ASIAN (PERCENT)	NATIVE HAWAIIAN/ OTHER PACIFIC ISLANDER (PERCENT)	TWO OR MORE RACES (PERCENT)
Nursing baccalaureate 2016 (71)	9.9	10.4	.5	8.1*	N/A	2.7
Nursing master's 2016 (71)	14.3	7.2	.6	8.0*	N/A	2.2
Nursing PhD 2016 (71)	16.2	5.6	1.2	6.4*	N/A	1.5
Medicine 2016 (72)	6.3	5.0	.2	20.5	.1	7.8
Doctor of pharmacy (first professional degree) (73)	7.9	5.0	.3	25.0	.4	2.3
Pharmacy master's 2015 (full time) (73)	2.8	4.9	.1	9.0	.4	1.2
Dentistry 2014 (30)	4.3	8.5	.3	23.4	.1	3.0
General postsecondary enrollment 2014 (74)	14.5	16.5	.8	6.3	.3	3.3
General population 2015 (75)	13.3	17.6	1.2	5.6	.2	2.6

*Includes Native Hawaiian or other Pacific Islander

TABLE 2. Racial and Ethnic Composition of Health Professions Faculty Relative
to US Higher Education and the General Population

US HEALTH PROFESSIONAL SCHOOLS	BLACK (PERCENT)	LATINO/A (PERCENT)	NATIVE AMERICAN/ ALASKA NATIVE (PERCENT)	ASIAN (PERCENT)	NATIVE HAWAIIAN/ OTHER PACIFIC ISLANDER (PERCENT)	TWO OR MORE RACES (PERCENT)
Nursing 2016 (18)	7.2	2.7	.4	2.9	.4	1.3
Medicine 2015 (19, 72)	3.0	2.2	.1	14.6	.1	5.3
Pharmacy (full time) 2016 (20)	4.5	2.9	.2	14.7	.1	1.0
Dentistry (full time) 2013 (76)	4.9	8.6	.3	12.2	3.4	.4
Postsecondary faculty 2013 (77)	5.6	4.2	.44	9.0	.15	.7
General population 2015 (75)	13.3	17.6	1.2	5.6	.2	2.6

not fared much better. From 2008 to 2016 black and Latino/a faculty decreased from 5.6 to 4.4 percent and 3 to 2.9 percent respectively, while Native Americans improved slightly, from .1 to .2 percent (20, 80). Dental education showed the greatest improvement among the professions, increasing the total URM full-time faculty from 561 in 2010 to 699 in 2014 (81).

Since passage of the 1964 Civil Rights Act, health professions education has garnered significant achievements in education, research, and practice while at the same time failing to diversify the faculty. This might suggest that lack of racial and ethnic diversity in health professions faculty is an intractable problem, but that is not so. Health professionals of color are underutilized in academia, and there has always been a talent pool available to develop to increase the supply. What is needed are leaders with the heart to prioritize a comprehensive array of robust diversity efforts above other competing interests, such as leading a strong political movement to increase funding to support racial and ethnic diversity in the health professions and implementing educational policy changes.

Thinking Errors That Obstruct Hiring and Advancement of Faculty of Color

Pervasive inequities have created an undersupply of faculty in the health professions. Given this reality, one would expect academic institutions to aggressively recruit health professionals of color for faculty positions. Yet available evidence suggests otherwise. As described by Smith, "many . . . believe that the academy's commitment to diversity, combined with a limited supply of minority-group scholars, has created a bidding war that favors faculty of color over white men" (82) p.21. Such views are often used as an excuse for not taking the necessary steps to increase racial and ethnic faculty diversity. In a study of the academic job market, Smith found only 11 percent of URMs were sought out by an institution. Further, Turner and Myers's analysis of PhD degrees conferred by US institutions from 1977 to 1990 found the supply of URMs was underutilized. Low salaries had a greater effect on representation of faculty of color than availability of those with PhDs (83).

Hiring and advancement of faculty of color is also hindered by the common concern that candidates of color are less qualified than their white counterparts (84). Many participants shared stories of whites questioning their qualifications and expertise. In the post–civil rights era, arguments for such beliefs are sometimes based on the unsubstantiated view that affirmative action (assumptions are made about candidates regardless of whether or not they actually benefited from affirmative action) yields substandard faculty. But the real basis for this belief has much deeper roots. America's scientific and medical communities have reified claims of whites' intellectual superiority over racialized others for centuries (85, 86); discussion of historical and new claims of innate racial differences continues today (87, 88). Research reporting racial differences in IQ is ongoing, and although interpretations of these differences are mostly different now than in the past, scholars are still working from the same old constructs (89–93). In her remarkable book *Breathing Race into the Machine: The Surprising Career of the Spirometer from Plantation to Genetics,* Lundy Braun pointed out "cultural assumptions about race and ethnicity are informed by 'normal' or routine scientific and technological practices" (94) p.xx. Thus, those who dismiss claims of whites' intellectual superiority as pseudoscience while comfortably embracing the "real" science of today as divorced from political and social forces should reconsider. From the time they began, the US health sciences have explored new knowledge based on an ideology of racial difference. As members of the scientific community, faculty take in and perpetuate this taken-for-granted explanatory framework of racial difference. Hence, faculty are steeped in biases affecting their perceptions of the competence of people of color. Perceptions of faculty of color as struggling (95, 96), weak, deficient, or less than whites must be stringently challenged to ensure health professions education fully accesses the available supply of racial and ethnic minorities prepared for the faculty role.

Minority-Serving Institutions and the Health Professions Pipeline

Until the implicit bias of white gatekeepers is addressed, increasing the number of health professionals of color alone will not sufficiently improve representation of racial and ethnic minorities among health professions faculty, yet attention to supply is nonetheless critical. Minority-serving institutions, which are a major source of URM college graduates, are central to efforts to nourish the pipeline for faculty of color in the health professions. *Minority-serving institution* refers to historically black colleges and universities, Hispanic-serving institutions, tribal colleges and universities, and Asian American– and Native American/Pacific

Islander–serving institutions. These institutions evolved in response to historical inequity, lack of access to predominantly white institutions, and increases in US racial and ethnic minority populations (97).

The nation's 105 historically black colleges and universities are the only institutions created for the sole purpose of educating blacks. In 2011 historically black colleges and universities represented only 3 percent of higher education institutions in the country, but they enrolled 11 percent of black students (98). *Hispanic-serving institution* refers to degree-granting institutions with an undergraduate Hispanic full-time equivalent student enrollment of 25 percent or higher coupled with a substantial enrollment of low-income students. In 2013, 409 institutions were eligible for the Hispanic-serving designation (99). In 2011 Hispanic-serving institutions made up only 6 percent of all higher education institutions but enrolled nearly 50 percent of Latino/a undergraduates. Hence, as a group these institutions play a critical role in making college accessible to Latino/a students (97, 100). Tribal colleges and universities are chartered by their respective tribal governments. Currently there are 37 tribal colleges and universities; 34 are fully accredited, and 12 offer baccalaureate degrees. In 2012, 78.5 percent of all associate's degrees and 88.4 percent of all bachelor's degrees conferred by tribal colleges and universities were awarded to Native Americans (101). *Asian American– and Native American/Pacific Islander–serving institutions* refers to degree-granting institutions with an undergraduate Asian American/Pacific Islander full-time equivalent student enrollment of 10 percent or higher coupled with a substantial enrollment of low-income students (102). In 2016, 133 higher education institutions were eligible for this designation (103). Although Asian American– and Native American/Pacific Islander–serving institutions comprised only 3.4 percent of higher education institutions in 2010, they enrolled 41.2 percent of Asian American/Pacific Islander undergraduate students and conferred 47.3 percent and 25.3 percent of associate's and bachelor's degrees respectively awarded to this population nationally. Like other minority-serving institution student populations, a large proportion of Asian American/Pacific Islander students attending such institutions were from low-income backgrounds, were the first in their families to attend college, and struggled to pay for school (102). Hence, Asian American– and Native American/Pacific Islander–serving institutions play an important role in expanding Asian American/Pacific Islander students' access to higher education.

Minority-Serving Institutions and
Health Professions Education

Because of the large numbers of URMs they serve, minority-serving institutions are critical to efforts to increase racial and ethnic diversity in the health professions. Fifty percent of the top twenty schools conferring science, technology, engineering, and math (STEM) degrees on blacks and Latino/as are historically black colleges and universities and Hispanic-serving institutions. One tribal university is among the top twenty institutions conferring STEM degrees to Native Americans, and seven Asian American– and Native American/Pacific Islander–serving institutions are among the top twenty institutions conferring STEM degrees on this group (97). A substantial number of URMs with doctoral degrees in STEM fields received their undergraduate education at a minority-serving institution (104, 105). But a sizable proportion of minority-serving institutions are two-year colleges, including 12 percent of historically black colleges and universities, 54 percent of Hispanic-serving institutions, 67 percent of tribal colleges and universities, and 55 percent of Asian American– and Native American/Pacific Islander–serving institutions. Two-year colleges' open door policy and relatively low prices provide an important educational pathway for working-class racial and ethnic minority students (106), highlighting the need for robust pipeline programs that target these institutions.

Despite their importance, minority-serving institutions are underresourced and underutilized. In medicine and dentistry the need for practitioners of color has been recognized for decades, yet prospective students can apply to only three historically black schools of medicine and two of dentistry (107). In my review of tribal colleges and universities, I identified seven registered nurse and seven practical nurse degree programs. In addition, I found associate's degree transfer programs with titles specific to health professions careers as follows: seven prenursing, two premed, one pre-prepharmacy, one predentistry, and one preoptometry. Other tribal colleges and universities also offer associate's transfer degrees designed to prepare students for a health sciences career using general titles such as biomedical science, life science, and allied health. Some tribal colleges and universities also offer associate's transfer degrees and certificate programs in areas such as emergency services, human services, social work, chemical dependency, dental assisting, and vision care technology. I also found five programs conferring social and health-related bachelor's degrees and one master's program in human services. Given their track record of educating Native Americans and the cultural integrity they provide, building capacity at tribal colleges and universities, which currently offer mostly two-year health-related degrees or certificate programs, is an important strategy to increase representation of Native Americans in the health-care workforce. Tribal colleges' and universities' current limited capacity and lack of higher degree health professions programs prevents them from graduating desperately needed clinicians in local areas.

The contributions of Hispanic-serving institutions in developing the Latino/a health-care workforce and faculty pipeline are major. In 2013, of the top twenty-five institutions where Latino/as earned associate's, bachelor's, master's, and doctoral degrees in health, fourteen, sixteen, eleven, and five, respectively, were Hispanic-serving institutions. Moreover, nine Hispanic-serving institutions were in the top twenty-five institutions where Latino/as earned their first health professions degree (108). In addition, the Hispanic-Serving Health Professions Schools consortium was developed in 1992 in response to President Bill Clinton's Executive Order 12900, "Educational Excellence for Hispanic Americans," and Health and Human Service's "Hispanic Agenda for Action: Improving Services to Hispanic Americans" initiative (109). There are currently thirty-one US-accredited schools and colleges of nursing, medicine, public health, pharmacy, and dentistry in the consortium. The consortium offers training opportunities for students, academic and career opportunities for professionals, support to faculty and students seeking academic positions, and support for member institutions seeking research funding to promote Latino/a health (110).

Collectively, minority-serving institutions offer students of color opportunities for education at multiple levels in culturally supportive academic environments, opening the door to a possible future as a health professions faculty. In a primer on minority-serving institutions, Gasman and colleagues described tribal colleges and universities as being defined by "sensitivity to students' varied levels of preparation and time constraints, relevant degree programs and teaching, support for developmental education, and highly supportive faculty" (100) p.133. Students of color who are educationally or economically disadvantaged face barriers to admission and graduation in health professions programs; because most institutions are predominantly white, all students of color face obstacles that white students do not. For students of color who are educationally or economically disadvantaged, attending institutions with the philosophy and supports described by these authors can make the difference between dropping out and becoming a future faculty member.

About the Study

I enlisted the help of two co-investigators to complete this study. Dr. Ann Beckett, a black faculty member with experience working at both a historically black university and a predominantly white institution, and Dr. Kristin Lutz, a white faculty member, both contributed to development of the interview guides, conducted interviews, and assisted with data analysis. Dr. Beckett's contribution to conducting interviews was particularly substantial; she collected data from thirty-six participants. The knowledge, expertise, and perspectives Drs. Beckett and Lutz brought to the study were invaluable. Dr. Edward Junkins, a medical school faculty member of color, served as a consultant and also contributed to the integrity of the analysis. We interviewed faculty from nursing, medicine, pharmacy, and dentistry schools by profession, completing our work with each school's faculty before going on to the next profession. We then incorporated all of the data into our analysis. This allowed us to compare data both within and across professions.

PARTICIPATING FACULTY

We interviewed one hundred us health professions faculty who self-identified as people of color. Ninety-six came from predominantly white institutions, and four came from historically black colleges and universities. There were forty men and sixty women in the sample. Some 58 percent of the participants were black, 20 percent Asian, 14 percent Latino/a, 5 percent Middle Eastern, and 3 percent Native American. Twenty-four percent of our sample was foreign born. I use these racial and ethnic categories because they emerged organically from the data, reflecting their everyday use; I also recognize that the concepts of race and ethnicity themselves are Western ideological inventions (111–113). Participants came from a variety of specialties, such as psychiatry, community health nursing, pharmaceutical science, and pediatric dentistry. Some 21 percent of participants occupied formal leadership positions, including one dean and several department chairs, and the sample included all academic ranks: instructors (15 percent), assistant professors (33 percent), associate professors (32 percent), and professors (20 percent). Participants were sampled from different types of institutions, including research-intensive (n = 78) and teaching-focused (n = 22), small and large, religious and secular, and public and private schools. Because we recruited our sample through educator listservs and word of mouth, I was not able to calculate how many faculty of color viewed the study announcement but decided not to participate. With the exception of dentistry, the disciplines were well represented. We had great difficulty recruiting dental school faculty, who make up just 10 percent of the sample. When we encountered this difficulty, we asked participants why this might be happening. One participant answered: "[In dentistry] we are ultraconservative . . . and what you may be experiencing is that some of the faculty members' academic careers, their retirement—everything is depending on them staying at that school . . . so some of what you are getting is a fear of people being outed . . . they don't want this to get back to their schools. If you remember I asked you about identifiers [whether participants would be identified in our published work]. Because there are only so many battles even I want to fight." A number of participants asked fearfully whether they would be identified. One medical school department chair said, "I'm just going to trust you. You're not going to hurt me, okay?" Many participants expressed a level of fear that likely affected recruitment for our study and in itself reflects a major problem in health professions education.

INTERVIEW FORMAT

We conducted semistructured interviews ranging from 30 to 120 minutes long; most interviews lasted 90 minutes. *Semistructured* means that we used a set of questions, but the questions were open-ended to allow for personal responses and elaboration. The length of interviews varied depending on the amount of information participants had to share and the time they had available for participation. Interviews were done in person (15 percent) and by telephone (85 percent). All interviews were audio-recorded and transcribed verbatim. During the interviews we asked participants to share their stories, including aspects of their careers that stood out for them. We asked when they had felt most respected and valued and when they had felt most disrespected. We also asked if they had ever experienced racism and about their relationships with students, mentors, and leaders. The questions were nonleading to allow the participants to share their stories in the ways most meaningful to them. Recognizing the intersectional nature of human experience, we also asked about the influence of gender and considered the influence of contexts such as type of school and discipline on participants' experiences. We used grounded theory as described by Glaser and Charmaz to guide our analysis and collected follow-up data with 20 percent of interviewees by repeat interview or written correspondence (114–116). We followed up in order to clarify meanings, learn more about emerging themes, and ask participants whether or not we were accurately capturing the meaning of their narratives in our analysis.

Although narratives from all of the professions are substantively represented in the book as a whole, including the strongest quotes for corresponding themes was my primary concern. Therefore, narrative representation of the professions throughout the book is not uniform. I also converted some qualitative data into numerical data to supplement the analysis. In presenting the findings, I have endeavored to offer a rich, thick description to enable readers to transfer findings relevant to their contexts. The concept of transferability is based on a philosophical assumption that the multiplicity of contexts in which complex human phenomena occur precludes the possibility of generalizing research findings from the human sciences homogeneously across settings. At the same time, the study is grounded in the assumption that faculty of color possess a privileged view about their own experiences and the workings of racism in academe. Hence, faculty of color will be able to assess the transferability of findings most accurately; white faculty must guard against distortions wrought by white privilege and racial bias when taking on this task.

All participants gave permission for their narratives to be used in this research, and we pledged to do our best to protect their identities. For this reason, I removed identifying information from all the examples in this book. I avoided identifying cities and states and have referred only to regions of the country. All the names in this book are fictitious, and I have changed any details that could identify a participant while remaining true to the meaning of the text. I deliberately omitted a table listing individual demographic characteristics to minimize the likelihood of participants being recognized.

Overview of the Book

Chapter 1 presents findings about racist processes in health professions education. From these findings, you will learn about the manifestations and consequences of white privilege in health professions education and strategies you can use to change the status quo. The enactment of Eurocentric norms and white privilege devalued participants' individuality and facilitated their exclusion from social and professional life. Participants who were underrepresented, had darker skin, and were more outspoken about racial equity experienced greater marginalization. Although most of the institutional leaders described by participants touted the value of diversity, their experiences suggest that these words lacked substance. Inequity in pay, workload, and access to leadership opportunities was commonly reported. Many participants were also supervised more closely and disciplined more harshly than white colleagues. Some described being afraid to assume the full authority of their faculty role because of lack of leadership support should someone complain about them, such as might occur if they failed a white student. Although most of the racism experienced by participants was covert, overt racism was also reported, including physical attack. I discuss the consequences of racism for participants, including isolation, inequities in promotion and tenure, feeling the need to prove oneself, and harm to self-confidence.

From chapter 2 you will gain tools and strategies to assess and improve the diversity and equity climate at your institution. The chapter presents a model of institutional climate that portrays an institution's recruitment and retention, faculty and student racial and ethnic diversity, diversity programs, reports of racism, dialogue, and leadership based on level of inclusivity across four stages (ranging from least inclusive to most inclusive). Participants in inclusive institutional climates were the most satisfied and enjoyed the greatest opportunities for success. The chapter offers specific positive and negative examples of institutional practices and a rubric for institutional climate assessment that can be used by individual faculty and leaders to inform decision making. I conclude the chapter by reviewing current accreditation standards in academic nursing, medicine, pharmacy, and dentistry and calling on accrediting bodies to play a more aggressive role in mandating meaningful and measurable change toward educational equity in the health professions. Current standards fall short of the educational reforms needed to prepare a sufficiently racially and ethnically diverse health-care workforce to meet the health needs of the US population.

Chapter 3 presents findings about the importance of strong and committed mentors and leaders as keys to change. From these findings you will learn about the mentoring needs of faculty and leaders of color and programs, as well as strategies that will help ensure that their needs are met. The support of mentors, preferably at the same institution, was vital to participants' satisfaction and success; many cultivated these relationships. The presence of a leader who strongly supported diversity and equity and protected and nurtured faculty of color was also important. These mentors and leaders could be faculty of color or white faculty; the key characteristic was their strong support. As I present these findings I discuss the role of leaders in implementing institutional policies and practices supportive of the mentoring needs of faculty of color and highlight their responsibility for mentoring faculty of color into leadership positions. The chapter concludes by exploring mentorship needs specific to faculty of color.

Chapter 4 describes common strategies used to thrive in academia reported by participants. If you are a faculty member of color, learning about these strategies may enhance your satisfaction and will increase the likelihood of your achieving success. Thriving in academia required a fine-tuned awareness of personal and academic values and of the institutional climate, strategic approaches to dealing with interpersonal and institutional racism, and proactive management of professional opportunities. Chapter 4 reveals these skills and approaches, systematically outlining examples shared by successful participants.

Chapter 5 documents the significant and unique impact that participants had on health professions education. In this chapter you will learn about these vital contributions and what changes are needed to better recognize and reward the work of faculty of color. Participants' work in teaching, research, service, and practice was both excellent and varied, including contributions to educational and health equity. Participants' unique positioning led to a striking connection to students, patients, and communities of color. Through their life experiences and community connections, participants brought diverse perspectives to their academic positions. These experiences included coming from a nondominant culture, facing discrimination, and in some cases coping with extreme economic disadvantage. Participants were able to relate to people who were different from themselves while also understanding the experiences of people of color from similar backgrounds. This chapter shows how this strength grounded participants' contributions, such as mentoring students of color; teaching about the social determinants of health and cultural humility; serving on admissions committees with an eye toward increasing racial and ethnic diversity in the student body; and providing respectful, culturally congruent care to minority and medically underserved communities.

Chapter 6 examines differences in experiences among participants by gender, class background, foreign-born status, and race/ethnicity. The inherently artificial nature of separating people into such groupings makes it inevitable that various social identities are threaded throughout these sections. In this chapter you will learn about the differences in experiences within and across these groupings, with a particular focus on the impact of sexism, classism, migration, xenophobia, and racism on participants' experiences. To contextualize the data, I frame findings with information obtained from US population surveys and historical reports. This chapter also describes participants' experiences at historically black colleges and universities. Although all minority-serving institutions make important contributions to health professions education, this book focuses exclusively on historically black colleges and universities, which have the longest history of educating health professionals of color in this country.

The study raises important issues about the experiences and contributions of faculty of color in the health professions. When faculty of color succeed in health professions education, they add perspectives that strongly support the traditional tripartite mission of teaching, research, and practice while promoting educational and health equity. Listening to the voices of faculty of color provides an opportunity to understand their experiences and learn from them. This book shares lessons learned from the courageous faculty who participated in this study, in the hope that it will contribute to the satisfaction and success of faculty of color, foster equity in health professions education, and promote improvements in the nation's health.

CHAPTER ONE

Swimming Upstream

EXCLUSION AND CONTROL

OF FACULTY OF COLOR

Dr. Christian Head, a black surgeon and faculty member at the UCLA School of Medicine, was subjected to ongoing racism, including threats and harassment by administrators, faculty, and residents within his department. Despite his reporting this behavior and seeking assistance from university channels, the racist behavior continued unabated. A particularly disturbing and public example occurred in a racist slide show at a resident roast attended by faculty, graduating residents, and their spouses:

> [A] series of 20 slides, describing me as a poor doctor . . . then the final slide
> was a photo of a gorilla on all fours with my head photo shopped onto the
> gorilla, with a smile on my face, and a Caucasian man, completely naked,
> sodomizing me from behind, and my boss'[s] head photo shopped on the
> person, smiling. I could feel the pressure in my chest, listening to them laugh.
> I waited until the laughter subsided, and then I approached the podium, and I
> pulled my boss aside, Dr. Gerald Berke, and I said to him, "How could you let
> this happen? How could you do this?" And he just smiled and chuckled, you
> know . . . "What's the problem?" (Dr. Christian Head, quoted in an interview
> with The Root) (117)

In the West people of European descent have historically been viewed as superior, while people of color have been viewed as inferior and labeled as "Other" in society (118–121). This belief is the basis for racism, a system of racial domination that confers unearned privileges on whites while excluding people of color in all areas of life (122, 123). Maintenance of racialized hierarchies governing resource distribution is the hallmark of this oppressive system (124). Despite tangible and persistent evidence to the contrary, many Americans believe systemic and institutional racism is a problem of the past, citing the election of President Barack Obama as evidence of a postracial turn (123, 125). Indeed, a recent study documented common perceptions among whites that antiwhite discrimination in the United States is a now bigger problem than antiblack bias (126). Similarly, dominant views in higher education now take for granted the existence of a postracial academy (127). The ideology of color blindness, which pretends indifference to race and ethnicity while leaving structural inequalities in place, perpetuates this problem (123, 128). Institutions that assert the value of diversity while failing to engage in discussions about the importance of race and ethnicity reinforce the invisibility and hence the hegemonic power of whiteness in higher education (129, 130).

Although the civil rights movement removed the most visible and blatant means of producing and reproducing racial inequality in US education, another layer of racism and discrimination remains beneath the surface. Identifying, analyzing, and understanding the mechanisms through which racial inequality persists is critical to addressing this problem (131). Many participants experienced racism, sometimes overt but more often covert, occurring through processes I have named *exclusion* and *control*. Exclusion and control co-occur and are interrelated and mutually reinforcing systematic processes, rooted in the overlapping effects of individual, interpersonal, institutional, and cultural racism. Together, these processes constrain the important influence that faculty of color bring to health professions education.

Evidence suggests that modern and aversive racism, forms of individual and interpersonal covert racism, are often caused by implicit bias (132–135). *Implicit bias* refers to the attitudes or stereotypes that affect our understanding, actions, and decisions in an unconscious manner. Such bias provides a foundation for institutional and cultural racism. Theorists have suggested that modern racists express bias indirectly through their attitudes, such as opposition to equity measures, rather than directly, such as support for segregation. Aversive racists espouse egalitarian values and thus only discriminate when other non-race-related factors, such as perceived lack of performance, can be used to justify discriminatory behavior. Rather than creating out-group hostility, aversive racism creates prosocial behavior toward whites. Hence, aversive racists discriminate in favor of whites (136). Some participants in this study rejected implicit bias theory, believing that people know when they are being racist. Critiques of implicit bias theory in the literature raise similar questions about personal accountability for racist acts. Participants were not always able to determine the intent behind racist acts, and their efforts to discern the true nature and intent behind acts of covert racism were often exhausting.

Because racial and ethnic stereotypes vary by group, participants' experiences sometimes differed by race and ethnicity. Among participants, black faculty experienced the most frequent and severe exclusion and control; however, participants from all racial and ethnic groups reported these experiences. For women, gender intersected with race and ethnicity, creating a raced-gendered experience. This is consistent with the concept of intersectionality, which describes how various aspects of social identity such as race and gender interact to shape the multiple dimensions of the human experience (137–142).

This chapter presents examples from participants' stories that describe their experiences with exclusion and control. The exclusion strategies identified in this study are invalidation, being treated like an outsider, and unequal standards and access to resources. Control strategies are silencing, using, and being put in your place. I also transformed qualitative data to quantitatively examine the effects of race, ethnicity, gender, and institution type on participants' experiences. I conclude by considering the consequences of exclusion and control.

Invalidation

Many of the participants experienced invalidation of their individuality, knowledge, and cultural values. Dehumanizing perceptions of faculty of color as "Other" are the result of long-standing social norms that view whites as superior and maintain whites as the standard against which all other groups are judged.

Participants experienced invalidation of their individuality when they were viewed as members of a racial, ethnic, or gender group first and as individuals second, if at all. Professor Rice, who worked in an inclusive department, did not experience invalidation in her unit. Her humanity, with all of its uniqueness, was intrinsic to her experience, which in turn allowed her to feel a sense of belonging:

> I just felt like I fit here. And no one has treated me overly special because I'm black, because . . . they're not walking on eggshells. They treat me as though I'm just me. [medical faculty] (143) p.4

In contrast, other participants felt their skin color rendered their individuality invisible, as described by Professor Meriwether:

When you read the book *Invisible Man*, the . . . opening says, "I'm invisible simply because you refuse to see me." . . . Not because I'm not there; you refuse. That is really what I think a lot of minority faculty go through. [nursing faculty] (144) p.318

PROFESSOR CLARK: Ultimately . . . it's simply your skin color [that] will determine . . . how you're treated. [medical faculty] (143) p.4

PROFESSOR BLAKELY: We have lived with educated people who are racists . . . People look at us and the first thing they see, they see this black male. They see this black female . . . [W]hen someone looks at me, they don't look at me as Dr. Blakely, director of the nursing program. They look at me as a black person. [nursing faculty] (144) p.318

A focus on skin color led to perceptions of innate difference, as described by Professor Hayes. Greater phenotypic divergence from common European traits such as white skin or blue eyes placed faculty at greater risk for being perceived this way:

Instead of seeing me as a . . . colleague, as an American, even as a woman, I think what they see me as first being black and I think . . . with the face of being black, they automatically assume that we are just completely different. [medical faculty] (143) p.5

Invalidation of individuality was also manifested through treatment of participants according to racial and ethnic stereotypes by faculty colleagues, students, and staff. Professor Belmont's disturbing story of campus police harassment reflects stereotypes of black men as intellectually inferior and criminal:

I came into the office and we had a security guard who was down in the lobby . . . I went up to my office and was there for . . . twenty minutes just checking e-mails and then was on my way home . . . There were . . . campus police cars out in front . . . As I was walking to the parking lot this police officer yelled out to me, "Hey, you . . . you hear me talking to you?" . . . He was talking to me . . . and they questioned me . . . I told them that I work in the building . . . They didn't believe me because . . . I didn't have my faculty ID, . . . just my driver's license. I didn't intend to stay long . . . I gave them my name because I knew they could check for me in the system if they called the security office . . . I gave them my name, and the . . . officer from my understanding called the head office and said, "They came back and said they never heard of you." I said . . . "I have a key, I can show you my office." . . . This officer went up the stairs . . . shouting at the top of his voice . . . calling me . . . names and just cursing . . . And I was scared . . . He was very intimidating. He kept getting in my face . . . like he was going to grab me . . . I opened my office and showed him my degrees . . . my pictures . . . so he could see it was me . . . He said, "This can't be you . . . you are stupid and . . . ignorant just like the rest of them" . . . going on and on . . . I looked at him . . . I said, "You know who I am now. I would like you to leave my office." . . . He said, "I will leave when I want to leave." I said, "Then I would like to leave." "You will leave when I tell you to leave," he said . . . He . . . was about two inches away from my face . . . He . . . was literally spitting in my face as he was talking to me, pointing his finger in my face. I just stood there. He stayed in my office for about half an hour terrorizing me . . . He was going to arrest me . . . I was going to prison . . . He was trying to provoke me . . . I just sat there and listened to him, and he finally left. [nursing faculty]

Although Professor Belmont's harassment by campus police was the most egregious example of racism shared by participants, it was rooted in the same stereotypes fueling covert racist acts experienced by others.

A common example of students' invalidating behavior toward participants was a difference in their use of the title "Dr." when addressing white faculty compared to faculty of color. Although this behavior was viewed as disrespectful by all concerned participants, the driving stereotypes differed by race and ethnicity. Professor Chen provided an example:

I have one of my peers who is an Asian female who said they [the undergraduate students] are calling her by her first name . . . They think they can get away with it more if you are an Asian woman because you are expected to be kind of a pushover and mousy, and if you are not that way they don't react well. Because I am not that way. [pharmacy faculty]

Examples of racial and ethnic stereotypes shaping the perceptions of colleagues were also shared by Professors Belmont and Ahmed. Stereotypes of black men as violent criminals influenced how some women faculty interacted with Professor Belmont:

Some white faculty . . . women were afraid to ride in the elevator with me. They were afraid I was going to rob them or attack them. [nursing faculty]

Professor Belmont learned of the perceptions of the white women faculty from a third party. In contrast, faculty members spoke to Professor Ahmed directly:

Oftentimes a lot of people will say, "Well, you are too nice to be Palestinian." [pharmacy faculty]

Because many faculty of color experience stereotypical treatment throughout their lives, they are aware of the raced and gendered lenses through which they may be viewed. In response, some feel a sense of responsibility to represent their social group favorably. Professor Bailey described this experience:

I've spoken to other professionals who have it in the back of their mind[s] that if you do something wrong, people won't just say, "Oh, so and so's just a turkey." They'll say, "Oh, it's a black person who did that . . . That's something I carry with me . . . if somebody has blond hair and blue eyes and does something really idiotic, people say, "This guy is an ass." If the person is black then "black men, blah, blah, yak, yak, yak," instead of, "This guy's an ass." It's never just you. It's sort of you are holding the banner for your race or your entire gender. It makes me feel like I should always mind my p's and q's. [medical faculty]

Fear of confirming negative stereotypes about one's race or ethnicity is referred to as *stereotype threat*, a phenomenon associated with anxiety and under-performance (130, 145–147). Race-related stress has also been demonstrated empirically to result in decreased research productivity in faculty of color (148).

Participants whose professional skills and abilities were challenged on the basis of racial, ethnic, or gender stereotypes experienced invalidation of knowledge. This form of invalidation occurred when biases about participants' race, ethnicity, or gender caused concern that they were less competent than a comparably trained white male. This suspected incompetence generated a host of disrespectful behaviors that participants endured. As medical faculty member Professor Chavez said, "What I hear from my colleagues who are African American is that people pass judgment on their ability before they open their mouth[s], because of the way they look" (143) p.5. Professor Rice's experience supported this observation:

I've had other physicians also call . . . and question my diagnoses . . . and I think they have some apprehension based on their typical imageries of people of African descent in this country . . . To have someone in my position that looks like me is atypical . . . Unfortunately, the way that blacks are personified in this country particularly . . . speaking of black females, it's been ornery and typically not very well educated. [medical faculty] (143) p.5

Likewise, Professor Balewa felt her clinical judgment was often ignored because of her race:

[I say] this is actually going on with the patient and they say, "No, that's not what's going on with the patient." And two days later they say, "Oh, yeah. That's what was going on with the patient." So it's . . . a matter of not respecting [my] judgment. [medical faculty] (143) p.6

Faculty colleagues frequently challenged Professor Zahra to assess her content knowledge and teaching abilities:

I was always challenged with what I knew. In other words, they [other faculty] were always in some obscure way challenging me . . . trying to see if I really knew what I knew or if my knowledge base was up to par with . . . where they thought it should be and making me feel less than, which in turn made me work harder to show that yes, I am capable. Yes, I can coordinate this course. Yes, I am capable of being in charge of a course. I can manage the group of students. Validate that I can do it. [nursing faculty] (144) p.319

Professor Zahra went on to describe how difficult it was for her to be recognized as a faculty member when doing rounds with her students in the hospital:

There is stuff like "Who are you? You are the teacher?" kind of questions. I have to have my white coat on . . . and . . . I have to buck myself up with a lot of other things saying . . . who I am, what I do here . . . There is nobody that you can talk with . . . who would respect you . . . [give you] the respect that you deserve. It is almost like you are fighting for who you are . . . And that is hard for me . . . and I see that every day. (144) p.318.

Invalidation of knowledge was summed up by Professor Zahra's statement that "you are fighting for who you are." Faculty are qualified for their roles as academicians and clinicians because of what they know. For the majority of faculty, it takes several years to gain the requisite knowledge needed to be hired for an academic position. In those moments when assumptions are made that faculty of color have less educational preparation or are incompetent, they are robbed of their status as knowledge workers, and part of their identity is denied.

Higher education has been described as a culture that values rationality; devalues emotion; and rewards individualistic, competitive, aggressive, and self-promoting behavior (149). Participants who differed from this standard were vulnerable to cultural invalidation (150). Cultural invalidation occurred when an important part of a participants' culture was devalued. Participants' experiences of cultural invalidation often included lack of respect for values such as interdependence, humility, and the importance of family.

Turner and Myers noted that in academia persons of color are treated as "'guests in someone else's house'" and that guests should "honor their hosts' customs without question'" (83) p.84. Participants shared examples of implicit Eurocentric Christian norms, with white faculty in effect expecting them to act, talk, and look like them. Professor Hamid's refusal to attend a dance was met with hostility:

Maybe because I'm from the Middle East and a different religion, it sometimes becomes a conflict. I remember they invited me at the pharmacy school [to what] they call . . . a formal; it is dancing for our students who graduate . . . The dean told me, "You need to attend, you and your wife." And I told her, "With respect, this is different for me, I don't take my wife dancing in public," and the dean was upset with me. She knew she couldn't force me to attend, but she expressed how upset she was . . . I told her, "My religion, my culture—I don't feel comfortable attending these kinds of events." [pharmacy faculty]

Professor Yazzie described her experience with invalidating communication:

They were confrontational. Some of the faculty [who] were with me . . . violated my sense of self. I don't know how else to say it. I don't mean punitively or anything like that, but in Native culture we don't tell people what to do. And they would tell me what to do about anything. My research, my service, my—it is hard to capture it exactly. A Native person does not tell another person how to do it . . . You respect the other person and [her] decision making and autonomy. That is what tribal sovereignty is all about. And it is kind of like, "I don't respect your tribal sovereignty," and I want you to respect mine. And they didn't . . . It was uncomfortable for me. [nursing faculty] (144) p.318

Professor Noble reported hearing negative comments about the appearance of blacks:

There's this one administrator who will say things like she doesn't like people with natural African American hair. She makes comments all the time. [pharmacy faculty]

Many of the values that imbue academic culture in health professions schools are rooted in a history of exclusion. The nation's colleges and universities were originally established to educate white men (151, 152). Although social movements and presidential and judicial decisions have made it possible for women, people of color, and working-class people to access the health professions, academia is slow to change, and strong traces of the foundational culture linger. Continued dominance of whites in total numbers and in leadership positions perpetuates this restrictive culture, demanding conformity. Thus, invalidation of culture requires that faculty of color "perform their social identities carefully and selectively to avoid being criticized, marginalized, dismissed, or rejected by colleagues and students" (153) p.8.

Invalidation of individuality, knowledge, and culture communicate messages that assault a person's sense of self. A person who is not recognized can be harmed, confining him or her to a false, disfigured, and degraded mode of being (154). Some authors have reported racial and ethnic stereotyping and cultural insensitivity in nursing and medicine (155–164); many have documented this problem in academia outside the health professions (21, 48, 83, 141, 165–181). This study is the first to document these assaults across health professions academe and to provide insight into the invalidating messages conveyed to health professions faculty of color at predominantly white institutions. Learning to see beyond stereotypes and honor diverse cultures requires valuing the various layers, nuances, and potential contradictions of a person. This human validation is the lifeblood of meaningful and sincere professional relationships (154).

Being Treated Like an Outsider

The tendency for members of a social group to view themselves as having similar positive traits and more diverse negative traits, while viewing outsiders as the reverse, is a common cognitive bias. This bias often results in within-group favoritism (136, 182). Because faculty of color are so often underrepresented, they are disadvantaged when treated like outsiders, placed perpetually on the margins. Participants shared experiences of being treated like outsiders, often involving exclusion from social and decision-making processes. This experience was summed up by Professors Chavez and Belmont:

PROFESSOR CHAVEZ: There's not a day that goes by that I don't look at myself in the mirror and remind myself of who I am, meaning that, "Hey, remember, you're Latino . . ." And . . . I found myself feeling very marginalized, feeling very isolated, being very alone even though I'm in the Department of Family Medicine. [medical faculty] (143) p.6

PROFESSOR BELMONT: In my . . . faculty position, it was clear . . . that I was . . . the outsider . . . I had an office. I had all those things that a faculty [member] has. But . . . as an individual faculty member, I felt that there was a clear, sometimes subtle, covert message being sent that my role was to be quiet and stay in a corner and not say too much and . . . like I didn't have colleagues and often faculty didn't speak to me. They wouldn't say hello or make me feel welcome or take me out to lunch. There was one person on the faculty who did, and she and I became close. But the others wouldn't have anything to do with me at all. [nursing faculty] (144) p.319

While US-born participants attributed being treated like an outsider to their race or ethnicity alone, some immigrant faculty felt that being foreign born also contributed to their out-group status. Professor Kapoor shared his experience:

I think the success contributes to that. The feeling that I am taking away something that is theirs [US-born faculty's] . . . There are a small number of colleagues that I work with now who don't even acknowledge my presence in the room. [pharmacy faculty]

Being treated like an outsider also meant exclusion from meetings, which precluded participation in decision making, as described by Professors Jones and Pope:

PROFESSOR JONES: The two of us—supposed to be co-directors of our fellowship program. We were going to do the education and help with the fellowship program . . . It turns out they started having meetings, and I wasn't included. I wasn't invited . . . I found out because we'd be in faculty meetings and they'd say, "Oh yeah, this is our plan . . ." And I'd say, "When did you meet?" I wasn't included; I wasn't invited." "Oh yeah, we forgot, but don't you worry, we took care of it. But we'll include you in the next one." I was never included. And so that kind of thing kept going on . . . Because it's about the race . . . It's not about anything else . . . the sheer fact that people still see me as an outsider. [medical faculty] (143) p.6

PROFESSOR POPE: We have monthly meetings of the chairs of all departments, and I remember . . . when my dean got together with me, and he said, "You know, you don't have to come to these meetings. Technically, I'm the chief diversity officer, so I will attend these meetings, and if I need you to come in and talk about some matter of diversity, I'll let you know, and I'll have you come." And I've come to those meetings periodically over the years, but only as I have been requested to come. So there are lots of people sitting around the table making decisions and having influence, but not me. [medical faculty]

In addition to being excluded from decision making, Professor Pope was physically isolated, further cementing his status as an outsider:

From the day that I came to this school of medicine I had an office [that] was immediately adjacent to the dean, and I was there probably for the first five or six years . . . And one day the dean said to me that he wanted to do some reorganization, that he had this particular person . . . that he wanted to become his assistant dean and that he wanted to bring that person over closer to him and he wanted me to go to an area, so that I could be closer to students, because it seemed that it had evolved, in his mind, that I was dealing more with students than I was dealing with administration. So he had me move my office to another side of the building, which is sort of an isolated area, and it's an area where primarily students are, but there are very few faculty members over here. So . . . I moved. This guy that he was talking about did indeed move into that office but still maintained an office in the original place where he was, as well . . . I had been in that spot from the very beginning. So I knew that, essentially, this was one of those things—I could use this analogy. Here's a black person who's living in our neighborhood; we need to get him out of here, and so they got me out of the neighborhood. And it was no big deal to me, not really, because, like I said, I've been black a long time. [medical faculty]

Professor Wakefield, who eventually went to a historically black university, described a climate of exclusion at a predominantly white institution. She was excluded from coauthor publishing networks and treated as an outsider at the simulation lab, where she had demonstrated expertise. Her experiences of exclusion eventually caused her to leave her position:

I did my dissertation and I wanted to publish, and so, despite one of the administrators actually being on my dissertation committee . . . when I got ready to publish she told me, "You go on and author it yourself, and then you can prove to yourself that you can do this." And . . . I was never asked to coauthor with anyone else. We had a dean change and we had a dean who was East Indian, and she was challenged as well . . . She was the first minority to have been a dean. She came with a stronger research background, but she was asked to step down . . . There was an IT person who was not a nurse who was doing a lot of favors for faculty, logistics and stuff, and she wanted the simulation lab. So she sabotaged me. I was the one who set the simulation lab up. I'm very tech savvy. And people from the university would come to see the lab, and I would consult with them, and she would try to get in the middle of that, and prevent my progress. And eventually she was given the lab. She was given the simulation lab. After being there four years, I decided that it was not in my best interest to stay . . . I expressed my concerns, and my concerns weren't addressed. I decided that I'm not feeling like an equal faculty person, so I need to move into an environment that's going to put me in the place I need to be. [nursing faculty]

Outsider treatment contributes to the creation of an unequal playing field for faculty of color by barring access to development of relationships with mentors and colleagues and limiting opportunities for guidance, support, and collaboration. Moreover, as social beings, humans are sensitively attuned to subtle cues signaling social exclusion, and racism as a form of social exclusion has been linked to poor health outcomes (183). This is an important concern considering that a full-time faculty member spends most of his or her waking hours at work.

Unequal Treatment

Several participants shared experiences of unequal treatment compared to white faculty. Common examples were unequal hiring processes, performance standards, supervision, and allocation of resources. Other examples were inequities in pay and workload. The extent to which unequal treatment affects the representation of faculty of color at specific schools or in health professions education generally is unknown.

Negative experiences during the hiring process placed participants at a disadvantage, setting the stage for the remainder of their appointments. Professor Belmont experienced unequal treatment during his job interview:

> I learned . . . after my interview process that they did something that they had never done before with a candidate . . . I was the first African American candidate they had ever had . . . Before I came there I got this phone call from someone there, and [he] had asked me to submit five years of my teaching evaluations. I said, "Really?" . . . For some reason someone on the committee couldn't believe that my evaluations were that high, and they shouldn't have been that high. They were questioning it, and so they wanted me to submit all of this to them. So I just happened to keep my records from day one, so I faxed them all to them. I never heard another word about it. But one of my colleagues who sat on the committee said he was highly disturbed. He had never seen them do that. He had been at that institution for a long time, and he said that this was the first time that they had ever required anybody to submit their evaluations . . . This was the first time they had ever done that, because normally they just get references and that would be it. [nursing faculty] (144) p.319–20

Professors Jones and Horne experienced unequal treatment when they were appointed:

PROFESSOR JONES: And going into medical school I had . . . a different set of views and values than other people . . . the traditional group that comes in . . . And I did my fellowship in geriatrics . . . So when I finished up I was joining the faculty, but they were not very open to me . . . joining the faculty. In fact, the first year they listed me as staff, not faculty. They courted a woman who was also a friend of mine, and I had encouraged her, she was a year behind me, to do the fellowship. And she did, and they actively courted her, and I called them on it. I said, "Look at what you're doing for her and you didn't do any of that for me when I came in . . . You . . . put me down as staff and I was actually faculty." Oh well, that's going to impact you [faculty of color] long term. [medical faculty]

PROFESSOR HORNE: If I wasn't of color I probably would've gone straight to the hygiene department. But because I am of color they wanted to start me at the lower end of the totem pole. That's how I feel. I had to prove myself. I was able to move because the department of dental assisting closed down. They didn't have a choice. But I still deserved to be where I was—the hygiene department, but I had to prove myself . . . They hire new graduates. They just graduate, and they hire them to teach. I at least had experience when they hired me. I was a hygienist already eight years when they hired me. But they hire people not of color straight from graduation, like, "Here's a job. Come to the department." [dental faculty]

Professor Said's unequal treatment began when she was first appointed and continues today:

I was part of a group of postdocs that was hired . . . When I interviewed they told me that they were offering multiyear contracts until tenure track positions opened up. But when I got a job offer it was for an annual contract. I knew the others had been given multiyear contracts, and I when asked why . . . the administrator . . . said, "I am all out of multiyear contracts." There was no reason to treat me differently because . . . I had an NIH [National Institutes of Health] grant and published my dissertation findings and had actually done really well . . . In my first year they gave me way more courses to teach than the other new faculty, even though 50 percent of my time was grant funded, which was not the case for anyone else. A few years later I found out I was being paid $10,000 less than the lowest paid of the group. I was so mad I was ready to walk over that, and I wrote a letter to the dean and she gave me a $10,000 raise . . . When I was ready to go up for tenure—because our contracts had been switched over—they said that I couldn't do it. I had received a letter appointing me to the tenure track a year before, but my record keeping is not so good—luckily I was able to find it [the letter] and . . . they had to honor it. When I asked them what happened they said, "We had no record of the letter." That hasn't happened to anyone else in the school. If I hadn't found that letter, I would not be tenured right now, because they were not going to give me the opportunity. Now I am a tenured full professor with a good track record of funding, and I have never received anything other than outstanding annual reviews. But I am the lowest paid in my rank, and there are assistant and associate professors who are paid much more than I am. My history here has been demoralizing, and I take it as a message that I am not valued. I have thought about leaving. [nursing faculty]

Many participants shared their belief that faculty of color must perform better than whites to receive the same benefits. Professor Sewell summed this up, saying, "Faculty of color cannot afford to be average" (143) p.6. He explained:

I think some of my majority colleagues cruise . . . and that's tolerated. I know that won't be tolerated for me. I cannot be perceived as average. That won't go. So I got . . . awards last year . . . I need that . . . just to stay in the game. There are other folks that I think cruised, they're not engaged in the full gamut of research, community service, patient care, and teaching. But they are de facto allowed to cruise because they are part of the ruling class. I am not allowed to cruise. And so I get frustrated. [medical faculty] (143) p.6–7

Professor Kone described the same unequal performance expectations:

PROFESSOR KONE: People don't just accept you just as you are . . . They want to find out what your weak areas are . . .

INTERVIEWER: What if you are an average performer?

PROFESSOR KONE: I believe that I need to perform 90 percent for me to be recognized at 70 percent.

INTERVIEWER: So you cannot afford to be average?

PROFESSOR KONE: For sure. Yes. If I showed up and I . . . had a bad day and I skipped something, it would be a disaster. [pharmacy faculty]

Unequal performance standards were associated with unequal scrutiny and supervision, as described by Professors Barnes and Belmont:

PROFESSOR BARNES: Just having to justify maybe my question writing, or maybe lecturing, whereas some of my other colleagues who[m] I started with at the same time . . . There were three of us that started at the same time, and I just find that . . . with some of my material . . . it's like, okay, "Well, we want to see your materials like an extra week early." Or, "We want to sit in on your lecture, so on and so forth." And my other colleagues probably don't have as much experience as I do. This is my first time being here, but I came from another state university before, and I did an extensive academic fellowship with them. So I have pretty good experience in terms of academia, where the other new colleagues just came straight out of practice and didn't have that background. So it was strange to me that I was having to go through this extra surveying process despite the fact that I was pretty well credentialed . . . It's small things like that, like in terms of both academic and also clinical practice. Just . . . extra shadowing, extra checklists. I had to go through . . . an extra-long background [check], and I'm not sure if [I don't notice racism because] . . . I'm used to that extra process of having to jump through a little bit more hoops . . . I obviously have been African American my whole life. [pharmacy faculty]

PROFESSOR BELMONT: I would have this feeling of being constantly micromanaged, being constantly under a microscope all the time so that each word I spoke, each sentence I wrote with respect to students, grading a student, everything was scrutinized. So there was a sense of not having any freedom to be a full-fledged faculty member. In that setting at that time, I was the only minority . . . It was difficult. [nursing faculty] (144) p.321

Professor Wakefield described her similar experience:

I was challenged about the way I was grading and the manner in which I was teaching. And I just wasn't prepared for that. So after a semester, I was just like, "I don't need this." [nursing faculty]

Not only were many participants expected to perform at higher levels; they were also subjected to greater scrutiny by supervisors than were white faculty. Some participants also reported inequities in acknowledgment of their contributions and achievements. Professor Horne experienced this in her communication with colleagues:

I feel like because I am of color they don't recognize anything that I do. They don't acknowledge—they don't even care to see—they just do not appreciate me at all . . . For example, they send out an e-mail. They want someone to volunteer and help out with the student organization. I'm the first to respond . . . to say, "I'll do it. I'm interested, yes" . . . Only one response . . . giving me an attitude, "Why don't you do Thursday?" Well if it was someone not of color, they would say, "Great, wonderful. You're going to do this? Awesome!" How about saying, "Thank you for responding. Thank you for helping out." It's just like, "Oh, do it this week," we set a date. Being pushy. I feel I don't get the same respect as . . . someone who is Caucasian, "Oh, great, wonderful, oh look who's here," and all of that. But it's me and it's just, "Oh, whatever." [dental faculty]

Professor Hamid's experience provided a more overt example of inequitable acknowledgment:

Normally they decide who gets the Teacher of the Year Award by deciding who gets the most votes . . . I got the highest number of votes . . . and the one who was number four, they decided to put him as Teacher of the Year. And because the students told me, "We elected you" . . . I had access to the results of the survey, and I looked at it and I saw that I got the most votes, so I talked to them. And the dean got very upset, because she said, "You can't see this information." I said, "It's there in the faculty folder. It is not something I need a password to access" . . . Anyway . . . she wrote a very harsh letter to me because I looked at that information, and she forgot what the actual problem was, and then she tried to tell me, "Maybe this is okay in your culture . . . Here this is something very serious." [pharmacy faculty]

Participants also described unequal distribution of resources. This was often manifested as denial of protected time, affecting their ability to engage in scholarship, as experienced by Professors Griffin and Meriwether:

PROFESSOR GRIFFIN: I was . . . promised one thing and then it didn't turn out that way . . . [I've] been added a lot more clinical time since I've been here . . . I've been told things I felt were not fair to me. And . . . that if I didn't have a publication then my . . . research time wouldn't be supported, . . . which I have found not to be equally true for other members of the division. [medical faculty]

PROFESSOR MERIWETHER: I said I need at least a year or two to get my practice up and going, and I need to see how I am going to integrate my research into my practice . . . Now mind you, they were letting other people come and [do] their research. They are supporting them, reducing teaching loads, giving them research money, and saying, "We are going to give you three or four years to figure out how you are going to get your research up and going." Whereas with me, they are expecting me to go out there and immediately start doing research.

INTERVIEWER: So the standards seemed to be different?

PROFESSOR MERIWETHER: They seemed to be different. [nursing faculty] (144)
  p.320

The health professions education literature has begun to document unequal treatment of faculty of color, including unequal representation at the higher ranks, which is likely both a sign and a result of controlling racist processes (16, 34, 184, 185). Research outside of health professions education has also documented that faculty of color receive less support for teaching and research and experience a more challenging path to promotion and tenure than do white faculty (165). This study supports these findings and suggests these inequities are common in health professions education.

Silencing

Silencing strategies attempted to control the voices of participants. Although it is likely this happened on a one-on-one basis, participants shared experiences of being silenced during group work. Examples of silencing tactics included targeting participants, refusing to engage with them, and obfuscation. Professor Belmont described his experience of being silenced:

> They had two African American females . . . but we all three [faculty of color] felt like we were singled out. We all three didn't feel safe to speak in this environment, that we couldn't trust the environment . . . We had to constantly be looking behind our backs. We were not allowed to speak during meetings; if we did it seemed like it was creating a huge chaos. And one of the things that I remember with clarity was each time—and it didn't matter if it was me or one of them [who] was saying something—we could have said it in the most. . . kindest, [most] helpful way—it was as if the roof fell off the building. And I began to believe at one point that that was an attempt to keep us quiet, that if we said something and there was all this chaos ensuing because we said something, then maybe we would be quiet. And that had come to me because I had experienced that at my other position in a different part of the country, that this was a systemic attempt to keep us in our places so we would not learn about the power structure, we would not learn about the system, we would not learn about how to get ahead and move up, we wouldn't ask questions,

we wouldn't go to people and talk with them, and that way we would never be in the know. [nursing faculty] (144) p.320

Silencing occurred most often when participants challenged the myth of equal opportunity. Thus, participants in positions focused on equity were most vulnerable to silencing. As Professor Randolph said, "I can't talk about any people of color, about myself, and not feel targeted" [medical faculty].

Likewise, Professor Jones shared her experiences of silencing and her determination to speak the truth no matter the cost:

If you raise real issues, critical issues about racism, they will try to work around it and reframe it in a way so it is more palatable for them ... and I will tell people the truth. I'm not going to lie, and I tell them it doesn't matter what level—I'm not going to participate in your lies. I keep waiting and watching to see if they are going to fire me, but so far, I'm still here. [medical faculty]

Professor Jones's quote highlights the burden that faculty of color who speak out against racism bear. Professor Pryor's hesitance to bring up the topic of diversity reflects this burden as well as the disillusionment that can occur when the voices of faculty of color are repeatedly ignored:

I remember sitting in a [meeting] room debating whether or not I was even going to bring it [student diversity] up, because I was playing out what was going to happen in my head. And it was almost like a joke. And almost like a game for me ... My image was throwing a bone, dogs devouring it, which is what happened. So I threw it. I said, "What about diversity?" And immediately, "Well, why are you bringing that up? What are you talking about? Are people complaining? What examples do you have? Can we operationalize diversity?" ... I just sat back and said nothing more than that. And ... everyone was going on about this issue. And eventually it got quiet and they were like—I guess I wasn't talking anymore—and someone said, "Well, Professor Pryor, could you elaborate?" And I said "No, forget it, I withdraw. I withdraw the point." [nursing faculty] (144) p.320–1

Harris and Gonzalez described the contradictory culture of academia: "On the one hand, the university champions, encourages free expression and the search for truth, and prizes the creation of neutral and objective knowledge for the betterment of society—values that are supposed to make race and gender identities irrelevant. On the other . . . higher education reflects and reproduces—yet also sometimes subverts—the social hierarchies that pervade American society" (153) p.1. Silencing the voices of faculty of color flies in the face of claims of meritocracy, free speech, and objective knowledge—claims that health professions education clearly makes (186–189). Silencing probably occurs because the voices of faculty of color have the potential to subvert social hierarchies (190).

Using

Participants were used when they were exploited for the benefit of others who would not otherwise include them. Common examples included tokenism and diversity work. Professors Achebe and Phillips described being used as tokens for photos:

PROFESSOR ACHEBE: When you are always the only one, it kind of gets tiring after a while . . . I think having one is like having a token, so we have a token and then we don't need to look anymore. I think it would be nice to have a couple in this department . . . That way if they'll be needing a picture that they want to show a black face [in], they don't have to call me; you know [laughing]? [pharmacy faculty]

PROFESSOR PHILLIPS: When the first dean was here when I came, we went to the same conference . . . And the school had two tables of people. And I was invited to be at one of the tables. And I knew then . . . that I was a token. I knew I was to be there for show. And a picture was taken . . . They used it for [an academic program pamphlet] . . . So you play that part. [nursing faculty]

Professor Cleary experienced using when she was asked to take part in grant applications and teaching because of her race:

I think it's a continual struggle actually just on my mind because it happened last week. Being asked to be on grants just because they're American Indians–specific, but not even as a co-investigator, because there should be key personnel being asked to write and contribute to the grant. Expected to even though it's not my subject area has come up . . . being asked to write and it's not my grant. It doesn't go toward my tenure and being expected to research or know about American Indian education, for instance, which is not my area at all. [pharmacy faculty]

Professor Jones described being used for diversity training and likened this experience to being a minstrel, a performer on display:

> When they talk about diversity, cultural competencies, whatever it is—they want you to be the minstrel, to do your song and dance. But at the same time they're saying you have to acculturate to what we want . . . [at these sessions on diversity]. I should not be dancing in front of you . . . [The] last time I was asked to do something on diversity, which was earlier this month, I actually agreed to do it, and I was the only one . . . So I went into this group; it was the leadership people doing the leadership training thing the university has, and I basically sort of introduced myself and told a little about myself. I said, "First of all, for the record I have no training in diversity. I have as many skills to discuss diversity as you do. I am in here talking because I'm the darkest person in this room" . . . As far as decision making goes, I'm included only if it's a problem with the African American community against the institution. That's the only time. Otherwise decisions are made about me without me, so they won't bring me to the table unless the African American community is up in arms about something . . . So it is sort of, "Okay. I get it." [medical faculty]

As these examples show, using does not benefit faculty of color and does little to promote institutional diversity and equity. Rather, using may cover up the absence of genuine diversity and equity efforts. At its worst, using is an exploitative practice (191).

Being Put in Your Place

Being "put in your place" occurred when participants were demeaned, reprimanded, or otherwise punished for enacting the authority of their roles. This commonly occurred when working with students. Despite being a senior faculty member, Professor Sewell was constrained in his ability to exercise his full authority:

> I feel kind of threatened . . . I am very reluctant to go to my faculty and say, "What's with this resident?" . . . I'm the chair, so I kind of put up with it . . . I had a bad experience in another medical center, where I gave a bad grade to a female resident that I thought was abusing our system and I ended up getting reprimanded. I'm very reluctant to give a resident or a student feedback

on [his or her] behavior because I'm concerned that it will work against me. [medical faculty]

Similarly, Professor Belmont was reprimanded for attempting to hold students accountable for poor performance:

The students I had . . . abandoned . . . patients who were critically ill. These students . . . [who] were white . . . went shopping for about three hours . . . We had policies clearly in our school that if students did that, that was grounds for automatic dismissal and failure. Well, I tried to execute those policies, and I repeatedly was slapped on the hand for disciplining the students. I was slapped on the hand for trying to fail them; I was not even allowed to fail them . . . In fact, I was told to apologize to them for being so harsh . . . I came to the agreement where they could only get a C and that was it, but these students should have failed. I have seen them fail students of color who had done far less egregious acts than that. [nursing faculty] (144) p.321

Professor Zahra was reprimanded for helping a student, an act that was perceived as upstaging the lead faculty:

[I was told that] I need to leave because the faculty felt . . . the student might think I was the [lead] instructor when she should be the lead . . . And I'm thinking, all I did was give some feedback to the student . . . so she would learn from the mistake. It was not about you, it was about the student . . . And it was "no, no, no . . . I was running the show. I was the lead faculty . . . We didn't have the time for that. And you didn't need to bring it up." They [white faculty] sat and listened, and fought kind of on her side . . . "What she's trying to say is [. . .] ." And I'm thinking what she's saying is, she didn't want me to know more than her. [nursing faculty]

Being put in your place decreases the influence of faculty of color. It is a means of enforcing an unspoken and at times unconscious raced-gendered hierarchy that continues to haunt academe. For participants who experienced it, being put in your place was a powerful reminder of this hierarchy and the arbitrary nature of its boundaries. It was also a humiliating experience that was not soon forgotten. This process, along with the other exclusion and control processes described in this chapter, contributes to a web of constraints that faculty of color must learn first to understand and then to cut through as they make their way in academe.

The Influence of Institution Type, Race/Ethnicity, and Gender on Faculty Experience in Predominantly White Institutions

The data suggest that race, ethnicity, gender, and type of school influenced participants' experiences of exclusion and control in predominantly white institutions. To examine these contexts, I counted the frequency of reports of positive experiences, such as receiving support from leaders and mentors, and negative experiences of exclusion and control. Participants with a preponderance of positive or negative experience were categorized into groups (see table 3). Participants from historically black colleges and universities were not included in the analysis because the racial climate at those institutions was markedly different than at predominantly white institutions.

Type of institution was a context that affected participants' experiences. In the study, 33.8 percent of faculty at research-intensive universities ($n = 74$) reported negative experiences, compared to 22.7 percent of faculty at predominantly teaching-focused schools ($n = 22$). It is possible the large number of Asian participants (36.4 percent) in the teaching-focused sample affected the results, because this group was most likely to report positive experiences. Although it is possible that the absence of constant pressure on faculty to bring in external funding can lead to more positive experiences in teaching-focused institutions (192), it seems unlikely that the absence of pressure to secure grant monies would relate directly to race-related negative events.

I saw clear trends when examining race, ethnicity, and gender. Black participants reported higher rates of negative experiences and lower rates of positive experiences than Asian and Latino/a participants. In addition, Asian participants reported higher rates of positive and lower rates of negative experiences than Latino/a participants. Although I have included data for Middle Eastern ($n = 5$) and Native American ($n = 3$) participants in table 3 to avoid excluding these groups completely, their numbers were so small even for a qualitative study that I do not report them here.

I asked the participants I interviewed to rate their job satisfaction on a 1–10 scale (other interviewers did not consistently use this scale) ($n = 55$). Social hi-

TABLE 3. Percentage of Positive, Negative, and Mixed Experiences
at Predominantly White Institutions for Each Racial and Ethnic Group

RACIAL/ ETHNIC/ GENDER GROUP	OVERALL SAMPLE n = 96	OVERALL POSITIVE n = 33	POSITIVE RESEARCH INTENSIVE n = 24	POSITIVE TEACHING FOCUSED n = 9	OVERALL MIXED n = 33	MIXED RESEARCH INTENSIVE n = 25	MIXED TEACHING FOCUSED n = 8	OVERALL NEGATIVE n = 30	NEGATIVE RESEARCH INTENSIVE n = 25	NEGATIVE TEACHING FOCUSED n = 5
Asian	n = 20 20.8%	n = 12 60%	n = 7 35%	n = 5 25%	n = 4 20%	n = 2 10%	n = 2 10%	n = 4 20%	n = 3 15%	n = 1 5%
Black	n = 54 56.2%	n = 12 22.2%	n = 9 16.7%	n = 3 5.6%	n = 22 40.7%	n = 17 31.4%	n = 5 9.3%	n = 20 37%	n = 17 31.4%	n = 3 5.6%
Latino/a	n = 14 14.6%	n = 6 42.8%	n = 5 35.7%	n = 1 7.1%	n = 5 35.7%	n = 4 28.6%	n = 1 7.1%	n = 3 21.4%	n = 3 21.4%	n = 0
Middle Eastern	n = 5 5.2%	n = 1 20%	n = 1 20%	n = 0	n = 1 20%	n = 1 20%	n = 0	n = 3 60%	n = 2 40%	n = 1 20%
Native American	n = 3 3.1%	n = 2 66.7%	n = 2 66.7%	n = 0	n = 1 33.3%	n = 1 33.3%	n = 0	n = 0	n = 0	n = 0

Note: Percentages in columns 2–10 were calculated using the total number of each ethnic and racial group
as whole values and the number in each column as part values.

erarchies related to race, ethnicity, and gender are reflected in these ratings. The average satisfaction level for the sample was 7.8. Asian men reported the highest level of job satisfaction at 8.75, followed by Asian women at 8.5. Latinos and Latinas reported average satisfactions of 8.4 and 7.8 respectively. Black men and women both reported an average satisfaction of 7.4. Middle Easterners and Native Americans reported average job satisfactions of 8 and 6.5 respectively. Allen and colleagues reported similar patterns of racial and gender disparities in faculty satisfaction in their study of faculty from six colleges and universities (n = 1,166), which included 35 black faculty members (193).

Consequences of Exclusion and Control for Faculty of Color

Exclusion and control of faculty of color, combined with lower pay relative to practice environments, lack of mentoring for academic roles, and a host of other concerns, contribute to the underrepresentation of blacks, Latino/as, and Native Americans in health professions education (4, 16, 18, 20, 76, 194). This underrepresentation means that faculty may be the only members of their racial and ethnic groups in their departments and schools. The absence of a critical mass of faculty of color helps perpetuate exclusion and control, isolates faculty of color, and contributes to promotion and tenure inequities (4). In addition, the messages embedded in exclusion and control implicitly require that faculty of color prove their academic worth beyond what is expected for whites, while simultaneously damaging their self-confidence. I briefly describe these consequences—isolation, inequities in promotion and tenure, proving, and lowered self-confidence—before concluding this chapter.

Isolation

Participants frequently mentioned the importance of seeing "someone who looks like me" in their departments or schools. In most cases there were few faces that fit the bill, and often there were none. The lack of faculty of color resulted in feelings of isolation and loneliness and created a canvas against which the actions of a few faculty of color were highly visible. Such visibility created pressure to avoid mistakes and to do more than was required of others, contributing to increased stress. Professor Achebe described his experience of isolation:

I think the main real issue most of the time [is that] you are always the only person . . . Let's take who I am right now. You have in pharmaceutical sciences [in my school] I think four people of Indian descent . . . three [who're] probably Chinese, and you have people who would consider themselves Caucasians. I'm the only person that will encode as black. And the other minorities that would identify with you, like Hispanics or [those of] Arab descent, the people who are minorities in the sense of true minorities in the sciences, there [are] none. So I think that's the key issue. The thought that you're usually the only person . . . which means that all your actions are quite visible and in most cases . . . anything bad about you is always quite noted. I'll give you an example. If there is a department meeting, and if I'm there everybody will know. If other people come, people may or may not know. So those are the issues that make someone less comfortable . . . Something that you still feel . . . [is] lonely. You know the Indians have their own group. The Chinese get together and speak Chinese. I'm always all by myself. Of course you try to strike up friendships and things like that, but it's not quite the same. I would say that's the main negative . . . You're not part of any caucus. I think that's my whole experience. I'm not part of any caucus. [medical faculty]

Professor Achebe's experience is consistent with the greater scrutiny that other black faculty members reported in their narratives and suggests that because of their visibility, any mistakes faculty with darker skin make are more easily identifiable and perhaps also more memorable, further reinforcing the need to mind one's p's and q's.

Promotion and Tenure

Qualitative data from this study shed light on findings from previous quantitative studies documenting racial and ethnic disparities in faculty promotion in the health professions (16, 34, 35). There are benefits in belonging to a larger group that can help faculty successfully navigate the process of promotion and tenure. These benefits include receiving help through mentoring, advocacy, and more lenient interpretation of promotion and tenure guidelines. Professor Achebe described the unacknowledged benefits that faculty receive when they belong to a larger group. He also commented on stereotyping of black faculty members. These covert processes converge, disadvantaging black faculty relative to their peers who belong to larger groups:

> There was a meeting that we had on promotion and tenure for one of the Indian candidates, like a fourth year, something like that. Okay, now everything is supposed to be confidential, but I also know that a lot of discussions that were supposed to be confidential get through to the candidate through the Indian caucuses. The Chinese [caucus] also is the same thing. There was a candidate that came up for promotion that really should not even be considered ... Those individuals, in my opinion, really did not merit the promotion, but in one case it was granted. In the other case it is still pending ... Those to me are very clear examples [of inequity]. If both individuals had been black or had been from other minority groups, two things would [have] happen[ed]. One, nobody would have told them what's going on because nothing would leak. Two, it would have been considered negatively, ... whereas other minorities benefited from being part of a caucus ... Or if a black person [received a similar break], it would have been considered affirmative action. It's the syndrome where if a black individual gets a break, it's viewed as affirmative action. If a nonblack gets the same break, it's seen as he was lucky or he was smart, some other word is used that is not negative [about] that individual. [pharmacy faculty]

The promotion and tenure review process judges the legitimacy and value of a candidate's scholarship, placing him or her in a vulnerable position (192). Professor Achebe described some of the opportunity differentials in academic culture that are unacknowledged, yet very real, that mitigate this vulnerable position for larger groups. These breaks are extremely advantageous to those who receive them. For members of underrepresented groups, there is no protective cohort, or "caucus" as Professor Achebe called it. This leaves faculty members isolated and without the unofficial benefits that others may receive. In turn, this contributes to an uneven playing field that remains unacknowledged in the context of hegemonic notions of a color-blind, meritocratic, objective academy and to disparities in promotion and tenure of faculty of color.

Professor Achebe described his own experiences with uneven interpretation of the rules. Though this inequity did not prevent him from earning his full professorship, he did so on an unequal footing:

If the rules say you must publish five papers, I have to have six or more . . . If I have four, I'm going down. So I'm always thinking that in the back of my head, because there is no supposed godfather that would look out for me. So I have to look out for myself, because they will give me the harshest interpretations. The rules are not different for me. The rules are the same, and everybody will agree they are the same. But they are enforced very differently . . . The enforcement of the rules, the interpretation of the rules—you will not benefit from it [as a person of color]. And the few that benefit from a . . . more general interpretation, they are the majority . . . Somebody's not going to come and say, "I hate you because you're black." No, that doesn't happen. But we're all human beings, and our comfort levels are different between races. For example, where two people of Indian descent meet each other, their comfort level between each other is different from when an Indian person meets a Chinese person or maybe somebody of white origin. The only disadvantage of being a black person is that you don't have that colleague that you can have a high comfort level with, that you can let down your guard and share your frustrations, your hopes, your fears, your weaknesses, your strengths [with]. So you've got to be official in all of your dealings . . . I earned my promotion, I earned my tenure, and I did receive it. No ifs, ands, or buts, but anything where there is opportunity for interpretation, I have not benefited [from]. [pharmacy faculty]

Professor Achebe's reference to a "godfather" implies a powerful figure who looks out for the well-being of a protégé. This speaks to the importance of mentors being aware of the reality and impact of exclusion and control on faculty of color generally and promotion particularly, and acting to counteract these effects. The fact that faculty of color are disproportionately represented at the lower professorial ranks speaks to the impact of exclusion and control on some academics' ability to progress in their careers and meet promotion criteria. It also raises questions about the fairness of academic decision-making processes.

Proving

Because of racial, ethnic, and gender stereotypes implicit in the dominant culture, many people consciously or unconsciously believe white males possess abilities superior to others (195). For this reason, many faculty of color feel the need to prove themselves (149, 196). While this is also true to some degree for white faculty members, the stories shared by participants reflect a clear bias. Professor Kendall described how she was warned as a student at a historically black university that she would need to prove herself in predominantly white institutions. She continues this tradition, warning her students of the same concern:

> Well, I remember something that was told to me when I was at a historically black university is, "For a lot of places you're going to go, because of your color, you are going to have to prove yourself more than other people in some races." So I have definitely told some people that. [pharmacy faculty]

This perception was echoed by several participants who felt they needed to work harder than others to prove their worth, as described by Professors Ames, Hassan, Kadam, and Jordan:

PROFESSOR AMES: I feel when you are a minority you're always scrutinized that much more and you're expected to—you always feel like you have to do that much better for yourself. I think you're always having to prove yourself. [dental faculty]

PROFESSOR HASSAN: You really have to prove yourself over and over and over and over. [nursing faculty]

PROFESSOR KADAM: I do feel that . . . I have to work harder. And there is a sense of wanting to prove myself more. [pharmacy faculty]

PROFESSOR JORDAN: I feel like I have to be . . . at the top of my game, beyond the top of my game . . . I don't feel like I'm competing on the same level [as whites] . . . It just keeps me pushing to be my best . . . I get the sense that, when people see me, they may not appreciate what I have to offer until I show them what I have to offer. [pharmacy faculty]

Professor Ortiz, a light-skinned Latina faculty member, passed for white, not revealing her ethnicity until after she had proven herself:

> Four years after becoming a faculty member I am starting to connect to that side of myself [her ethnicity] professionally . . . I felt that I had to keep it quiet . . . I proved myself before they discovered I was Hispanic. [dental faculty]

Many participants anticipated the burden of needing to prove themselves beyond what is expected of whites before accepting an academic appointment, while others, naïve to this possibility, learned this unspoken expectation on the job. Participants' perceived need to prove themselves is consistent with the problem of racially biased performance standards that penalize faculty of color who do not outperform white males in higher education generally (55). Expectations for faculty of color may include greater quantity and quality of publications, heavier teaching and advising loads, diversity-related service, and visibility when it is in an institution's best interest to have a scholar of color on display (55). This double standard, along with institutional refusal to acknowledge it, adds burden to an already stressful junior faculty role.

Decreased Self-Confidence

Invalidating messages negatively affect self-confidence. When this happens, faculty's ability to advance and contribute to health professions education may be damaged. Professor Belmont internalized the negative messages he received over several years:

> After a point—you can be as strong as you are—but when you are in an environment like that, it's like being hypnotized almost; you are just not consciously aware of how much stuff is going into your subconscious. I didn't appreciate at the time how much was going into my subconscious, that my mind was taking in all these messages; it was storing them there. And even though I consciously thought I was doing a good job ... navigating through all this stuff and keeping it at a distance, it was affecting me subconsciously. So at one point ... I called this the tipping point for me ... I started to doubt myself that I wasn't good enough, and I became so paranoid that I was afraid to even get up in front and talk or say anything. Whether it was giving a report, or whether it was giving a lecture in front of my ... peers. I think it was just the years of feeling these subtle, sometimes very covert messages that I wasn't good enough and I didn't deserve this and I wasn't smart enough, and that is what I kept getting ... I realized at that point that I was in trouble, and I needed to get some support ... And here I was going from top student of my class, going from that to this person who no longer believed in himself [or] believe[d] that I could speak and be smart or any of those things and lost my confidence ... That was when I knew I was in trouble ... and that the environment had gotten to me ... I believe in myself, I got my strength back again. But not for a moment do I not think that the scars are there. The scars are still very there and very real. They are never going to go away. [nursing faculty]

The negative messages Professor Belmont received created feelings of self-doubt. Eventually he reached a point where he began to invalidate himself—"the biggest lie":

> What I learned through all of this was the biggest lie that I think . . . was ever told to me in an indirect way was that I wasn't as smart or that I couldn't write or I wasn't articulate . . . compared [to] my colleagues. And that was the biggest lie that I was ever told within this environment and [that] I bought into. That was the other thing that was bad: I bought into the lie. The other thing that also . . . became pretty apparent to me, too, when I look back at all of these experiences, there was one thing in common in all these places: that was somehow to get me to invalidate myself . . . to get me to invalidate who I am as a person, to get me to not believe that I'm smart. To get me to not believe that I earned my PhD, and I deserved it, to get me to buy into all these things about me. And if they could get me to believe it, then they were successful, because that's all they had to do was to get me to convince myself that it was all true. To beat me down to the point where I would give in and believe it. And looking back I really believe that that was sort of the systemic attempt to get me to self-doubt. Because the minute that that door opened up, then I allowed all the other stuff [to] come in and destroy who I was as a person, and that was what it was about. [nursing faculty]

A lifetime of subtle devaluation in the context of a racist society, combined with the indignity of having to defend one's ideas and prove one's legitimacy as a faculty member, may lead to feelings of insecurity in faculty of color (197). Andrews referred to the struggle to counter dominant constructions of what it means to be a scholar in predominantly white institutions as psychic taxation (198). Such burdens unjustly handicap faculty of color in academia, where confidence and competitiveness are at a premium.

Summary and Recommendations

Exclusion and control were experienced by participants across racial and ethnic groups, by both genders, and in all of the health professions. Moreover, exclusion and control affected participants at all ranks, although participants at higher ranks were more likely to have developed sophisticated coping strategies than junior faculty. Participants' experiences of exclusion and control were not minor, nor did they take place in a vacuum; they were embedded in contexts of institutional racism (199). The racial and gender hierarchies that pervade American society were reproduced in the sample. Participants' stories reflect the often subtle nature of exclusion and control and suggest avenues for change. We have seen that exclusion and control is characterized by ongoing marginalization of faculty of color that negatively and systematically affects opportunities for satisfaction and success, reduces institutional influence, and inflicts psychological harm. Participants' stories present issues of psychological and cultural safety, equitable and respectful treatment, and the unacknowledged advantages that accrue to white faculty in promotion and tenure.

Participants' stories reflect the need for behavioral change in white faculty. Although many participants shared examples of exclusion and control, there were no cases in which white faculty intervened. Perhaps this is due to the mostly covert nature of these incidents, making it difficult for white faculty to see what is going on, or to conscious or unconscious collusion. In addition, research on aversive racism suggests that whites are less likely to help a person of color in a group setting, when responsibility for action is diffused (136). Whatever the reason for this inaction may be, it is vital that white faculty learn to interrupt and actively combat exclusion and control of faculty of color. White faculty outnumber faculty of color, and whites have the privilege of speaking against the operations of racism without being accused of playing the race card. In contrast, faculty of color who speak out against racism risk being accused of focusing too much on race (200).

Training white faculty to engage in real-time direct intervention when incidents of exclusion and control occur is vital. Such training must be part of an organizational development effort that reflects an integrated institutional commitment to diversity and equity and uses expert trainers to increase effectiveness and minimize backlash (201). Long-term interactive training that promotes development of antiracist consciousness and behavior is most likely to be successful (201, 202). Additional skill development for mentors and leaders is also needed to advocate, nurture, and support faculty of color, who must learn to succeed despite these obstacles. White faculty assuming primary responsibility for antiracism (203) and equity work, and leaders prioritizing equity and cultural safety, are also crucial steps to countering exclusion and control.

What is even more striking than the incidents of exclusion and control shared by participants in this chapter is the silence and inaction of whites who were uninvolved or peripherally involved in these incidents. By choosing to be silent and inactive, whites who did not personally harm participants provided tacit support to those who did. Without whites' widespread silence and inaction, exclusion and control in health professions education could not occur. Hence, to stop exclusion and control of faculty of color, white faculty and leaders must act. If you are a white faculty member or leader, this section is for you.

Accept responsibility. In *Privilege, Power, and Difference,* Johnson coined the term "luxury of obliviousness" to describe how whites are often blinded to their racial privilege, a phenomenon that reflects such privilege (204). Because white privilege is conferred by a system of power, whites cannot give away their privilege. But it is important for you to recognize that through no fault of your own, you receive substantial benefits from being white. On the other end of the stick are faculty of color, who are penalized because of their race and ethnicity. This does not mean only whites will succeed and or that whites cannot fail. But it does mean whites have an unearned advantage that has created and continues to maintain their dominance as a group in the health professions. If you want the status quo to change, you must accept responsibility for your white privilege and use it to dismantle the system that sustains it.

Educate yourself. Racism has a complex historical legacy and continues to manifest throughout all societal sectors. Each racial and ethnic group has its own history and unique experience with racism while also sharing commonalities with others. Learn as much as you can about the various forms of racism from books, documentaries, YouTube videos and other films, and community and scientific reports. Take Implicit Association Tests at Project Implicit (205) and seek training and development to help you not only identify and address your own biases, but also skillfully navigate difficult conversations about race. The more you understand about the complex workings of racism, the more effective you will be at identifying and responding to exclusion and control. Don't make faculty of color your first source of information. It is not their job to educate you.

Be comfortable with discomfort. Because the United States is an individualistic society, whites often take it personally when racism is discussed (204). As a result, denial, minimization, defensiveness, and complaints of being tired of talking about racism are frequent responses. Get past your white guilt. It is not doing anyone any good. Denying or minimizing racism in health professions education, blaming people of color for the disadvantages they face, seeing yourself as a victim, or refusing to talk about the problem are signs that you have more work to do.

Recognize human similarities and differences. All human beings have common needs for social inclusion and respect. We all have feelings, hopes, and aspirations. At the same time, cultural and societal differences create variations in human experience. When a white person says "I don't see color," he or she is denying this reality. Hence, a person of color should be recognized as a unique person whose life is influenced by the social contexts of race and ethnicity. Moreover, systems of oppression such as racism, sexism, classism, heterosexism, and disabilism intersect and shape people's experiences and opportunities in different ways. Therefore the experiences of Asian men differ from those of Asian women, the experiences of black women with and without disabilities differ, and so forth. Understand that everybody is an individual with his or her own unique personality and life story and that the effects of systems of oppression are complex.

If you see or hear something, say something. There is no such thing as being neutral or removed. Every second of the day, social life involves you. Be mindful of yourself in circumstances in which privilege comes into play. For white privilege to operate, whites need the compliance of other whites (204). If the majority of white faculty strongly objected to the lack of racial and ethnic diversity among faculty and students at every opportunity and took significant action, underrepresentation of faculty and students of color could not continue. If a lack of progress on institutional diversity goals was considered unacceptable by the majority of white faculty, leadership would shift its priorities. Similarly, if the majority of white faculty and leaders insisted on a more diverse leadership, change in leadership representation would occur. Hence, it is imperative that white faculty who are supportive of greater racial and ethnic diversity in the health professions speak out loudly and take action every day. It is not enough to say you support racial and ethnic diversity and equity goals privately in a group of like-minded friends or colleagues. It is not enough to make indirect, mild, or infrequent references to "diversity" in larger groups but avoid talking about racism and white privilege. It is not enough to express dismay about inequities without doing anything. Your voice matters. Your actions matter. The silence and inaction of whites is required to uphold the status quo. If you do not speak up and take action against racism and inequity, others will interpret this as agreement with the status quo of white racial dominance.

Organize others who are willing to speak up and act with you. If faculty are unprepared to talk about race, ask for faculty development. If a leader, faculty member, or student makes a comment with racist overtones, seize the moment to provide accurate information and challenge false beliefs. Do so calmly, gently, and respectfully to avoid creating a negative experience. If a faculty member of color is trying to make a point at a faculty meeting and is being silenced or ignored, speak up to offer support. To gain confidence and skill, practice with supportive white colleagues what you will say and do to respond to the processes of exclusion and control described in this chapter. Do not remain silent during incidents of racism and then come to faculty of color later to commiserate in private. You are needed when other whites are in the room. By speaking up and taking action, you are serving as an antiracist role model for faculty and students (206). Conversely, by remaining silent and inactive in the face of inequities in student and faculty representation, recognition, and power, you are role modeling support for white racial dominance.

Tune into your empathy. Listen to and validate faculty and students of color who share their experiences. You don't know what it is like to face racism on a daily basis, but you can try to imagine what it would be like to be in that person's shoes. Do not ignore faculty of color who share concerns about racism, whether they are personal or more broadly related to the institutional climate. The absence of a response is a response that says you don't care. Similarly, if you address an incident of racism in class, be sensitive to the feelings of students of color, who are almost always outnumbered. Check in with students when appropriate.

Integrate your social circle. Your life will be enriched by a more diverse social circle. You can begin by saying "Hello" and being friendly to faculty and students of color just as you would to anyone else.

Engage in antiracist action. Support leader and faculty candidates who endorse equity. Let existing leaders know you expect them to be accountable for diversity and equity goals. Work to make sure faculty and student policies address racism. For example, codes of conduct need to be explicit and concrete; violations should be associated with consequences. Develop a Courageous Conversations group using well-prepared facilitators by adapting the work of Singleton and Linton for use in higher education (207, 208). Engage in antiracist pedagogy to educate the next generation of clinicians and academicians in ways that challenge white racial dominance. Acosta and Ackerman-Barger described the eagerness of medical students to talk about race and the simultaneous reluctance of faculty to engage in these discussions. They called on faculty to break the silence and change the environment: "No longer can we afford to ignore racism; no longer can we avoid talking about its real and damaging effect on all of us" (208) p.4. Be willing to endure the discomfort of speaking and acting against racism in health professions education every day, and you will be part of the solution, not part of the problem.

CHAPTER TWO

Institutional Climate

In America there is institutional racism that we all inherit and participate in,
like breathing the air in this room—and we have to become sensitive to it.

Henry Louis Gates (209)

You have to act as if it were possible to radically transform the world.
And you have to do it all the time.

Angela Davis (210)

Climate includes features of the institutional environment that are most easily observed, such as leadership composition, communication patterns, and organizational structure. Culture, which gives birth to institutional climate, includes more unstructured features of the environment, such as values and beliefs (211). In an analysis of a nationally representative sample of 29,169 faculty, Victorino and colleagues found a significant and substantial relationship between faculty satisfaction and perceptions of positive racial campus climate. The authors also found that faculty of color held significantly less positive views of campus racial climate than did whites (212). These findings are disturbing because institutional climate plays a major role in determining whether or not faculty of color will receive the nourishment they need to grow and achieve their career goals (213, 214). Hence, improving institutional climate is vital to the satisfaction and success of faculty of color in the health professions.

Participants described a spectrum of racial and ethnic inclusivity in the departments, schools, and/or larger institutions where they worked. Participants were most affected by department and school climates, but for the purpose of simplicity I use the term *institution* to represent different units in this chapter. A strong understanding of their institutional climates enabled participants to strategically manage their environments (197). Assessing climate also helped participants seeking new positions by increasing the likelihood of a good institutional fit.

Participants' descriptions of their experiences within a variety of institutional climates allowed me to identify a climate spectrum with four stages, ranging from exclusionary to inclusive, which are reflected in the "Diversity and Equity Climate Stages Rubric" shown in table 4. Research team members and participants both reviewed and gave feedback on this assessment tool. This spectrum is connected to the processes of exclusion and control described previously. The four stages range from covert exclusion (stage one = covert but high exclusion and control) to real inclusion (stage four = minimal if any exclusion and control). In covert exclusion, participants were surreptitiously and systematically excluded from full participation in their institutions and were constrained in their roles. They were only allowed to advance to the extent that they played by the "race rules" of their institutions. Participants sometimes did and sometimes did not follow these rules, often at great cost to themselves. Stage two was indifference, in which participants continued to experience some exclusion and control, albeit at lower levels than at stage one. At stage three, beginning inclusion, participants had better experiences overall and were hopeful that their institutional climates would improve. Acts of exclusion and control were fewer, and white colleagues had a sincere and budding interest in diversity and equity. Finally, at stage four, real inclusion, cultural pluralism and structural and informal integration of participants existed at institutions. Institutions had made sustained efforts to recruit and retain a racially and ethnically diverse faculty and student body. The climate was safe, respectful, and nurturing.

Six major elements make up the institutional climate. In this chapter I use the climate spectrum to rate these six major elements: recruitment and retention, faculty and student racial and ethnic diversity, diversity programs, reports of racism (formal and informal), dialogue, and leadership.

Climate Element One: Recruitment and Retention

The value an institution places on faculty of color is reflected by ongoing and often aggressive recruitment and retention efforts to ensure a racially and ethnically diverse faculty. At stage one, candidates of color were less likely to be hired, and retention was a problem. At stage two there were no intentional recruitment efforts. At stage three, active recruitment and retention efforts were in place. Faculty of color were moderately valued at these institutions. Finally,

TABLE 4. Diversity and Equity Climate Stages Rubric

ELEMENTS	COVERT EXCLUSION	INDIFFERENCE	BEGINNING INCLUSION	REAL INCLUSION
	Stage One	*Stage Two*	*Stage Three*	*Stage Four*
	High to moderate exclusion and control	Low exclusion and control	Low to no exclusion and control	No exclusion and control
Recruitment and retention	FOC candidates less likely to be hired. Retention is a problem. FOC may be tolerated.	No active, intentional recruitment.	Beginning active intentional recruitment and retention efforts. FOC are moderately valued.	Aggressive recruitment and retention efforts. FOC are highly valued.
Faculty and student racial and ethnic diversity	Lack of faculty and student diversity. FOC face barriers to promotion.	Some diversity in students and residents but not faculty. FOC promotion is not considered.	Greater racial and ethnic diversity among faculty and students. Some FOC are represented at midlevel professor ranks or above.	Diverse presence across faculty, students, and postgraduate trainees. FOC are at senior levels. FOC are overtly highly influential. Broader conceptions of scholarship and merit promote and reward diversity and equity teaching, research, practice, and service.

Diversity programs	No program or unsupported diversity programs.	Beginning interest in diversity.	Support for diversity programs.	Diversity is a high priority. Ongoing and successful diversity programs. Desire to share ownership with diverse partners.
Reports of racism (formal and informal)	High to moderate faculty, student/postgrad trainee racism reports.	Some faculty and student/postgrad trainee reports of racism.	Few faculty or student/postgrad trainee reports of racism.	Rare faculty, student, or postgrad trainee reports of racism.
Dialogue	Isolation, silencing, lip service. High resistance.	Beginning conversation. Some resistance.	Active conversation about diversity and equity issues. Pockets of resistance to open dialogue.	Open, respectful communication. Discussion of systems of oppression and historical inequities is part of diversity dialogues.
Leadership	Leadership action or inaction counterproductive to diversity.	Leadership indifferent or neutral.	Opportunity for real leadership extended to FOC.	Leadership is visionary. FOC are represented at all levels of leadership. Zero tolerance for racist attitudes and behavior, including covert racism. Commitment to diversity and equity is genuine.

^aFOC = faculty of color

at stage four, aggressive recruitment and retention efforts had long been under way, and faculty of color were highly valued.

RECRUITMENT AND RETENTION AT STAGE ONE: COVERT EXCLUSION

At stage one, powerful white faculty used their influence to hinder recruitment and retention of faculty of color. Keeping faculty of color out kept the academic environment comfortable for those whites who felt uneasy being around people who were different from them. This finding suggests that the subjective criterion of "fit" commonly used in faculty searches should be questioned as potential subterfuge (4). Professor Singh provided an example:

> [The good old boys] make a focused effort to recruit the right fit. So the fit is much more important than anything else . . . So do you think like me? Are you going to be able to work with me? Are you going to be my friend? Are we going to have a good relationship? That's more important than skills and ability to teach and things like that. So it's more: how do you fit into our group and are you going to dispute me publicly? . . . That's why . . . they've always recruited people they knew, right? So then [they] never had to face this diversity issue. [pharmacy faculty]

Professor Singh referred to senior faculty having an investment in the status quo. This was a consistent theme in participants' responses, with terms like "good old boys," or in the female-dominated field of nursing, "good old girls," being mentioned frequently:

PROFESSOR MERIWETHER: As long as those good old girls continue to sit around the table, you're not going to have change in nursing. [nursing faculty]

PROFESSOR CHOPRA: In the younger generation, there's more of an even mix of gender and color. I think when they arise, then it'll make a difference and improvement . . . But it's going to take time—another fifteen years, I think . . . [Now] it's a boys' club. It's really . . . this very archaic feeling. [medical faculty]

PROFESSOR WOODS: I would say in academic pharmacy that it's more of the good old boys. I think it's changing because more pharmacy students—like Pharm D students, they're more female in the Pharm D program across the country. So I think it's changing. But in terms of academic pharmacy . . . it's more of the . . . good old boy's club. [pharmacy faculty]

The good old girls' and boys' club had a negative influence on racial and ethnic diversity, as described by Professor Mansfield:

INTERVIEWER: Participants have brought up that faculty who have been around for a long time and have sort of grown older in their profession may be very hesitant to make any changes. So if I don't want to make things different, I am not going to take the risk of stepping out and saying, "Okay, let's do this because this will help us recruit and keep students and/or faculty of color." . . . Any thoughts about that?

PROFESSOR MANSFIELD: I think there are a lot of faculty that actually feel that way. And then I also get the sense that a lot of the faculty—particularly faculty that [have] been at the school for a while—kind of felt that they want to keep the faculty the same. [nursing faculty]

Often participants perceived senior faculty as more resistant to diversity and equity than junior faculty; many cited this as a generational issue. Professor Green, however, also expressed concern about younger faculty:

INTERVIEWER: Many participants have described a need for more faculty born after the civil rights movement to make progress. What are your thoughts?

PROFESSOR GREEN: The old boys' club is still around, and white senior faculty want to keep their power. But many of the younger faculty pretend not to see race. They whitewash inequities by saying they are color-blind, and this is a barrier to progress. [pharmacy faculty]

Strategies to influence existing senior faculty and leaders include requiring participation in carefully chosen, long-term equity training as part of a larger institutional initiative and holding them accountable for equity goals. Without such measures, senior faculty and leaders may offer lip service to diversity, but their actions may be superficial and insincere. Professor Dillard described insincerity at his institution:

The administration and the environment tend to marginalize faculty of color with no real demonstrated support for diversity . . . no true academic appointments . . . In the many years I have been at this school, [there have been] only two African American faculty members, and I was the third. In forty years! And there's no interest whatsoever in hiring. When it comes to diversity, we pull files out of the cabinet [and] dust them off at . . . accreditation time. Once accreditation is over, they go back into the files to collect dust. So there's absolutely no demonstrated interest, no support, no programs, nothing to attract faculty of color. [dental faculty]

Professor Dillard used the words *real* and *true*. These terms suggest that surface efforts to support racial and ethnic diversity may be made for appearance's sake, but they have no substance. Participants easily recognized lip service and were frustrated by this disingenuous approach. Insincerity was also evident in the use of coded language such as "we only want the best and the brightest." Such statements were commonly used to shoot down proposals to target recruitment of URM faculty. Professor Morgan explained:

When we were hiring people, I was the one who said things like, "Are we actually interviewing a diverse pool? What are we doing to make sure?" There was some disrespect there, because some of the faculty members were of the opinion, "We're just trying to get the best and the brightest. We don't need to worry about diversity." So there was some disrespect there for me, I thought. Because you really do have to go and find—in this specialty there are some very bright African American or underserved population folks, however you want to define it—but you've got to go find them. They don't just show up at your door. [medical faculty]

Lack of a diverse talent pool was another commonly used excuse for poor recruitment and retention of faculty of color. Professor Adams commented on this barrier:

And saying that they don't have enough qualified people out there to seek them out. Well, I mean you have got to think outside the box, you have to be more proactive, in that people aren't going to just land in your lap. You have to be actively engaged . . . and when you find them and make a really big effort to get them to come, and when they come, [make] sure that they interact with the people that look like them and see that they have some sort of social base, and try to improve your recruitment efforts. [medical faculty]

Participants' concerns about recruitment of faculty of color reflect long-standing resistance to hiring racially and ethnically diverse faculty at predominantly white institutions. More than thirty years ago Harvey and Scott-Jones noted that although the supply of PhDs of color had increased substantially, many searches for new faculty still concluded with "a thoroughly remorseful committee chair explaining that the position is not being offered to a black person because, 'We couldn't find any'" (215) p.68. Thus, the statements described by participants, such as "we only want the best and the brightest" and "there aren't enough qualified people [of color]" were long ago recognized as meaning "we don't want any." Although there are more white than minority candidates to choose from, evidence does not support claims of an insufficient talent pool to increase racial and ethnic faculty diversity in nursing, medicine, and pharmacy. Representation of URMs among faculty in these health professions lags behind national graduation rates for PhDs, DNPs, MDs, and PharmDs. In nursing, URMs make up 21.1 percent of PhD and 18.2 percent of DNP graduates but only 11 percent of faculty (18, 71). In medicine, URMs make up 10.3 percent of MD graduates but only 5 percent of faculty (19, 216). In pharmacy, URMs make up 20 percent of PharmD and 10 percent of PhD graduates but only 8 percent of faculty (20, 217). We found no mismatch between URM graduates and faculty representation in dentistry; blacks, Latino/as, and Native Americans were poorly represented among dental school graduates and faculty alike. Health professions schools also have the option of hiring faculty of color with doctoral degrees in related fields.

Studies of scholars of color have reported bias in candidate selection and difficulty finding faculty positions, with some resorting to industry positions after being turned away from academe (4, 218). Coded language thinly disguises concerns about the qualifications of candidates of color as compared to a pool of white candidates. Such statements also reflect assumptions about what qualifications are valued. Although abilities to effectively relate to and mentor faculty and students from diverse backgrounds are critical skills for improving diversity and equity outcomes, these qualifications are rarely required for faculty positions (83). Moreover, what counts as excellence in a field is defined by the field and affects who is hired and retained. The lack of diverse perspectives in the health sciences and continued presence of white faculty as the gatekeepers of academe has led to a narrow view of what qualities are commonly identified as most desirable in faculty, fostering conformity and homogeneity in the professions. Lack of commitment to recruitment, covert discrimination during the hiring process, and undervaluing of candidates of color converge, negatively affecting racial and ethnic faculty diversity. These problems continue when leadership fails to recognize and address these patterns, as described by Professor Said:

Our dean says she values diversity, but we don't have diversity. She says diverse faculty won't accept our job offers because of the lack of minorities in this state. Now why would minorities come here to interview if they had completely ruled out this state? And what kind of fool would believe that every time we offer . . . a job to . . . diverse candidates they *all* decline for the same reason, and it has nothing to do with the climate at this school? Good grief. The reality is there is racism at this school, and people pick up on that when they come for an interview. Are they going to say that to our dean? Of course not. So she's failed to recognize an obvious problem, and we haven't made any progress hiring minority faculty at this school. [nursing faculty]

The stage one climate, highly exclusionary and controlling, leads to turnover of faculty of color, as described by Professor Balewa:

I mentioned that it's very difficult to be black in that area, which is true. I mean, I've been there ten years and what progress have we made? How many more [faculty of color] have we hired? Very few . . . People who come always run away. I told you, there was a guy in pediatric endocrinology. He lasted one year. One year! He was gone . . . I never asked what was the issue. I just noticed. And that bothered me. I wondered, what was it about this place? [medical faculty]

Professor Balewa never asked what happened to the missing pediatric endocrinologist, but she noticed his departure. This is consistent with the scanning of the environment we observed with other participants. Participants were keenly aware of how their colleagues were faring. This highlights the effect retention of even one visible faculty member of color can have on perceptions of institutional climate.

RECRUITMENT AND RETENTION AT STAGE TWO: INDIFFERENCE

In contrast to stage one, in which resistance to recruitment and retention efforts was marked, diversity and equity were just not institutional priorities at stage two. Professor Jennings provided an example:

That's [recruitment and retention] just not on the radar screen at all. We just recently had our strategic planning retreat, where we're thinking of over the next five to ten years, what are some goals . . . that we want to do and . . . to prioritize . . . As a whole, the faculty created these lists of things, and we got together and prioritized what would be most important to do in the immediate years versus later. And recruitment of students, diverse students and faculty, was on the low, low priority list. There were comments made that we're in the Midwest, so why should we make that a priority? We're not going to get students of color or faculty of color. I definitely said that I disagree. I feel like we have to be intentional, and I think that it should be a priority. If we continue to feel that way, then it will continue to stay the same. I definitely did not like the comment. [pharmacy faculty]

Although lack of racial and ethnic diversity in higher education is a concern generally, for faculty of color in the health professions, this concern is tied directly to the nation's health. Professor Bailey expressed her frustration:

PROFESSOR BAILEY: This is ridiculous. We're training all of these residents to work in a community where everybody's black or Latino, and there's hardly anybody who's from that community or has roots in that community.
INTERVIEWER: What would need to happen for that to occur?
PROFESSOR BAILEY: It would have to become a priority, because there's lots of good people with lots of good grades and resumes, but if you're not thinking along those lines, then it's very easy not to happen. I suspect that people aren't saying, "Oh we don't want this person because [he or she is] black." I think what's happening is they aren't saying this is an important thing that we need to address. And that effort to make sure that there are people who are black or who are Latino . . . It doesn't feel like a conspiracy, but it does feel like, let's use that old expression benign neglect . . . If you don't make that effort, it's not going to happen just by coincidence. It has got to be worked on. [medical faculty]

Professor Bailey spoke of the importance of recruiting students and residents of color, yet our findings suggest that faculty of color, who are also underrepresented, are essential to this effort. There are good candidates at the student level, but these students will not necessarily choose academic careers over lucrative clinical practice without good mentoring and support and improvements in institutional climates. These are "leaks" in the pipeline that must be repaired.

At stage two, participants also reported indifference to retention of faculty of color. This meant that institutions made no effort to retain faculty of color. Professor Garcia described the negative impact:

PROFESSOR GARCIA: If someone said "Anna, you are a good role model for the few minority residents we accept into our internal medicine program, can you please stay?" I would say, "Pay me more and help me pay off my student loans." Or "mentor me," or something, because I have no incentive to stay.

INTERVIEWER: So you are thinking about leaving?

PROFESSOR GARCIA: Oh, yes. I think about it all the time. I can't tell you the number of times I have thought of leaving. I could make twice as much and work less anywhere else. Private hospital. I mean, that's what I would say, for retention. [medical faculty]

Professor Garcia was the only Latina in a teaching hospital with a large Latino/a patient population, yet she received no mentoring or support for her interests. Because of this, she frequently considered leaving her institution. Because she supported an extended family and had student loans, the lure of a more lucrative clinical career was difficult to resist. Yet her presence was critical for the care of many of the indigent Latino/a patients at her hospital. Another participant, Professor Suparmanputra, commented on a lack of concern for the needs of faculty of color:

Like I said, at any one time they're [faculty of color] there, and then next thing they're gone . . . The faculty [member] that I recruited . . . she needed certain things and couldn't necessarily get the answers. And I would get a call from her—she's not here anymore. But [she] would call me and ask me what I thought about this, and thought about that, and how do you go about getting this and whatever the case might be, and what should I do in this situation? . . . But they [faculty of color] don't get what they need. [nursing faculty]

Professor Suparmanputra described a revolving door for faculty of color at her institution, despite her own efforts to bring in diverse candidates. Participants' experiences reflect what is documented in the literature. Faculty attrition is a serious problem affecting health professions education, in which faculty shortages continue to be a concern. A study examining attrition rates among full-time US medical school faculty from 1981 to 1997 reported that 43 percent of first-time assistant professors left academia (219). In addition, although one study found no differences in intent to leave faculty positions (220) between URM and white medical school faculty, others have documented actual disparities in attrition, with faculty of color in nursing and medicine leaving more quickly and at higher rates than whites (221, 222). Such attrition detrimentally affects institutions' ability to increase racial and ethnic diversity among the faculty even when aggressive recruitment hiring practices are in place. Moreno and colleagues reported findings from the twenty-eight colleges and universities that participated in the Diversity Campus Initiative (CDI). Although substantial increases in rates of hiring URMs occurred, only a slight increase in URM faculty overall was found after four years. To account for this, Moreno and colleagues devised a tool to determine the percentage of new faculty going toward replacement. The "Turnover Quotient" was derived by dividing the net change in core faculty by the total number of new hires during the period under study. Using this formula, 81 percent of overall new hires went toward replacement, suggesting that 19 percent of new hires could be considered new positions or true expansion of the overall faculty (223). These findings point to the importance of addressing attrition for building a racially and ethnically diverse faculty and the need for health professions schools to take attrition seriously, putting measures in place to retain faculty of color and track retention of URMs.

RECRUITMENT AND RETENTION AT STAGE THREE: BEGINNING INCLUSION

Institutions at stage three moved beyond the indifferent stage to actively recruit and retain faculty of color, particularly URMs. The importance of making a conscious effort and knowing how to search for black faculty was described by Professor Duncan, the dean of a nursing school in a state with a relatively small black population:

> I continue to think it's important . . . It's difficult for us to get black people in this state, and they say there's no black people . . . in this place . . . That's the perception, so it's difficult. I think in some cases where . . . the faculties aren't more diverse, it's because people have really not understood how to look for those faculty. And they don't find them, which is kind of understandable because they're not looking in the right place, or they're not using the right techniques. So I think if there's going to be a real commitment to bringing diverse faculty, there has to be more of a commitment to looking at some different methods . . . If you continue to do what you always have done, you will get the same results you've always gotten . . . Then if people decide they're going to bring diverse faculty, then they need to be prepared to support those faculty effectively, and that's another piece of it. It certainly does mean something to students, I think,

to have diverse faculty, and I continue to believe that. Clearly, it's going to be a different kind of knowledge base and experience that more diverse faculty . . . bring—[that] the white faculty won't necessarily bring. [nursing faculty]

As an academic leader, Professor Duncan was aware of what racially and ethnically diverse faculty members bring to an institution and knew the importance of purposeful recruitment and retention strategies for faculty of color in states where recruitment may be more challenging. She was a prime example of what racial and ethnic diversity can bring to leadership.

Effective recruitment requires search committee training to reduce selection bias. Professor Barnes described search committee members' awareness of the importance of the strengths that racially and ethnically diverse faculty bring to health professions schools:

> I've had an opportunity to sit in on [the] recruitment committee for this next upcoming, like our faculty season . . . So we'll have maybe five candidates come in, and of the five, one or two of them—well actually only one—one was of a different ethnicity. One was a woman that was of Indian descent. And she came in, and I saw on a lot of people's comments, they said, "Well, this will add to the diversity of our school, add to the diversity of the faculty pool." Some people commented on that on their sheets when they were turning them in. So I think that people are cognizant of the fact that they'd like to increase the diversity among the faculty and the student pool, if they can. Not saying that they are going to choose this individual solely because of that, but they did make notation of it. So I think that—again, I think they're cognizant that it would be a good idea to increase diversity. [pharmacy faculty]

In addition to awareness of the importance of diversity, targeted recruitment efforts for URMs are usually necessary. Professor Drake, a black faculty member, described her experience:

> I was at this other place and I got the call . . . that said, "When are you coming? We have positions. We want you to come now." And I said, "Well, I'll come next year. I'm not ready to come right now." Because things were going well with my research even though I hated the people I worked with. But my research was going well . . . so they asked me a couple times. And then I got a call, somebody said, "If you are coming, you better come now because we don't

have many positions." . . . So . . . I met with the dean and she said, "We have to move fast." And she said, "You are going to do this and this and this. And what is your salary now?" And I told her. And she said, "I can't do that. We are state supported and the salaries are posted, and I can't do that. But I can do this and I will give you this. And I can give you this. And what else can I give you? What else can I give you?" She just gave me everything. [nursing faculty]

In describing her experience, Professor Drake provided examples of many important recruitment strategies. First, she was identified as a promising recruitment target. Next, the timing of her move was negotiated, and she was offered as many supports as the institution had available, even though it was unable to match her current salary. Each of these actions clearly demonstrated that she was highly valued by top leadership.

Health professions education produces its own labor market, giving it a large degree of control over the faculty pipeline. Thus, "growing your own," or bringing graduates of color into faculty positions at their alma maters, was another recruitment strategy that participants reported their institutions used to increase diversity. Professor Hazelwood shared her experience:

I had completed my bachelor's and . . . the chair of nursing . . . said, "You know what, you need to go on to your master's." In fact, she actually grabbed my grandmother and my mother there at graduation to say, "We want her to go to graduate school. She has done well. She needs to get her master's." At the time I wasn't even thinking about it. But when I went back with the master's, they kept calling me to come teach, "We think you can do a good job teaching." And after that first year as an adjunct, the president called me in—they wanted me to go meet with them. I said, "What is this about?" And they told me, "You have done a fine job, you have faculty support. Faculty want you to come back, they want you in a tenure track, and you have excellent student evaluations." And so it was to tell me that they wanted me to teach, and that they wanted me to go to a tenure track position. And I really felt valued, then, because they said, "We will do what we can to make it possible for you to do that, if you are so inclined, by getting the support that you need." So that in itself was a wonderful piece for me, and to know that once I finally made the decision to go back to school. They accommodated me in terms of the scheduling so I could go to school and work on a full-time basis. [nursing faculty]

Professor Hazelwood is a good example of a faculty member who was mentored into an academic career beginning at the undergraduate level. She was identified as someone who should continue on to graduate school and later, in whom the school wanted to invest as a faculty member. In the end, the school gained a talented faculty member of color who became a leader. Professor Cleary also described the "grow your own" approach:

INTERVIEWER: Is there any evidence that the leadership is trying to place any emphasis on diversity for the faculty or the school?

PROFESSOR CLEARY: Yes, there is. Our dean actually hired me to increase our diversity on research and focus on indigenous research. Then the associate dean is also recruiting American Indian faculty. So we're increasing our . . . [number of] American Indian PhD students with hopes of hiring a couple in the future and increasing the diversity in our faculty . . . We are growing our own. They are . . . definitely making an effort . . . It gives me hope that I won't be placed on every committee that needs some diversity. It also [makes me] feel that they value me and value diversity. Overall, it is a more positive experience to know you're valued and others like you are valued. [pharmacy faculty]

Seeing the "grow your own" strategy in action not only gave Professor Cleary hope that her feelings of isolation would end soon; it also made her feel valued as a faculty member of color. She also described specific retention efforts: "They recruited me and have been very supportive. They've actually provided me with incentives and small funding to get going and time dedicated to do the Research Center. So they've been very supportive." The retention strategies Professor Cleary described benefited both her and the institution. By investing in Professor Cleary's interests, the institution gained a research center, and her funded research enhanced the school's prestige.

RECRUITMENT AND RETENTION AT STAGE FOUR: REAL INCLUSION

At stage four, institutional efforts to build a racially and ethnically diverse faculty had long been under way and had begun to bear fruit. Retention efforts promoted faculty of color's satisfaction and success; faculty of color were represented in the higher academic ranks and leadership. In these inclusive environments, participants were highly valued, and diversity and equity was a strong priority.

Visionary leadership was critical for institutions to reach stage four in recruitment and retention. Professor Meriwether described such leadership:

I had a visionary dean [who] fulfilled the need ... to recruit minority faculty ... She wanted ... minority faculty in order to recruit more minority students, and not only African American faculty, but an array of minority faculty. And what we were able to do in the first few years, we were able to really get the minority students involved. She had quite a few Hispanic faculty members who were able to have guest speakers from a Hispanic ... community come in and talk to students. [nursing faculty]

The result of this kind of leadership led to the development of a racially and ethnically diverse faculty, as described by Professor Morgan:

We have a couple of minority surgeons, which is hard to find. I mean again, I'm bragging right now a little bit, but we've recruited a couple of physicists, African American physicist faculty. You know African American physicists are like rare hen's teeth, and we've got two. Again, one of the surgeons is a black woman, we recruited her. I could go on and on and on, but I'm real proud of that legacy, in the sense I think once I sort of got there and showed people you could be successful and the good old boys died off, I mean ... that was a lot of it, the good old boys just went away. And the folks [who] came in behind them were willing to be more open-minded. So we now [in this department] have a very diverse faculty. I'm very proud of it, I'm very proud of it.

INTERVIEWER: So a major change?

PROFESSOR MORGAN: Major change, but again it took sort of me coming in and saying, "We're going to do this, and these good old white boys are going to accept it," but it also took the good old white boys just going away. [medical faculty]

Professors Meriwether and Morgan described visionary leadership and its positive effects on the academic climate. In particular, Professor Morgan described two milestones. First, a changing of the guard: the "good old boys" no longer controlled his department. Second, a black faculty member who valued equity had assumed a leadership role and took steps to build a diverse faculty. Similarly, participants reported that racial and ethnic diversity among students and postgraduate trainees was driven by leadership, as described by Professor Griffin:

The departments that do prioritize it ... within just the emergency medicine program the number of [racially and ethnically diverse] residents that they are able to pull each and every year, that has to be intentional. You don't just have that by accident. You know what I'm saying? You can't create eight spots out of like fifteen, or almost half of your spots, [for] minority candidates by accident. I'm sorry, [but] you have to be very intentional. [medical faculty]

Consistent with the overall findings, Professor Griffin aptly described the need to be "very intentional" to cultivate a racially and ethnically diverse faculty and student body. Only one of ninety-six participants from predominantly white institutions described a racially and ethnically diverse faculty body occurring by happenstance. Sustained, intentional, and strategic action was necessary to build a racially and ethnically diverse faculty, highlighting the importance of leadership that values and is committed to diversity and equity.

Climate Element Two: Racial and Ethnic Diversity among Faculty and Students

Sustained efforts to recruit and retain faculty and students of color, and in particular URMS, increase institutional diversity. Institutions at stage one lacked racially and ethnically diverse faculty and students. Furthermore, participants encountered barriers to promotion and assuming leadership roles. At stage two, institutions had some student racial and ethnic diversity, but little among the faculty, and promotion of faculty of color to the senior ranks and leadership roles was not on the radar screen. At stage three, institutions had a more racially and ethnically diverse body of faculty and students, and some faculty of color were in the higher professorial ranks and in leadership roles. At stage four there was racial and ethnic diversity among faculty and students, including URMS. Also, faculty of color were evident at the senior professorial levels and in leadership roles at various levels. At stage four, faculty of color were influential within the institution.

RACIAL AND ETHNIC FACULTY AND STUDENT DIVERSITY AT STAGES ONE AND TWO: COVERT EXCLUSION AND INDIFFERENCE

Because stages one and two had similar effects on faculty and student racial and ethnic diversity, I describe them together here. In both covert exclusion and indifference, there was a lack of faculty and student racial and ethnic diversity due to a dearth of recruitment and retention efforts. Participants attributed this situation to their institutions' lack of interest in racial and ethnic diversity, as described by Professor Jones:

INTERVIEWER: Another question for you has to do with the . . . lack of progress that's being made in having a more diverse faculty.

PROFESSOR JONES: The fact that people really don't want to have that. That's the bottom line. It is really the whole racism [problem]; people are afraid of what that might look like, what that means to them. In my mind, it's pure and simple. If you really wanted to do it, then we would be doing it. We can do lots of other things, if you can send, literally, let's think about this. If we actually have the capacity to send [people] to the moon and bring them [back], to outer space and bring them back, [but] we can't bring a faculty [member] of color in? Really? [medical faculty]

Professor Jones's belief was echoed by many of the participants: increasing racial and ethnic diversity in health professions education is not rocket science; it can be done if leadership makes the commitment. Health professions education will increase the racial and ethnic diversity of faculty and students when this goal becomes a high priority. Often diversity is touted by institutions as a value, and in many cases it is included in strategic plans, yet years later, little if any change is seen (224). Professor Dillard commented on the lack of progress at his school:

[For] the ten African American students who have graduated from the School of Dentistry over the past almost forty years . . . approximately sixteen hundred white dental students have graduated . . . The School of Dentistry has never admitted an African American to its orthodontic program and only one . . . to its general practice residency program. This situation exists despite the fact that universities across the nation have attracted African American dental students, students who have successfully attended and graduated, students who go back to underserved communities. I am not alone in my assessment that the School of Dentistry lacks any real commitment to inclusive diversity. [dental faculty]

Lack of racial and ethnic diversity, whether caused by covert exclusion or indifference, contributed to participants' sense of isolation and helped perpetuate lack of support for this group. In the words of Professor Swan:

I came to interview, it was very different because I am used to a little more diverse environment and this is not diverse in any way, I would say in ethnicity, race, or even I would say opinions, beliefs, and those types of things. It's a very conservative university, and so it was quite different. And so coming in it was very strange, because I really did not have—and still I don't really have—a big, strong support network here of other faculty. [pharmacy faculty]

Similarly, Professor King said:

I was the first African American male in a long, long time at this institution. There was an African American female [who] was there before me and essentially, there was nobody else . . . At the beginning it was . . . kind of a lonely experience. I was wondering when I was going to see another black faculty member in the department, but it never really quite happened. It's been kind of isolating. [medical faculty]

Professors Swan and King talked about feeling lonely and isolated without any support network, and there is a sense that they were waiting to see if the situation would change. When those circumstances did not change, disappointment set in for participants, which had repercussions for retaining them and recruiting new faculty of color. The importance of faculty of color for recruiting others was frequently noted, as described by Professor Smith:

Prospective faculty . . . will mention that they want to be in an environment where they feel like they are not the only person of color in their department. Also, when they see that there are no or few persons of color in leadership positions, that . . . seems to be a "red flag" that discourages someone from considering our institution. I can say that the negative reputation of an institution makes a difference. Even if efforts are being made to enhance or support diversity, the past reputation of a lack of attention to these issues is often difficult to overcome. [medical faculty]

Many participants described an informal network of faculty of color within health professions education. Sharing information about which institutions are and are not friendly to faculty of color is common. Participants who had negative experiences felt obligated to warn other faculty of color away from their institutions to protect them from experiencing the same fate. This suggests that when faculty of color are treated poorly, institutional reputations are affected and recruitment suffers.

In addition to the problems of isolation and recruitment challenges, participants were less likely to be represented at the senior professorial ranks at stages one and two. In some cases, this was due to lack of support. Professor Harding described her experience of being denied promotion:

> Someone usually who has been on board as long as I have [would] at least [have] been promoted to associate professor . . . For most jobs, if you do a good job and you have been told annually that you're doing a great job, essentially you're believing that by around the seven-year mark . . . you would be considered for promotion. So I have gone up for promotion, but I was denied promotion based on some deficiencies that I had in scholarship, well, writing . . . And I will say that I am in a very unique position within pharmacy practice. We now have about seventy practitioners [who] practice and teach, but I am the only one [who] has a practice setting that's like mine. So I have no peers. When I came on board I was told that I would have peers . . . and to me, I think that's a huge deficiency if you want to promote a person based on scholarship . . . You have to at least create the environment that's conducive to being promoted. [pharmacy faculty]

Indifference to Professor Harding's need for mentorship and scholarly development contributed to her difficulties with promotion. This is an example of how an indifferent environment can keep faculty of color from advancing. Although this problem can affect any faculty member, challenges to accessing mentorship and collaboration faced by faculty of color (225, 226) and underrepresentation at the higher professorial ranks document racial and ethnic inequities in the path to promotion and tenure (16, 34, 35). Given this reality, institutional efforts to support the advancement of faculty of color are necessary to address historical inequities and counter the effects of exclusion and control.

RACIAL AND ETHNIC FACULTY AND STUDENT DIVERSITY AT STAGE THREE: BEGINNING INCLUSION

At stage three, institutions had a nascent vision for racial and ethnic diversity and were taking steps to implement it. An example from Professor Pham illustrates this process:

Well, the fact with the mission of the school—they are trying to have diversity in students, but also in faculty, so in that regard knowing that that vision has already been put in motion because we are caring for it. We have always been caring for a diverse population; it just seems like now the school has a vision. [nursing faculty]

Professor Pham described "caring for" diversity. Achieving this vision required attention to recruitment and retention of faculty and students of color. In turn, successful recruitment and retention depended on the presence of some racially and ethnically diverse faculty to aid these efforts. Professor Morgan, a leader at his school, described how his presence helped his school recruit other faculty of color:

PROFESSOR MORGAN: I get asked this all the time ... "How do we increase diversity?" Well ... you've got to bring somebody in who looks different. Which is not ... a faculty of thirty or forty white folks who look at the one black person ... It makes you uneasy. I know it made me uneasy when I was interviewing for jobs if nobody in the room looked like me. So having me in the room, I think, gave Henry [his boss] some legitimacy ... I think it gave him some legitimacy to say, "You know, here's Oliver. I brought him in. He's done well. Don't be afraid."

INTERVIEWER: Another participant said that if there's someone [who] looks like you then you don't have to be the trailblazer and also that ... there's a "sense of safety" that that person is okay so maybe I'll be okay too.

PROFESSOR MORGAN: Yeah. I absolutely agree with that ... I can't say it stronger. That is absolutely the truth. I think once somebody gets in and who's done well—and again I'm trying to be modest but I think I did okay—other folks came in thinking it's a safe place to be. It's a big deal. White folks don't get that either ... being safe for us is a big deal. [medical faculty]

Professor Morgan's comments show that it is not enough for institutions to have racially and ethnically diverse faculty; their satisfaction and success are important in recruiting other faculty of color, who can see that their predecessors have done well. The concepts of trailblazing and feeling safe introduced by Professor Morgan also appeared in Professor Zeno's story:

PROFESSOR ZENO: I went online first—that was one thing that was in my mind as I was applying for jobs. To be honest with you, I didn't want to go into a department or into a university where everybody in that department or that college was white. So I looked online first, and I knew that there were two other professors, like faculty of color. So that's all I had in mind. It was just two, and I came with that in my head, and that's exactly what I saw, just two . . . and actually, when it comes to diversity among the faculty, I'm Hispanic, two blacks, and that's it. We don't have Indians, or we don't have other Asian or Middle Eastern, that's it. In terms of diversity, that's all we have right now.

INTERVIEWER: Did it make a difference to you that there were at least two African Americans?

PROFESSOR ZENO: Oh, yeah. Oh, yeah, like I said, I wouldn't have come here if I would have been the only one. Definitely.

INTERVIEWER: It sounds like it really made a big difference then if you wouldn't have come at all.

PROFESSOR ZENO: It actually did, and the person who was running the committee for my position, she was one of the African American faculty [members] that we have, and she was the one who was sent to pick me up at the airport, so pretty much the first face that I got from this college, from my university was her face, and it was a black face, you know? . . . One of the very first questions I asked as we were driving to have dinner . . . was, "Can you tell me about diversity, can you tell me about, not only diversity. Clearly, I don't look like everybody else in this city, is that okay, outside of work?" I want to make sure that I live in a city where it's going to be okay, that people are not going to be looking at me weird because they have never seen something like this. She assured me that it was going to be okay. [pharmacy faculty]

Professor Zeno described the comfort he felt seeing a faculty member of color at his interview and being greeted by a diverse faculty member at the airport. This first impression set the tone for Professor Zeno's interview visit and provided information about the community. Having the opportunity to ask frank questions of another person of color in order to assess the safety of the situation was an important part of his positive experience.

In summary, stage three was characterized by a growing institutional vision of racial and ethnic diversity. Steps taken toward progress included recruitment and retention efforts that created some racial and ethnic diversity among faculty and students. In addition, there were early efforts to support the advancement of faculty of color. Consequently, stage three institutions had some faculty of color at the middle and senior academic ranks and in leadership.

A racially and ethnically diverse body of faculty and students, including appropriate proportions of URMs, was characteristic of stage four. This stage was the product of sustained recruitment and retention efforts. Professors Chavez and Singh provided examples:

PROFESSOR CHAVEZ: The literature shows and also best practices show at the institutions that if you create a healthy environment, a diverse environment, an environment in which your organization becomes a multicultural organizational community, and it's obvious and it's very visible and you actually do that by increasing your minority faculty, . . . students, and residents, then that's going to feed and that work is going to reward you in the future by being able to get to where you want to get, as far as the diversity [in] workforce. [medical faculty]

INTERVIEWER: If you were looking for another school . . . what type of qualities would you be looking for?

PROFESSOR SINGH: Someone who's used to the diversity—in a true sense. A group that has worked with this for a long period of time . . . It's second nature to them, they all just get along. And understand each other and have fun with each other's cultures . . . And they all participate in events together . . . totally diverse. [pharmacy faculty]

Professors Chavez and Singh emphasized visible diversity and comfort with difference as elements of a truly inclusive climate. As Professor Rangan noted, this kind of climate can positively shape the faculty interview experience:

When I came for an interview, it was very surprising to see there were a lot of other faculty [who] were of different colors. They were black, they were Asian, they were brown like me, they were Caucasian, so there was a big mix so that—that made me really confident that there is a lot of diversity. So okay, I thought if I can get a job here it would be nice. [pharmacy faculty]

Professor Rangan's experience underscored the desirability of visible faculty diversity, as well as its positive impact on recruitment of additional faculty of color. When visible diversity was part of the institutional climate, participants noticed:

PROFESSOR RODRIGUEZ: I see faculty members who are African American. I see faculty members who are Asian . . . I think all kinds of people are represented: Muslims, African Americans, Hispanics for sure. [medical faculty]

PROFESSOR CHEN: I would say that it's very diverse and open . . . The school that I first started teaching at was not as diverse as this school is. I think that makes a difference. [pharmacy faculty]

At stage four, participants were appreciated for who they were and what they brought to their institutions. This included their diverse perspectives, scholarly interests, and connections to communities. White faculty recognized the importance of visible diversity and had taken the steps needed to ensure full representation of different racial and ethnic groups among faculty, students, and leadership. Faculty and leaders were well informed about equity, which included information about oppression and historical inequalities; attention was paid to remedying current inequities among groups in the institution. The climate was supportive and nurturing, enabling faculty of color to maximize their contributions and thrive.

Climate Element Three: Diversity Programs

A third element in an institution's climate was the status of diversity programs. These programs could be centers, committees, mentoring and faculty development programs, student groups, or other bodies. When effective, such programs could facilitate faculty recruitment and retention efforts and provide an array of additional assistance and resources for diverse faculty and students. Institutions at stage one either lacked diversity programs entirely or their existing programs were undermined and unsupported. Institutions at stage two had diversity programs with a fledgling commitment to diversity or more established programs that required additional investment to be effective. Institutions might use pro-diversity discourse, but no real efforts were made, and participants could easily see through such deceptions. Institutions at stage three had better-supported diversity programs, and at stage four, diversity was a genuine priority. Ongoing and successful diversity programs were in place, and leadership demonstrated a sincere desire to share ownership of the institution with diverse partners.

DIVERSITY PROGRAMS AT STAGE ONE: COVERT EXCLUSION

At stage one of the climate spectrum there was a lack of any meaningful diversity programs in the school or on the campus, even when problems such as underrepresentation of faculty and students of color were evident, as described by Professor Corbin:

> Ever since I've been here, generally we haven't had a large number of minority faculty. In fact, I've been one of the few . . . but the camaraderie . . . just really hasn't existed among minority faculty here . . . And we don't have a division of diversity or multicultural affairs . . . I think what would really need to happen is perhaps an office of diversity affairs, or however you want to label a multicultural affairs office. We don't have that—I've asked about it, and there hasn't been a clear answer as to whether or not we're going to have one. There is one on [the] main campus, but they're really not highly involved in what we're doing here. But I think there would have to be some support, there would have to be some funding, there would have to be a concerted effort to try to recruit more minority faculty. [medical faculty]

Professor Corbin linked the absence of faculty of color with the lack of a diversity office and noted that backing and financial resources would be necessary to create diversity programs. Professor Lang also spoke about a lack of diversity programs:

PROFESSOR LANG: I would say that I've had, maybe, over a hundred students, I have seen since I've been there. And I've only seen two African Americans or black people. So [it's] not just in pharmacy. I think this is something that is pervasive. Even nurses—it was shocking, when I came here—you don't really see many African American nurses. And I mean, granted the population of African Americans is lower than in other places, but it was still very striking when I first moved here. You don't see, really, African American physicians. You're not really seeing African American residency students. You're not really seeing African American nurses.

INTERVIEWER: So does your school have any programs to try [to] increase URM students in the pharmacy program?

PROFESSOR LANG: No. [pharmacy faculty]

Professor Lang was appalled by the lack of racial and ethnic diversity among trainees and health professionals at her institution. In addition, her institution's lack of plans or programs to address this inequity caused her concern. When diversity programs did exist in stage one climates, they were dysfunctional. Professor Chen described diversity activities at her institution:

> Our diversity efforts have been kind of sprinkled and spread out throughout campus. And we had sort of a half-time person who was sort of the director of diversity. But she really had no money and no staff, and it was just really incredibly halfhearted ... And even in our own school we do not have a diversity committee. We just now have a diversity plan. The diversity committee has not met. It [was] ... formed like over a year ago. We have not had a single meeting. [pharmacy faculty]

Diversity programs in stage one climates consisted of a single individual who had responsibility for the entire program but lacked the budget, staff, and buy-in from administration needed for work to be effective. Professors Pope and Pryor described the lack of support they experienced in their diversity-related administrative roles:

> PROFESSOR POPE: One thing that I really lament is that there was no mentoring system for me ... I had to learn everything on the job. That was difficult for me. And I never had anyone that I could turn to, [to] tell me whether I was right or wrong because, essentially, this was an office of diversity, and I think the office was probably formed grudgingly to begin with. One of those situations where if Dr. Pope makes it work, that's fine, but if he doesn't, it's not our fault. And so I was left to my own devices to sink or swim, and the way this system has been structured here—and this is something that I don't like— ... most of the programs that I have developed for the school ... [are] voluntary ... Well, that's not threatening. Because you can nullify what I'm doing by simply ignoring me. [medical faculty]

Professor Pope described being left to "sink or swim" and being placed in a position in which his efforts can be "nullified." His school's investment in the diversity program was superficial and likely had little leadership support. Professor Pryor was similarly expected to champion diversity at her school without institutional backup:

PROFESSOR PRYOR: My role . . . was to do diversity development. So . . . I came in . . . a position that automatically pushed buttons and challenged people about the climate of the nursing school, which from talking with other faculty members and talking with students was one that felt very racist and sexist . . . They bring you in singing a song: "We want it. We will encourage you. What do you need?" And . . . it's like leading you down a dark alley and there's twenty thugs back there wanting to beat the tar out of you. Because they lull you, even the people in positions of authority will lull you in and throw you to the rest of the wolves who are here, who aren't buying into it, who aren't reprimanded for anything, who aren't called on anything, and who can act any way they want and treat you any way they want. And then when you go to the people who said, "Come, make a difference," bleeding, they're like, "Don't give up!" While they sit back and do nothing. They don't say anything. They don't talk to anybody . . . They leave you out there to dry. That's crazy. [nursing faculty]

Professor Pryor's use of violent metaphors reflected her perception of being repeatedly attacked by white faculty when she brought up the topic of equity, which as diversity officer was her job. Her school's assertion, "we want it [diversity and equity]," was insincere. Professor Pryor's position as a diversity officer created the appearance of interest in diversity and equity, covering over a racist climate. Similarly, in some cases when participants offered to implement diversity and equity programs, they were unsupported or faced resistance, as described by Professor Garcia:

I started my mentorship program for [disadvantaged] undergraduate students . . . After its second successful year it was shut down by the hospital, which is very frustrating to me . . . It was shut down because they wanted me to have 20 percent of my time funded through a grant or through some channel . . . to cover my time that I was spending with these students. With all volunteered work on my part, and I was willing to do it, but they wanted it to provide funds. I'm not sure why . . . Reducing health disparities, one way to promote [it] would be the success of future brown people [in] education, and I just did not feel the support at all. I was providing a super cool free program for their students. [medical faculty]

Professor Garcia, who volunteered her time, provided another example of how lack of institutional support for diversity efforts negatively affects faculty of color. This could result in participants becoming disillusioned and in decreased job satisfaction. Professor Duncan, who was invited to guide activities for Black History Month, experienced a more passive form of resistance:

> We were asked to be the faculty advisors for the Black History Month program. And that is where, I'm telling you, it [racism] was just really blatant. We found out after we got there that in previous years, during . . . Black History Month they had burned a cross at the school. And so I said, "Oh my goodness." Coming from the north, you just don't expect that. And so then some years passed before we were asked to lead the history week program . . . And I remember one of our friends from the family came over and told us—I think Sally worked in the music department—that they were supposed to have the risers set up for them for the program. And she came over and told us later that she had been over there and found that they hadn't done a thing . . . Because she was over there late and got those risers set up. But it was just that kind of passive nastiness . . . I remember that . . . it was—like, everything that happened, it was just like a big hassle. [nursing faculty]

Because of her experiences, Professor Duncan declined to be involved in Black History Month in future years. Busy faculty are hard pressed to engage in service activities and are much less inclined to do so when they face resistance to their efforts.

Many participants spoke about the lack of support for diversity programs in institutions at stage one. In turn, lack of effective diversity programs became a barrier to recruiting faculty of color, as described by Professors King and Kapoor:

INTERVIEWER: Based on your experience, would you recruit other faculty of color to come to work at your school?

PROFESSOR KING: Probably not . . . because . . . there's not a lot of support here and you kind of have to go on your own . . . Some of the places I have been before, they seem like they have an actual structure that somehow supports diversity, and there [are] faculty members at multiple levels where it feels like if you had problems, you [could] get help with [them]. Here it seems like you're kind of off on your own, and if you did have problems, you'd feel like maybe you would just be screwed. [medical faculty]

INTERVIEWER: Are there any diversity programs at your university or your school?

PROFESSOR KAPOOR: I do not know of any.

INTERVIEWER: Okay. It sounds like you're pretty clear from what you said before that you wouldn't recruit faculty of color to come to work at your school.

PROFESSOR KAPOOR: No, I wouldn't. [pharmacy faculty]

Professors King and Kapoor described how faculty of color at institutions lacking diversity programs or with ineffective programs often felt unsupported.

In summary, diversity programs at stage one were either nonexistent, despite obvious underrepresentation of faculty and students of color, or if present, they were dysfunctional, existing only for show. In these contexts, participants were wary of recruiting other faculty of color to their institutions.

DIVERSITY PROGRAMS AT STAGE TWO: INDIFFERENCE

At stage two, institutions had made early progress toward developing diversity programs or had more established programs that needed more investment to be effective. Professor Ibori described the early development of a diversity program:

Well, we started an initiative, maybe three years ago, to write a diversity plan. The school had never had a diversity plan ever, and it's fifty-something years old now. So we sat down and started writing a diversity plan and eventually got a group together to do this. And the group has kind of grown to ten people or so. And the chancellor then got involved—got interested and involved. And so we're coming to the point where we're now going to present our diversity plan to the university in the next month or so, and that's been pretty exciting. We've had lots of fights, and it's taken three years to do this, but I think that's been really rewarding . . . So, that's been really, really good. [pharmacy faculty]

Professor Griffin described the importance of involving multiple stakeholders:

I wanted to create a minority resident association because I felt like, okay yeah, we all have like small resources. We might have small numbers, but together we can just pool our resources together and provide that sense of community. To that group of residents. Then maybe it'll make it easier for other people to come in and see themselves here. And so I mean it got to the point that one of the residents who has been very instrumental . . . was like, "Why haven't you been doing this?" And I was like, "Because it's going to take a resident taking the lead on this," and so she presented it. It started out with our internal medicine department. They started it as a diversity strategy committee, which the chair of the department at the time then asked me to be on because he had heard about me . . . So they started this and then subsequently the GME [Graduate Medical Education] took it over, and now they're actually starting to work on an actual committee, a subcommittee under the GME, to try to recruit. I mean like they're going to the national SNMA [Student National Medical Association] meetings. Like, last year was the first year that our university, from the residency side of things, has actually gone to the national meeting. [medical faculty]

Professors Balewa and Jennings also described fledgling efforts:

Professor Balewa: Well, the current president is trying his best . . . I have to say he's trying his best. They didn't really go back to the way it was . . . the lip service they had been paying . . . At least for the first time this year they . . . celebrated black contributions in the medical college, which is the first time they'd done that, at least they . . . recognized a couple of other black physicians who are in the medical college . . . They've made some progress. [medical faculty]

PROFESSOR JENNINGS: I honestly . . . would love to be over some type of diversity initiative because it's such a great passion of mine.
INTERVIEWER: And how well developed are those programs right now?
PROFESSOR JENNINGS: Not very well developed. I think they're starting to come around, but there's not a ton of them. I think many universities, and even here, the different schools, they're starting to get them. [pharmacy faculty]

Professors Balewa and Jennings noticed their institutions' new diversity efforts and hoped for more. Many other participants were passionate about equity and seeing institutional buy-in was motivating.

At stage two, beginning efforts were made to address diversity and equity; however, these efforts were not usually associated with significant investments. These efforts might involve beginning development of a diversity plan or forming student groups or diversity committees. In general, however, diversity efforts were nascent and had not yet borne fruit.

DIVERSITY PROGRAMS AT STAGE THREE: BEGINNING INCLUSION

At stage three, institutions had made substantial investments in diversity initiatives and made significant progress. As Professor Davidson described:

I have been at this institution now since I started my residency in 2000 and I have been here ever since. I've certainly seen more action instead of just words in terms of, I think, values that support—that suggest the institution values diversity, and it's been my opinion or my assumption along the way that there has always been talk about diversity, but no one knew how to do it. And not only not knowing how to do it—the institution wasn't applying resources to try to know how to do it. And I think that I have definitely seen change for the positive. [medical faculty]

Leadership support for diversity programs characterized institutions at stage three. Professor Singleton described such support at her institution:

I guess as well they're trying to recruit . . . and the university in general because we're a small university, some of the things that you might think would be in the school [are] in different places in the university overall. I know they're talking about definitely a mentorship program for faculty retention. Like I said, that whole area of a diverse faculty is a big thing at our university level with our current president. I know they're trying to do things there. I think they're making an effort. That's a plus. The president is very supportive. That's part of the reason I liked his philosophy. [nursing faculty]

Like other participants, Professor Singleton described the importance of leadership to advance a diversity agenda and linked diversity programs with recruitment and retention of faculty of color. Consistent with what would be expected at stage three, faculty diversity was an emerging priority at her institution.

The creation of chief diversity officer positions within health professions institutions and ardent support for these roles was mentioned as a sign of real progress toward strong diversity programs. Professors Chavez and Adams commented on this feature:

PROFESSOR CHAVEZ: I was promoted to becoming the chief diversity officer for the school of medicine. So now I have direct reporting to the dean. I'm just three months into it, but it's made a difference. [medical faculty]
PROFESSOR ADAMS: We are kind of at this real interesting tipping point right now because our dean has . . . made a huge decision by creating this new [diversity] position . . . and also creating the brand new center for diversity and inclusion. And the specific task we have is to enhance our minority faculty.

So it's a huge tipping point, only because [we] have put this certain element in place including the new minority faculty affairs committee ... So there is part of me that says this is the momentum and it's real. [medical faculty]

Professor Adams referred to the creation of a chief diversity officer position as a "tipping point" in the movement toward supporting diversity at her school. In contrast to earlier stages, institutions at stage three provided diversity officers with the support required for such offices to be successful.

In summary, at stage three there was some institutional investment in diversity programs, and fairly well-supported administrative structures were often in place. Institutions might go beyond focusing on student programs to also address faculty needs. Although leadership showed genuine support for diversity programs at that stage, pockets of resistance among some leaders, faculty, and students still existed.

DIVERSITY PROGRAMS AT STAGE FOUR: REAL INCLUSION

At stage four, diversity and equity was integrated into an institution's climate and was a high priority. Faculty and students of color felt comfortable and safe. Professor Chavez described faculty experiences at stage four:

There are institutions that embraced us, engaged us, and there's not even any question that you instantly will feel embraced. People who really have gone a long way in creating that environment, that safe environment, that welcoming and embracing environment for minority faculty, for diversity. [medical faculty]

Professor Chavez used the terms *embrace, engage, safe,* and *welcome* to describe an environment in which diversity programs have real power. Professor Hazelwood detailed the structures and events at a school in stage four:

There are resources there, there is a blacks for government, whatever that student group is. We have someone [who] will communicate with multicultural affairs and that type of thing. And they are a powerful group because one of the things they do is they invite the [university] president there at the meetings ... to talk about what might be issues for students of color. It's a watchdog experience. [nursing faculty]

Professor Hazelwood's use of the phrase "watchdog experience" suggests leadership interest in and accountability to diverse constituencies within the institution. At stage four, diversity programs were supported with appropriate budgets, as Professor Tehrani described:

> My university gives a project to any minority to have their own social event ... So ... they gave us a budget, and they keep telling us, "Use this budget." So we used to go [in] together ... We had some tool or some project ... We use the budget, or we get together—have lunch or dinner—and they pay [for] us. And so it's great. And I don't think the other universities have this program, but this one has a budget for each group, each minority, and if you do this, the next year they give you a little bit more of a budget. [dental faculty]

Professor Tehrani's example suggested a value of supporting diverse cultures at her institution. In turn these programs resulted in changes in school culture, as described by Professor Rodriguez:

> To me ... training and programs result in more respect for women ... more appreciation of other ethnic groups . . . all of these things probably came together to induce these changes in culture. [medical faculty]

Because training is most likely to be effective when it is long term, integrated with institutional initiatives (202), and skillfully implemented, it requires significant institutional investment (4).

To summarize, at stage four, diversity programs were well developed and had been sustained, contributing to institutional change. Participants described the climate with words like *safe*, *embracing*, and *welcoming*. True appreciation for differences and support for faculty and students of color were part of these climates, and diversity programs were backed at the highest levels of leadership.

Climate Element Four: Reports of Racism

In the study reports of racism were mostly informal, made to trusted colleagues behind closed doors. At stage one, reports of racism were pervasive among faculty and students of color. At stage two there were fewer reports. At stage three, reports of racism became infrequent, and finally, at stage four, reports of racism were rare. Because the nature of racism reports overlap across stages, I combine stages one and two below.

Participants' stories included many descriptions of felt and observed racism, from off-color remarks to subtle but systematic marginalization and blatant removal of equal opportunities. As noted, participants rarely reported racist incidents to anyone but sympathetic friends, colleagues, or family members. This was often because the racist incidents were subtle and insidious and thus difficult to substantiate. Most often, participants picked their battles and chose to ignore such events.

I detailed the nature of some of these racist behaviors when I described exclusion and control processes and do not repeat them here. In this chapter I discuss how participants perceived and responded to reports of racism from students or colleagues. Professors Pryor and Said described reports of racism:

PROFESSOR PRYOR: It's lip service, and it's the inability to see that they [whites] hold the racism that's within each of them. And they keep trying to say, "we're fine." Either you people of color go get them [students of color], work with them, and deal with them, or, "Oh, well we don't have the resources," and it's a way of excusing themselves [from] any kind of personal accountability. Because even when we had the resources . . . when the last dean put money toward actually recruiting people of color, their [students of color] experiences were so horrible they left. Okay, so now what's the reason? . . . Because you're the problem. But they don't want to see that. They don't want to see that. There are people here that hold racist attitudes and don't want to be different, don't want [to] allow themselves to be different and take in anything that is different or change who they are, and you're not going to lose your job. What are you going to lose for it [racist behavior]? Or being in a classroom where students have told me that students are saying racist things and the teacher doesn't say anything about it. [nursing faculty]

PROFESSOR SAID: I have taught diversity courses, and I have mentored minority students, and the racism here is very pervasive. I remember a white student in one of my diversity courses saying something about black men and how they like to sleep around. I corrected the student immediately, not in a harsh way, but I was clear, and after that class the student who made the racist comment gave anonymous feedback that she didn't feel safe to speak . . . There was a black student in the class when the racist comment was made, and she didn't say anything in class . . . but gave anonymous feedback about how the comment made her feel. I feel like as faculty we are supposed to respond to student feedback, but I'm not going to let racist comments just go unaddressed in the classroom, which unfortunately from what I have heard from students of color is kind of the norm around here . . . Most of the students of color in our graduate program have chosen to work with me, and I know about the racism they have experienced here. I have done everything I can to fight for them when something comes up. Sometimes it makes a difference, and sometimes it doesn't. [nursing faculty]

White faculty's lack of accountability for addressing racism was a consistent theme in the findings. With nowhere else to turn, students of color often went to participants for help and support. This was also true for racism experienced by colleagues. Thus, participants were often the repositories for reports of racism at their institutions. For junior faculty, this sometimes proved challenging, as explained by Professor King:

Our school has kind of been having a history of having a hard time retaining residents, fellowships, and other staff . . . from the experience that the residents had had and everything, residents that tried to get me involved in somehow being a champion or some sort of mentor, I think like probably the first year I was here. I think . . . a lot of the residents feel that . . . other coresidents have made racist comments or said disparaging things about the patients . . . where I work, [who are] predominantly black, African American and Puerto Rican, Asian population. The people said other residents have experienced, the black residents have experienced other residents saying disparaging comments or making comments about the community that we serve but not always directly at the residents themselves, but at the people that look like us, but that stuff is said and additionally some of the residents feel that their treatment has not been equal . . . I actually talked [to] previous mentors and essentially, the unanimous position was you have to take care of yourself, try to learn how to say no . . . Without any seniority or power you really can't do much. And if you spend a lot of time or energy on trying to defend people, then it can potentially hurt you and make it harder to be there. So essentially, I tried to do some [advocacy] but not actually take a leadership role. [medical faculty]

As the confidants of students of color, participants sometimes became reluctant champions, placing themselves in positions of vulnerability. At stages one and two, leadership did not support participants when they intervened on behalf of students. This perpetuated a climate of exclusion, as expressed in the following account by Professor Balewa, who intervened on behalf of medical residents:

I had gone to the chair of pediatrics and I said "You know, it's extremely difficult to be black in this place. As a resident, you're always dumb. They're always putting you down, saying you don't know what you're talking about. They're hard on you. I mean, you see the difference in interchange between when it's a black person presenting and when it's a white person presenting. You know?" And I said to him, and I gave him this example of this patient that I had . . . And I gave him other examples. And do you know what he came back to me and said? That he talked to the black residents and . . . there was no evidence of racism in the hospital. [medical faculty]

Insensitivity to power dynamics and refusal to address racism were characteristic of white leaders at stages one and two. Professor Dillard reported that institutional leaders were not interested in hearing about students of color who declined admission because of a racist climate:

We are to the point where the student experiences for students of color are not very good here. Case in point, we had a young lady who is from this state, born here, had a 3.8 GPA and she also had a 24 on her DAT [Dental Admission Test], and she was accepted here but selected to go out of state, pay an additional $100,000 to be an out-of-state student because of the racial politics at our school. She talked to students here and they told her, "Do not come here." And I've pointed that out to the dean, to the chancellor, that if we can't even keep our own in-state students of color, we have some significant problems. They want to dismiss it. [dental faculty]

Professor Dillard pointed to the impact reports of racism can have on an institution's reputation and how this can ultimately affect student recruitment. Such reports could negatively affect enrollment of students of color, but this reality rarely reached official channels. Professor Dillard also described his experience with a formal complaint of racial discrimination made by a colleague:

My dean had a screaming fit at me. There were only three African American faculty members at this school. And one faculty member filed a notice of claim against this state school . . . based on his racial treatment . . . And I had heard about the notice of claim—it had hit the paper and I had been able to get an exact copy . . . My dean calls me in and says, "There [is] someone I want to schedule a meeting for you to talk with." And I said, "Whom do you want me to talk with?" [She said,] "Well, it's a university person and I'm certain you are aware of the notice of claim that Dr. Douglas filed and I want you to talk to . . . the university attorney. Well, people will be asking you questions and I want you to know that the university attorney will be there to help you." And I said "No, the university attorney is appointed to protect and works for the university. The university attorney does not work for John Dillard." [She said,] "Well, that's true." I said, "So therefore the university attorney will not be protecting John Dillard." And I said, "Dean, what is this really about?" [She said,] "Well, what Dr. Douglas said wasn't true, this and that." And I said, "Well if it's not true, then let the claim stand on its own and the facts will come out." And she went freaking berserk. "Are you saying that you won't support me?" I said, "I'm getting the impression that you were trying to tell me what you want me to say." And I said, "Dean, we have huge racial problems here at this school. And they do need to be addressed." [She said,] "Are you saying this is a racist institution?" I told her, "Well yes, as a matter of fact it is." [dental faculty]

Despite Professor Dillard's concerns about racism and the fact that a black faculty member had filed a formal complaint of discrimination, no subsequent efforts were made to improve the racial climate at that institution.

To summarize, at stages one and two, reports of racism were frequent. When racism was reported openly, it usually involved participants advocating for students. The racial climate did not support such advocacy, placing participants in vulnerable positions. Leadership's response was to ignore, minimize, and dismiss the concerns, perpetuating exclusionary climates.

Climate Element Five: Dialogue

Participants frequently mentioned dialogue about diversity and equity, including racism in the institution and profession, as an important factor in creating a climate for growth and change. At stage one, participants were isolated and silenced. Only lip service was paid to diversity and equity, and resistance to addressing racism was high. At stage two, conversations were beginning to take place, but they were in the very early stages, and resistance was still a major problem. At stage three there were active conversations about diversity and equity, and racism was a safe topic, although pockets of resistance to such dialogue still existed. At stage four, open, respectful, and safe communication was the norm.

DIALOGUE AT STAGE ONE: COVERT EXCLUSION

At stage one it was not safe for faculty and students of color to speak out about diversity and equity, particularly on sensitive topics such as racism. Professors Chen and Hazelwood described this problem:

PROFESSOR CHEN: So I do think it is the institution, kind of, because I think some institutions . . . they're not as open about it [diversity and equity], and I think at those institutions, that's where you can get more challenges. [pharmacy faculty]

PROFESSOR HAZELWOOD: I heard from my other colleague that I am working with on this, I have heard her say how white students will make ridiculous remarks in class with black students and minority students around. It's just so— and she can sort of see the expressions—a lot of the black students here may not say anything. They just sort of, sometimes, let a lot of things go by. I know as a faculty member she would try to bring discussions up or get them—but she said the students wouldn't even discuss it. They wouldn't even allow it to come to a point to talk [about] anything about racism or inequality or—even as it related to health care sometimes that was very difficult. [nursing faculty]

Professor Hazelwood's example shows how the power imbalance between faculty and students is often reversed in favor of white students when faculty of color are teaching. This silencing was the opposite of what participants felt was necessary for institutions to promote diversity and equity, as described by Professors Jones and Patel:

INTERVIEWER: What changes do you think your school could do to improve the academic environment for faculty of color so that you'd have better recruitment and retention?

PROFESSOR JONES: Participate in some honest truth telling and conversations about what the real issues are. And try to have people come up with ways to resolve the hurt and the pain and to not ignore it. [medical faculty]

INTERVIEWER: What changes could your school make to improve the academic environment for faculty of color and promote recruitment and retention?

PROFESSOR PATEL: I think that open dialogue about these issues, acknowledging that there is subtle discrimination, and openly discussing [it]. And taking actions against instances of such [discrimination]. [pharmacy faculty]

As Professors Jones and Patel noted, dialogue is a critical element for improving the inclusivity of institutional climates. Yet at stage one, speaking out about diversity, and particularly about racism, was not safe. Faculty and students of color who wished to engage in this kind of dialogue were silenced, reinforcing racial hierarchies.

DIALOGUE AT STAGE TWO: INDIFFERENCE

At stage two, dialogue about diversity and equity occurred occasionally, but it was not routine and was usually met with resistance, as described by Professor Singleton:

INTERVIEWER: To what degree do they discuss issues of racism? I mean, is there any opportunity to discuss those kinds of things at your school?

PROFESSOR SINGLETON: Probably not on an ongoing basis, and [they] often do not recognize that racism is a problem ... So I don't know, although certainly it comes up probably periodically. I think it comes up sometimes in some of the student appeals and whatnot. It is discussed, although I think people, students, or a lot of people deny that it still exists. A group of people always deny that it exists and [want to know] why are we talking about this? [nursing faculty]

Professor Singleton referred to the common problem of resistance to dialogue about racism and other "isms." Talking about racism is often uncomfortable for whites because it challenges denial and exposes white privilege. As stated by DiAngelo, "In racial dialogue, white silence functions overall to shelter white participants by keeping their racial perspectives hidden and thus protected from exploration or challenge. Not contributing one's perspectives serves to ensure that those perspectives cannot be expanded" (203) p.5. Hence, white silence may result in a systematic avoidance of discussions about race and ethnicity, as described by Professor Barnes:

INTERVIEWER: Is there any dialogue around issues of diversity?

PROFESSOR BARNES: Not really. We have a large focus on, like, interdisciplinary health care. And . . . we have a lot of Hispanic individuals, Spanish-speaking persons in this state, so to me, that was an outlet for diversity because it's like we should really help that community. But it was just kind of like, "Oh, that's not our focus right now." I was like, "okay." That's kind of how that went. [pharmacy faculty]

Despite resistance, fledgling efforts to discuss diversity and equity were present at stage two, climates when leadership took the initiative:

PROFESSOR BALEWA: When the dean came . . . and said, "You know, what is going on here? You don't reflect the population of this city. What's going on here? Why is it so?" And he made diversity an issue . . . But prior to that, nobody really cared. Nobody really cared . . . The current president is trying his best . . . they've made some progress. [medical faculty]

In most cases, however, participants initiated challenging dialogues, as described by Professors Chavez and Said:

PROFESSOR CHAVEZ: I felt that if I wasn't at a meeting then diversity would never be mentioned at the meeting because it just wasn't in the vocabulary. It wasn't even a consideration . . . And that's what I mean by it being on the back burner. It's on the stove, but the stove's not on . . . There is kind of . . . resistance I guess would be a good word. [medical faculty]

PROFESSOR SAID: You can count on me to be the one to bring up diversity at faculty meetings. Sometimes on a rare occasions a minority student falls conveniently into their lap and then they bring it up to take credit. But when things are not going well with student diversity, which is almost all the time, the faculty are silent. And when I bring up issues about support for minority students I always run into resistance. So I speak up and I feel like they kind of look at me and roll their eyes, sort of like, "here she goes again." [nursing faculty]

Active silencing of faculty and students of color was not as prominent at stage two as at stage one, although resistance to uncomfortable discussions continued. Without initiative from leaders, the burden of initiating dialogue often fell to participants, who were usually deeply concerned about diversity and equity and felt an ethical obligation to promote change. Yet when participants talked about diversity, and particularly equity, they were often branded by whites as people with problem personalities or as troublemakers. This tactic deceptively misdirected the focus of attention onto the participants, unjustly placing them in defensive positions while sidestepping equity.

DIALOGUE AT STAGE THREE:
BEGINNING INCLUSION

At stage three, regular conversations about diversity had begun. Professor Jones described how this happened:

> People call me and say, "Look, we need someone to talk about diversity" . . . and I say . . . "This is the ethics of truth telling. It's racism." I talk about it. I don't cover it. I am very blatant about what's going on, to the point that sometimes people don't want to hear me . . . and I say this over and over, the only way we're going to get rid of it is—in medicine we have . . . an abscess, it's just a pocket of nasty awful pus, and what you have to do is cut that thing open, let it drain out, rinse it out and let it . . . heal by secondary intention. You cannot cover it over. You can't sew it up, you can't, you have to leave it open and let it drain and heal. And the healing will be strong, but people are so afraid . . . I'm so frustrated with people not wanting to talk about it. [There is] a group of women, we meet once a month and we call ourselves the Race Women. It's a diverse mix of women and we get together and we talk about race . . . This is nothing but conversation . . . And it's healing and cleansing for all of us. We learn from each other. We share our stories. It's been really, really helpful to just have those conversations. [medical faculty]

Professor Jones described dialogue as "healing and cleansing"; however, it is important to note that her group's work was both informal and ongoing. When dialogue occurs in the context of formal training, it should be implemented skillfully as part of a long-term institutional initiative. Without such commitment, diversity training can have negative consequences. Thus, leadership investment in the change process is essential, as described by Professor Singh:

> I think that will help over the long run and then our dean is very good, he's very good. He's focused on diversity, and he's always trying to bring that

up with the people here, because he recognizes what the problem is here. [pharmacy faculty]

At stage three, uncomfortable conversations were allowed to occur with little resistance, as described by Professor Corbin:

We actually had a pretty tough discussion last year about whether or not it was a gender issue, because we had trouble retaining female faculty, and we still have trouble in retaining female faculty. But the few female faculty we had— and then also including myself in that discussion, really came to the conclusion that there's not any kind of gender discrimination; it had probably more to do with the lack of female mentorship. So that was our conclusion. I still believe that's true, even though I was really questioning whether or not there was some level of discrimination going on . . . I think that in some environments, it's very difficult to have those kinds of conversations . . . and it was difficult; there's no question about it, it was a very uncomfortable conversation. And there were some of us who really forced the issue to make sure that we did talk about this, and I'm glad we did . . . We need to have more of these conversations and be honest about it. So that's a lot of what I try to do in my teaching, is to bring up difficult facts, difficult situations, and have a conversation about it because that's the only way we're going to learn to think and act differently. [medical faculty]

At stage three there was a nascent willingness to engage in the crucial conversations about race required for change. Although these efforts typically continued to concern participants, as leadership involvement increased, dialogue about racism and other "isms" became more frequent and engaged more faculty.

DIALOGUE AT STAGE FOUR: REAL INCLUSION

Stage four dialogue was characterized by open, respectful communication facilitated by informed leaders. Professors Tolbert and Morgan, both department chairs, described this approach:

PROFESSOR TOLBERT: And with the faculty I am very open with them. If there is a student issue and it's related to a black person, I try to be objective and have open dialogue. And I think that I've allowed them to feel like they can say what they feel. They don't have to apologize to me, but they are respectful to me and I'll wait when they say things. I welcome open dialogue, and I give positive feedback and acknowledge when someone is just being ridiculous … if they're white or black or whatever, I am just trying to be objective … They can't be prejudiced in my presence and feel that I don't know it, because I have made it clear that I do … So I think I've created an environment, I've helped them to create an environment where we can have objectivity more than if I wasn't here. [nursing faculty]

PROFESSOR MORGAN: I think years ago when I first took over it was a very conservative, right-leaning department, which made it uncomfortable for people to speak their minds because people felt like, "If I speak my mind it's going [to] hurt me," right. And so I think now … people will speak their minds and that's a good thing … Absolutely. When I came to this university years ago, I was leaning left in those days, but nobody else was leaning left. And so when politics were being discussed I kind of kept my mouth shut, because I knew most folks didn't agree with me, not that I cared, but it made me a little uncomfortable and I'd like to think because I don't put my politics on anybody that folks can discuss stuff and have fun about it, and at the end of the day it doesn't usually matter. But I think we do have more open discussions than we did years ago, that's for sure. [medical faculty]

As in the other stages, leadership was critical at stage four. Faculty of color who were skilled administrators led significant and meaningful change at their institutions. These leaders had the ability to foster dialogue by creating a culture of safety and respect that was pervasive and cut across social groups. Faculty of color were in positions of power and served as role models of success, sending a strong message throughout the institution. These leaders dealt with diversity and equity head on, using dialogue as a tool.

Climate Element Six: Leadership

Leadership was both a reflection and a driver of institutional climate. Leadership directed the other elements by setting priorities, following through on initiatives (including providing adequate resources and ensuring accountability), and responding constructively to reports of racism, based on a larger vision for diversity and equity.

At stage one, leadership was counterproductive to diversity and equity in institutions. At stage two, leadership was indifferent or neutral. At stage three, leadership had an early interest in diversity and equity, and leadership opportunities were extended to some faculty of color. Finally, at stage four, leadership had a clear-cut vision for institutional diversity and equity. There was zero tolerance for racism and other "isms" and a strong understanding of the subtle manifestations of oppression.

LEADERSHIP AT STAGE ONE: COVERT EXCLUSION

At stage one, participants felt excluded from leadership:

PROFESSOR BALEWA: I'm not actually in leadership. And why I'm not in leadership at my stage of the game, I don't know. But obviously I've never been asked to be, even though I think I can do it. But I've never been asked. [medical faculty]

PROFESSOR SMITH: I would say that faculty of color have felt excluded from opportunities . . . if you look at our senior leadership here at the medical center it's, you know, overwhelmingly white and so, I've heard many people say, "Why is that?" . . . So, you know, most of the people openly question how is it we're in—it's 2012, and how can we as an institution have that little diversity at the senior level of the institute? People [in] the decision-making process. [medical faculty]

PROFESSOR SAID: I have been here quite a while, and as far as I know there has never been a racial or ethnic minority faculty administrator in the history of this school. They keep recycling the same old white women in these positions. Even when they can't fill positions because of retirements, they won't bring in minorities. They won't develop minority faculty, and they won't recruit them for leadership. They will bring in white men, but they won't bring in minorities. Diversity is part of the school's mission, and they have a so-called diversity plan, but what does it amount to? Nothing. It's just words on a page because there's no diversity and there's no accountability. [nursing faculty]

Some faculty viewed lack of influence as a reason for exclusion of faculty of color from health professions education, as described by Professor Dee:

INTERVIEWER: Is there much diversity among the leadership?

PROFESSOR Dee: Not really. It's mostly dominated by [people of] Italian and Caucasian [descent]. In fact, I don't know of anyone who is a different ethnicity [who is] either chairman of a department or an administrator.

INTERVIEWER: Okay, what do you think that the reasons might be for the lack of representation among the leadership of a diverse faculty? Because you're saying that there is a diverse faculty at the school.

PROFESSOR DEE: Well, I think it has to do, again, with the way people get to those positions is because of influence, right? For example, our chairman in our department—his family has been influential in terms of what they contribute to the school. And so the father was instrumental and a brother was instrumental. And so he's got into the position where he's at . . . and I'm sure that influence had a lot to do with it. And so, overall, that's how it works.

INTERVIEWER: So, do you think that maybe a privileged background may be a factor?

INTERVIEWEE: Yeah, I think it [is]. [dental faculty]

Professor Dee described an example of how historical inequities in wealth have contributed to the institutionalization of white privilege in health professions education. It is likely that if large numbers of wealthy people of color had historical connections to health professions schools, that would influence the balance of power. Current social inequities prevent this from happening. White leaders who have benefited from these inequities may be consciously or unconsciously reluctant to embrace robust change. This in turn negatively influences the willingness of leaders to promote dialogue about diversity and equity and do what it takes to recruit and retain faculty of color, as described by Professor Hsu:

One of my biggest frustrations is the fact that there are several people who don't want a conversation about racism and diversity to happen overtly, and that we don't really have an opportunity to aggressively recruit black and Latino residents to our program. Because the person who's in charge of recruiting and training the residents is very uncomfortable talking about race, and we've not had a chair of pediatrics who felt differently enough to sort of push the issue. And those are the two people who are really critical for just making that happen, those two positions, I mean. And this has happened [in] other places that I've been; the tone that those two people set determines what happens. That's a frustration for me just because I think that diversity is important, and I think that it's also one of the best ways to retain URM and faculty, right, is to have them actually come as trainees and to keep them. So I think that if that were different, if we were able to have a very open conversation and talk about how we could benefit from being a little bit more deliberate [with] our own diversity, that we'd be closer to achieving what I would think of as an ideal level of diversity in the department. [medical faculty]

LEADERSHIP AT STAGE TWO: INDIFFERENCE

At stage two, leadership could include racial and ethnic diversity, but this was not intentional. Professors Ahmed and Corbin described this climate:

PROFESSOR AHMED: We're in a large, diverse city, and so being here, there are quite a few African Americans. I mean, our IT program is run by an African American man . . . Putting even African Americans or even Hispanics in higher positions or higher level positions . . . others . . . see that. I do think, though, from an administrative level, yes, in the administrative officers' meeting when there's like maybe twelve administrators there for just the College of Pharmacy, there's only one or two that are black or Hispanic. So they're definitely in a minority, but there's no Asians . . . there are very few women as well. [pharmacy faculty]

PROFESSOR CORBIN: Essentially, leadership here are old white men for the most part. There are a few women in leadership positions, but very few. No real minorities in leadership positions when you talk about dean's office and department chairs and so forth. There's one female department chair. We have one surgery Hispanic faculty [member], who's the program director. But for the most part, most of our minority faculty tend to be more junior faculty. [medical faculty].

This lack of diversity in leadership detrimentally affected diversity and equity initiatives, as described by Professor Chen:

I think we sort of pay lip service to diversity. The administration doesn't think we have a diversity issue. I think we do. And I think the main problem is that the administration doesn't think we do because it's run by white males. It's run by white males. They don't think there's any problem. [pharmacy faculty]

As in stage one, lack of racial and ethnic diversity in leadership was a problem at stage two. Institutions at stage two, however, could have marginally more diverse leadership, although this was not intentional. This lack of racial and ethnic diversity negatively affected the institution's capacity for change.

At stage three, discussions about racial and ethnic diversity in leadership had begun, although more progress was needed, as described by Professor Morgan:

INTERVIEWER: Is the leadership at your school diverse?

PROFESSOR MORGAN: They're working on it, they're trying. You know, it's still a challenge for them. Yes, there is some diversity. Not as much as it should be. We talk about it a lot. [medical faculty]

Despite these challenges, leaders at stage three were attentive to the need for diversity and equity and made efforts to change. Professor Dillard provided an example:

You have a profession and it's so ultraconservative and where the racism is so deeply ingrained and that carries over into dental schools, not just here. So therefore, you have the profession as a whole that supports racism. That supports stereotypes, that African Americans [are] not as intelligent and we don't have the critical thinking and it's infused at many of our predominantly white dental schools. The only time you see some true change is if you get a really strong dean and somebody like Lydia Smith in a southern state, who made it clear that she was going to change things there, and she's a white lady. And she made it clear that those things were not acceptable. And she was strong enough that she told her admissions board that the admitting class had to be representative of the state. Well, you don't have many strong white deans who are willing to take up that cause and change their institutional environment. [dental faculty]

Professor Dillard described a dean who used her position of power to enforce a policy change in favor of diversity and equity in school admissions. As Professor Dillard suggested, faculty of color notice and appreciate leaders who use their power to change the status quo in favor of equity. Professor Chavez expressed similar regard for department chairs who were interested in diversity and equity:

I can think of two to three department chairs [who] are very open and want to learn as much as they can about the minority faculty and have done things proactively to retain them. And again, those are the ones who have retained our services from our [diversity] office, who basically come to me and say,

"We don't have enough minority faculty. Please help us recruit. Please teach us what we need to know, can you work together with us to do this sort of thing? And then once they're here, can we work collaboratively to do that?" That was, of all things, it was the surgery department. Pediatrics was the second one that did that. Not even my own department, family medicine, approached it, but those two other departments and also the department of anesthesia. And I think a lot of it had to do with leadership . . . The arrogance was totally absent. Because they got it. And I think they really understood the value of diversity, and I think the value of having a diverse workforce. And it wasn't just about having women . . . This was more of an inclusive kind of thing . . . This is important to us because if they look at the community we take care of, it is amazingly diverse. We speak fifty-four different languages in our hospital . . . and so these particular departments recognized that and [said] . . . we need to diversify our workforce because of the people we take care of. We want to reach them. [medical faculty]

Professor Chavez talked about administrators who "get it," suggesting that they understand the complexity of diversity and equity and its importance. Leaders who recognized the value of diversity and equity made special efforts to support and protect faculty of color in their institutions, as Professors Manning and Ames described:

PROFESSOR MANNING: In talking with the other faculty member who's African American, the one thing—our paths are slightly different, but I think the one thing that was a common denominator for both of us and reoccurred every time we discussed this was that we really felt that our chair was there to support us. That he was standing up for his faculty. We recently had a shift and had a new dean come in. Our chair really put her neck out there to support and protect and really look after us as faculty members . . . The dean's approach to the changes totally have to do with what her goals are . . . Some of her goals affected us, and the chair was very adamant about protecting us and making sure that we were evaluated under the criteria that we entered in versus some of [the dean's] newer criteria, [which] changed only months before we went up for promotion. Our chair has been very protective and supportive and encouraging. [pharmacy faculty]

PROFESSOR AMES: I think the dean is so very supportive of us [faculty of color] and what we do. I haven't had any issues. I mean he really wants us to succeed. I know he definitely makes sure I've been involved in some things on a professional development level. [dental faculty]

Professors Manning and Ames described the importance of deans and chairs protecting and nurturing faculty of color. Given the subtle inequities in promotion and tenure that faculty of color may face, this protection, guidance, and support was essential for creating a diverse senior professoriate. In addition, participants described leaders who went out of their way to recruit racially and ethnically diverse administrators. Professor Achebe described his experience of being recruited for a chair position:

INTERVIEWER: Okay, so are there any experiences in your career that have really stood out either in a good way or in a bad way in terms of your unique experience as a black man in pharmaceutical sciences?

PROFESSOR ACHEBE: Number one, to become chair ... Before I came, one would say, "Oh, you're not number one candidate," ... but it turned out that the dean really made it happen. So for me, that was refreshing. And he was a white male. And ... whatever the reasons were, I think he saw my prospects as a scientist, as a leader ... So that was very refreshing. That's why I came here. That's a very positive interaction. [pharmacy faculty]

Such changes pave the way for greater diversity in the organization as a whole:

PROFESSOR SMITH: Change is happening . . . just having more diversity . . . in senior level positions. We have right now, I mentioned we have one African American female department chair and . . . our VP of human resources is an African American female; both of those positions are high. Those positions came in within the last two years. We're kind of—looks like we're headed in the right direction, but I think still having more of that diversity at the highest level I think will be something that—I think people will see kind of that chicken and the egg thing. It's like okay, well, yeah, I don't want to come there because you don't have the diversity. Well, like we can't have the diversity unless you come here. So I think having people in positions of power will make a big difference. [medical faculty]

Professor Smith highlighted the importance having racial and ethnic diversity in top leadership for effective recruitment of faculty of color. This again underscores the importance of nurturing, protecting, and guiding faculty of color for promotion and grooming them for leadership roles.

At stage three, institutions recognized the critical nature of racial and ethnic diversity for excellence, and leadership was identified as an issue of concern. Efforts were made to protect and nurture faculty of color with the hope that in time they would be successful and advance to senior professorial ranks. In addition, efforts were made to identify faculty of color for chair and departmental positions. These efforts resulted in early change in favor of a more inclusive climate.

LEADERSHIP AT STAGE FOUR: REAL INCLUSION

Leadership at stage four had successfully followed an active and sustained vision for change. Professor Morgan described his experience:

> Well, the faculty within the department have changed over the years; when I first came it was pretty conservative except for my boss, who was Jewish, and me, who was black, it was pretty much you know, WASP. And over the years, because I'm chair now, it's really evolved. I've got an Asian person on my faculty. I've got more women on my faculty, though I don't have enough. As I mentioned, I've got a couple of African American physicists on my faculty, so it's really much more of a diverse-looking group. I love it when I have faculty meetings, because you know, it's exactly what I envisioned. You know, it's everything. There [are] women in the room, there [are] African Americans in the room, there [are] Asians in the room. So that's not the way it was when I came years ago. [medical faculty]

Professor Morgan described a visibly diverse faculty meeting—part of his vision for change. For stage four leaders, this vision may include significant investment in faculty of color. Professor Hazelwood described her experience with leadership investment:

> They funded me totally to go to college. Which was six months for administrative training for women in academe. That they would send me and pay for it fully; this was after I had the doctorate. And they said they sent me there knowing I might seek someplace else. [nursing faculty]

Stage four was also characterized by zero tolerance for racism and other "isms," as described by Professor Morgan:

PROFESSOR MORGAN: I think it [leadership] is absolutely critical. If people don't care about it [diversity and equity], then people can do what they want to do or say what they want to say. and I think people in my department . . . You know, if I would ever hear of anybody saying something to a woman or a minority or whatever that was inappropriate, I mean that wouldn't happen where I live because people know I'm sensitive to it. But if you've got a boss or a chair or whatever who's not sensitive to it, I think it's critical.

INTERVIEWER: So they tolerate behaviors and then the behaviors will continue in that case?

PROFESSOR MORGAN: That's what I suspect, and I'd like to think that we've moved past that here because most of the chairs that I know—it was kind of a turnover. When I came, there were a lot of good old boys. I'd like to say in the last five, six years there's been a real big turnover; . . . most of the chairs are in their forties, and I think that's helped because I think most of us in our forties understand those sensitivities. Where[as] guys who were in their sixties and whatever didn't get it. So there's less of that happening where I work, but clearly if your chairman doesn't really care or your boss, no matter what it is, doesn't care about that kind of thing, people can say things and do things. [medical faculty]

Professor Morgan described the importance of leaders' sensitivity to covert discrimination and of zero tolerance for such behavior in the institutional climate. Such a stance, by its very nature, required understanding of the subtle nature of covert racism, which administrators at stages one and two lacked.

At stage four, climates were highly inclusive. Leaders had a track record of strong efforts to increase the racial and ethnic diversity of faculty and student bodies, promote dialogue, set standards for appropriate conduct, and model sensitivity to diversity and equity. These efforts could occur at the school level or on a smaller scale, under the leadership of a chair or a department head. Participants had been mentored into leadership positions and were influential, both as role models for success and for the skills and value they brought to their institutions.

The Role of Accreditation Standards

Accrediting bodies have the authority to impose mandates that can change the landscape of health professions education and ultimately deliver a health-care workforce that matches the racial and ethnic diversity of the US population. Professors Ames and Said provided examples of this influence:

PROFESSOR AMES: It's [recruitment and retention has] been focused on the student side because of the new CODA [Commission on Dental Accreditation] . . . I don't think there's been any push on the faculty side . . . You have to have a representation of a diverse student population. There's no number, but they definitely want to make sure that you have a diverse student population . . . because there's a mandate—that's where the attention is. Because they don't want to get dinged obviously with accreditation. [dental faculty]

PROFESSOR SAID: A couple of years ago the university announced a budget allocation for diversity that was much larger than they ever had before. They hired a chief diversity officer and a recruiter and kicked off a university diversity plan, and every school had to have one. But the resources went to the school of medicine. Why? Because of an accreditation mandate. That was the impetus for the whole thing. The university didn't put it that way publicly when they rolled it [the diversity initiative] out, but the faculty knew what was really behind it. So the school of medicine got most of the money . . . Accreditation is obviously a big deal, and it will get them to move when nothing else does. [nursing faculty]

Accreditation standards for the professions mention diversity but in very different ways. Accrediting bodies for medical and dental education specifically address diversity in faculty, students, and staff in their standards. The Liaison Committee on Medical Education describes the benefits of diversity thus:

In a medical education program . . . having medical students and faculty members from a variety of socioeconomic backgrounds, racial and ethnic groups, and other life experiences can 1) enhance the quality and content of interactions and discussions for all students throughout the preclinical and clinical curricula and 2) result in the preparation of a physician workforce that is more culturally aware and competent and better prepared to improve access to healthcare and address current and future health care disparities (227) p.22.

In Standard 3.3, the Liaison Committee on Medical Education requires the following:

> A medical school has effective policies and practices in place, and engages in ongoing, systematic, and focused recruitment and retention activities, to achieve mission-appropriate diversity outcomes among its students, faculty, senior administrative staff, and other relevant members of its academic community. These activities include the use of programs and/or partnerships aimed at achieving diversity among qualified applicants for medical school admission and the evaluation of program and partnership outcomes. (227) p.4

Similarly, the Commission on Osteopathic College Accreditation has guidelines that require schools to "make every effort to hire" administrative staff and faculty from diverse backgrounds (in standards 2.8 and 4.3) (228) p.15, 17 and to "make every effort to recruit students from a diverse background to foster that richness while meeting its mission and objectives" (in standard 5.32) (228) p.15, 17, 18.

The Commission on Dental Education describes diversity as essential to academic excellence and has standards for diversity among students, faculty, and staff:

> Diversity in education is essential to academic excellence. A significant amount of learning occurs through informal interactions among individuals who are of different races, ethnicities, religions, and backgrounds; come from cities, rural areas and from various geographic regions; and have a wide variety of interests, talents, and perspectives. These interactions allow students to directly and indirectly learn from their differences, and to stimulate one another to reexamine even their most deeply held assumptions about themselves and their world. Cultural competence cannot be effectively acquired in a relatively homogeneous environment. Programs must create an environment that ensures an in-depth exchange of ideas and beliefs across gender, racial, ethnic, cultural and socioeconomic lines. (229) p.16

Consistent with this conceptualization of diversity, the Commission on Dental Education's standard 4 for institutional effectiveness states:

> The dental school must have policies and practices to: a. achieve appropriate levels of diversity among its students, faculty and staff; b. engage in ongoing

systematic and focused efforts to attract and retain students, faculty and staff from diverse backgrounds; and c. systematically evaluate comprehensive strategies to improve the institutional climate for diversity. (229) p.21

The Commission on Dental Education has similar diversity standards for dental therapy programs (230).

Unlike those for medicine and dentistry, the Accreditation Council for Pharmacy Education standards do not define diversity as it relates to faculty, students, and staff, although a definition of diversity specific to patient populations is provided. The Accreditation Council for Pharmacy Education focuses exclusively on diversity in students in Standards 16 and 25:

> The college or school develops, implements, and assesses its admission criteria, policies, and procedures to ensure the selection of a qualified and diverse student body into the professional degree program . . . The college or school regularly assesses the criteria, policies, and procedures to ensure the selection of a qualified and diverse student body, members of which have the potential for academic success and the ability to practice in team-centered and culturally diverse environments. (231) p.11, 18

Nursing education has five accrediting bodies: the Commission for Nursing Education Accreditation, Collegiate Commission on Nursing Education, Accreditation Commission for Education in Nursing, Accreditation Council for Nurse Midwifery, and Council on Accreditation of Nurse Anesthesia. The Commission on Nursing Education Accreditation describes diversity as a cultural value:

> A culture of diversity embraces acceptance, respect, and inclusivity . . . which can be along the dimensions of race, ethnicity, gender, sexual orientation, socioeconomic status, age, physical abilities, religious beliefs, political beliefs, or other ideologies. A culture of diversity is about understanding ourselves and each other and moving beyond simple tolerance to embracing and celebrating the richness of each individual. While diversity can be about individual differences, it also encompasses institutional and system-wide behavior patterns. (232) p.32

The Commission on Nursing Education Accreditation does not address diversity in faculty or staff, nor does it address admissions standards to promote diversity. Rather, it addresses student diversity as part of the learning environment, in standard IV:

A student-centered learning environment is cultivated within the program and student diversity is recognized and embraced within a supportive environment. (232) p.5

The Commission on Collegiate Nursing Education's accreditation standards are particularly weak, making reference to diversity only in the context of a "community of interest" to which nursing schools should be accountable:

The community of interest comprises the stakeholders of the program and may include both internal (e.g., current students, institutional administration) and external constituencies (e.g., prospective students, regulatory bodies, practicing nurses, clients, employers, the community/public). The community of interest *might* [emphasis added] also encompass individuals and groups of diverse backgrounds, races, ethnicities, genders, values, and perspectives who are served and affected by the program. (233) p.21

The Commission on Collegiate Nursing Education further weakens its standard for diversity by stating: "The community of interest is defined by the nursing unit" (233) (1-B, p.7). Even more troubling is the fact that the Accreditation Commission for Education in Nursing, the Accreditation Commission for Midwifery Education, and the Council on Accreditation of Nurse Anesthesia programs have no standards related to diversity in faculty, students, or staff (234–236). Perhaps reflective of such weak standards, participants from nursing disproportionately described stage one and two climates at their institutions compared to participants in the other professions. Considering nurses make up 2.7 million of the 11.8 million health-care workers in the United States, the profession's accrediting bodies' disregard for racial and ethnic diversity in nursing education poses a serious risk to the nation's health (237).

Summary and Recommendations

Consistent with what is documented in the higher education literature, participants valued a diverse climate grounded in equity; such climates improved participants' satisfaction and success (96). Many participants shared this perspective, but equity was particularly important to URM faculty. When diversity initiatives meant, "Come on in, but don't change anything," participants both received and were displeased by this message (83) p.220. Plaut and colleagues expressed concern about ornamental approaches to diversity that celebrate difference without making profound structural shifts in institutional power and administrative practices that avoid conflict. Because racial and ethnic inequality is so entrenched in health professions education, approaches to diversity that fail to address inequities will ultimately fail. Without equity, a tacit commitment to sameness remains (96).

Most participants described institutions consistent with stage two climates, suggesting significant change is needed in health professions education. Moving institutions out of the inertia of stages one and two, spurring progress toward stage three, and finally stage four, requires that diversity and equity be central to the mission and culture of health professions institutions. This finding is consistent with the diversity and equity literature in higher education, which requires diversity and equity to be at the core of institutional missions for change to occur (4). Thus diversity must not be a parallel mission at research-intensive universities, but rather be linked directly to the research mission (4). Improving institutional climate is the result of long-term engagement with principles, practices, and policies that are intentionally designed to address specific goals (238). Although important, diversity mission and vision statements, strategic plans, and policies are insufficient to address equity and justice at an institution. Diversity and equity documents are not a substitute for real action (224).

Participants were clear that institutional dialogue was essential to improving diversity and equity climates. Smith identified lack of institutional engagement in difficult dialogues as an obstacle to discovering and using talent in higher education and negative modeling for students (239). The Ford Foundation recognized the importance of such conversations and provided funding to selected higher education institutions to engage in "difficult dialogues." Yet it is imperative that leaders in health professions education recognize difficult dialogues, which engage "history fearlessly and truthfully" (4) p.15, are fundamental to institutional transformation, and hence must occur without the impetus of external funding.

Through their actions, language, priorities, and expectations, board members, presidents, provosts, deans, chairs, and other institutional leaders play a major role in determining institutional climate (240). Because institutional and structural racism exists independently of the actions of individuals, leaders must use their positional authority, resources, and networks to bring institutions to the stage four climate (7). Further, diversity and equity should be tied to administrative performance evaluation and reward structures. An important strategy for improving the quality of decision making, such as faculty hiring, is collaboration with an advisory board representing communities of color (241); this institutional strategy is currently underutilized by leaders.

Institutions that include diversity and equity in their mission statements or even identify diversity as a strategic goal must demonstrate meaningful progress. Diversity and equity initiatives occurring over several years without measurable gains leave institutions stuck in exclusionary climates (238). Identification of quantitative and qualitative indicators, measurement of progress, and use of strategic approaches to create change are essential. A prodiversity discourse without improved racial and ethnic diversity among leadership, faculty, and students is empty (4, 96). Finally, it is imperative that efforts to change not be reduced to counting people. Increasing the number of racially and ethnically diverse faculty and students will not be enough to effect change; the system that generates social and educational advantage for whites while disadvantaging people of color must be challenged and overcome to transform health professions education (9).

Accrediting bodies in health professions education have an obligation to serve the public good; not only do higher education institutions receive funds from public sources, but they benefit from tax-exempt status and enjoy the ability to generate tax-deductible contributions. All members of the public, including groups most affected by health inequities, have the right to know the preferred status enjoyed by higher education institutions is justified. Accreditation standards that mandate equity for faculty and students of color by addressing policies that address structural inequalities systemic to health professions are essential to change (242). Although equity at a single institution is important, structural changes in health professions education as a whole are required for the system to live up to its responsibility to successfully meet the health-care needs of a racially and ethnically diverse society.

CHAPTER THREE

Mentors and Leaders

KEYS TO CHANGE

> I didn't get here by myself . . . I have humility. Humility comes
> from inside out and it says, "Someone was here before me and someone has
> already paid for me." I have a responsibility to pay for someone else who
> is yet to come, there is no room in there for ego! . . . I am grateful to all my
> people who have helped me and all the ways they've helped me . . .
> and I try to help someone else as often as I can.
>
> *Maya Angelou (243)*

Strong mentorship and institutional leaders committed to the development, advancement, and protection of faculty of color were the two most important factors underlying the satisfaction and success of participants in the study. In this chapter I describe participants' common experiences with mentorship from the mentee perspective. These experiences are consequences of lack of mentorship, sources of mentorship, and unique mentoring needs.

Barriers to Mentoring for Faculty of Color

Recognition of the importance of mentoring for faculty satisfaction, research productivity, advancement, and retention is evident in health professions education literature (244–259). Despite the importance of mentoring, the percentage of faculty who have mentors varies, ranging from 19 to 92 percent (247, 257). Although most qualitative studies of the experiences of faculty of color in health professions education have not focused specifically on mentoring, findings across studies consistently identify mentoring as a major concern for this group (155, 159, 260, 261).

In a survey of 616 US-born tenure-track or tenured URM faculty conducted in

2015, 49 percent of participants reported that inadequate mentoring had significantly or somewhat hindered their career growth (262). Despite this disturbing finding from higher education generally, there is very little information about access and quality of mentorship for faculty of color in health professions education. With the exception of one study from nursing, what is known comes from medicine. The nursing study examined the experiences of black leaders using a sequential-mixed methods design. Key findings were the importance of mentors for motivating participants to seek leadership roles and support for the effectiveness of cross-race mentoring (263). Four surveys have explored mentoring in medical school faculty and included faculty of color in the analysis (162, 246, 264, 265). None of these studies has found any significant differences between the quality or rate of mentoring received by URMs and whites. Each study used different definitions of mentoring and sampled faculty of different series and ranks. Moreover, weaknesses in the design and methods of much of this work require that we interpret the results with caution.

Two of the four studies used nationally representative samples from US medical schools spanning all four regions (265). Given their importance, I discuss them in more detail here. Pololi and colleagues used four items from the 177-item C-Change Survey measure in their national study of mentoring in US medical schools. The four items were used to create a composite variable to assess whether faculty perceived mentoring as positive, neutral, or inadequate. In another article reporting results from the parent study, the authors reported that the study was powered with a sufficiently large URM sample for analysis (266). Although the C-Change Survey has good psychometric properties, the four items used to measure mentorship were not developed as a subscale, and the authors provided no information about the reliability and validity of this composite measure. Moreover, the extent to which this four-item measure was able to capture the nature and variability of mentoring of faculty of color in US medical schools is unclear. In a second national study, Palepu and colleagues used a 177-item measure to assess aspects of the work environment, including mentoring. No information was provided about the validity of the measure. The sample included 291 faculty of color and 129 URMs. The authors grouped URMs and Asians together and therefore did not conduct analyses for URMs, probably due to low statistical power (246). Future qualitative studies of mentoring of faculty of color across the professions are needed to explore this phenomenon in depth and provide a basis for instrument development. Rigorous development of a measure of mentoring for health sciences faculty grounded in data obtained from faculty of color is more likely to capture the concerns of this group. Moreover, longitudinal studies are needed to follow the patterns and effects of mentoring relationships over time.

Similarity-attraction theory suggests that commonalities among people such as race, ethnicity, and gender promote positive impressions and mutual attraction, while dissimilar demographic traits generate negative impressions and discomfort (267). This human tendency may explain in part why some faculty of color have greater trouble finding mentors and connecting with informal networks than do white faculty. Professor Adams voiced this concern:

> I think that people tend to gravitate toward those who kind of look like them, who[m] they feel that they have some commonality with. And if you don't have that kind of instant gravitational pull, then you're relying on other things to have you pair up with a mentor, either because you were assigned one or if you have to have one because somewhere in research you exchange your vision . . . things that probably are a little less natural, a little less innate . . . People like to be around people that are similar to themselves . . . If you don't have that to fall back on, then you're probably relying on other things to base your mentorship relationship on that may or may not have as much staying power. [medical faculty]

Race similarity preference and avoidance of cross-race mentoring by white faculty is most likely to occur among those who espouse a color-blind approach to diversity, are concerned about reverse discrimination, and/or believe faculty of color receive unfair advantages (268).

Underrepresented minority faculty are twice as likely as whites to focus their research on health equity; there is a need for senior mentors in this area (266). Yet in this study participants whose scholarship focused on educational and/ or health equity faced challenges finding mentors, as described by Professors Green, Pryor, and Balewa:

PROFESSOR GREEN: Some of the issues that faculty of color may be interested in may not be issues that others care to look at. I was just talking with another faculty [member] of color this morning, looking at some ethnic breakdown and success of minority candidates in the pharmacy school. I said, "Please do not expect widespread support, because the school doesn't necessarily want to know the answer" . . . So sometimes things that we are passionate about may not be shared because our life experience colors what we choose to research, write about, et cetera. [pharmacy faculty]

PROFESSOR PRYOR: The issue that has come up in terms of mentoring I would call out . . . is that my research focus is on race and ethnicity and disparities in health-care delivery and diversity in the health professions, and those topics are off the radar here. This is not a place where people focus a lot of attention on those things, and when I first got here and said, "This is what I want to do," there was sort of a blank stare: "Why do you want to do that?" . . . It is still sort of a blind spot for people. It is not something that senior faculty are involved with—mentors who could offer help aren't interested. [nursing faculty]

PROFESSOR BALEWA: Finding a mentor was a big issue for me . . . I found it very difficult to get by in the area that I was interested in . . . The clinical scholars program people would try to help. They tried to find me a mentor . . . to find what the barriers were. Because the clinical scholars program is a funded program. And then I did find one person who was willing to help me . . . with a minority NIH funded grant. But I could not get buy-in from the people I was working with in the idea that I was interested [in]. So it sort of discouraged me. [medical faculty]

The lack of support for educational and health equity research experienced by participants is consistent with reports from students and faculty of color found in the higher education literature (48, 55). Possible explanations include fewer senior mentors with programs of research focused on educational and health equity compared to other topics, differences in the conceptualization and design of educational and health equity research pursued by students and faculty of color compared to whites, and discrimination against faculty of color as principal investigators. The possibility that fewer senior research mentors are available in health equity than in other areas is plausible. The NIH Revitalization Act, which directed the NIH to establish guidelines for inclusion of women and minorities in clinical research, was not signed into law until 1993, and the National Institute of Minority Health and Health Disparities was only designated as an institute at the NIH in 2010. There is also evidence of discrimination against faculty of color as principal investigators. Ginther and colleagues' study of race, ethnicity, and NIH R01 awards found that black and Asian principal investigators were significantly less likely to receive an R01 award ($p < .001$) than whites, after controlling for demographics, education and NIH training, employer characteristics, previous NIH grants, and reviewer experience (269).

Although finding a mentor could be a challenge, some participants experienced disadvantages even when a mentor was identified. Racial, ethnic, and gender bias negatively affected the quality of mentorship some participants received. Professor Noble described her experience as an assistant professor:

PROFESSOR NOBLE: They assign us two mentors, one for teaching and one for research. My teaching mentor . . . at one meeting she said, "Well, when you meet the dean, you make sure that you dress well and make sure you have your hair combed nicely. You sit there and you fold your hands and cross your legs." I was like, okay, this is odd . . . My research mentor, who is Caucasian, and both of them are Caucasian, she seemed very uninterested in our meetings. I'll never forget our first meeting . . . She said, "There's a guy that they actually fired earlier last year. I hope you're not like him." I thought that was odd because I had just met her, and we hadn't really built a relationship or anything . . . [At another meeting] I was asking about promotion and tenure because I [was coming] up for my third-year review . . . and she's on the P&T committee. I said, "What should I do to plan for that and prepare?" She said, "You should come in there with thick skin because we're rough. We're going to say some hurtful things, so just brace yourself." I was like, "Okay, well can you tell me what to do to be best prepared?" She was like, "Just go over the criteria."

INTERVIEWER: Did race ever go through your mind as being a possible reason [that] your mentors were treating you that way?

PROFESSOR NOBLE: Yes, I have to say it did. With my teaching mentor, who spoke to me like I was a child, I did feel like maybe she was speaking to me that way because I was black. I wondered . . . would she still speak to me this way if I were the same color as her? She sees me as this extremely naïve person. It's just some of the comments she made. Then with my research mentor, I couldn't tell if she was treating me that way because of my race or because it was just her personality . . . She has some NIH friends, and she is very well accomplished, but I couldn't tell. Is she like this to everybody, or is she actually like this because of my race? [pharmacy faculty]

Professor Noble's mentoring relationships were not only of no value; they were harmful. She received no guidance and was left with the burden of trying to decipher the insulting behavior of her mentors. Efforts to understand her mentors' overt behavior and the subtle racial undertones manifested in their nonverbal communication and coded language created a mentally and emotionally draining process. Professor Chopra also experienced discriminatory treatment from her mentor:

> I had a mentoring committee meeting . . . And the plan was to update them about . . . my future plans . . . They first asked me what my goal is . . . and I said, "I want . . . to be scientifically independent." . . . And then this professor asked me this question. It was so unbelievable. He asked me, "So why do you want to be independent?" He asked me, "Is it an ego thing? Or is it really because you truly want to have your own lab?" And . . . he said that he has a woman faculty [member] under him, who is not independent. But he pays her salary. And she's non–tenure track under him and writes all his grants and writes all his papers and manages his lab . . . And so he was saying—referring to her, "Why don't you be like her[?] She goes—comes, does time. She goes home. She takes care of her kids . . . [W]hy can't you be like her?" I was totally taken aback . . . I can never forget that. It was pretty significant. He's a pretty internationally renowned person here at this university.
> INTERVIEWER: Are you on a tenure track?
> PROFESSOR CHOPRA: Yeah, I'm on a tenure track, but that's kind of the boys' club that I'm talking about. That's very visible here. So I don't know if [my mentor's behavior] was because I'm a person or color or . . . because I'm a woman . . . or both. [medical faculty]

Professor Chopra wondered whether it was her ethnicity, her gender, or a combination of both that made her a target for exclusion. Many women participants, particularly those from medicine, wondered about this same thing. In this example, Professor Chopra's gender played a greater role in marking her as a member of the out-group. However, findings in total suggest participants often experienced race/ethnicity and gender intersectionally (141). Professor Chopra was fortunate in that she had other mentors to support her development and was able to progress despite being stereotyped by her mentor, an internationally renowned researcher at her institution.

Consequences of Lack of Mentorship

The importance of mentorship for faculty satisfaction and success was recognized by every participant. Professor Adams described the consequences of a lack of mentorship:

> If you don't have appropriate mentorship, that sets you up for failure every step of the way down the road. So, your [poor quality] mentor is not going to tell you to steer away from some of these other stupid committee requirements that you've now completely filled your schedule up with. They're not going to tell you that it doesn't matter if you've seen fifty patients in clinic this week, what matters is that you haven't published anything in the past year ... Those things are important to both the majority and the minority faculty, ... but if you don't have a mentor who is telling you ... I mean if you don't have a mentor, you're just totally set up for failure. There's no way that you're going to succeed unless you're able to construct a real safety net around you that truly is going to prevent you from falling into pitfalls. [medical faculty]

Although participants understood the importance of mentoring for all faculty, many believed mentorship was more critical for the success of faculty of color than for whites. Reasons given for this difference included a greater proportion of faculty of color who are the first in their family to go to college, less access to informal networks and collaboration than whites, and the need to navigate exclusionary climates. These concerns are substantiated in the literature. A recent study of Harvard Medical School faculty found a positive association between coauthor networking and promotion from assistant to associate professor; URM faculty had significantly smaller coauthor network reach than white faculty at the instructor and assistant professor ranks. Asian Pacific Islander faculty had smaller network reach than whites at the instructor rank (270). A second study using national data found that faculty of color reported significantly lower levels of collegiality than did whites (271). Professor Balewa summed this up, describing academia as an "unequal playing field":

PROFESSOR BALEWA: If you are in an environment where you are in the minority ... you need someone who can encourage you and who can sort of look out for you and help you negotiate the system ... who can help you find the needed resources ... Because really, a good mentor helps you. He pushes you, critiques you, gives you good feedback so that you write better. That's what I needed!

INTERVIEWER: Wouldn't you say that those are the kinds of things that anybody can benefit from?

PROFESSOR BALEWA: Anybody can benefit from that, that's true. But I do think that people of color, because you're in the minority, you really need it . . . I've looked at people of color who are succeeding. They have had mentors who have taken them under their wings and said, "I will help this person succeed." Those are the people of color who have succeeded. It is a really critical factor! I'm not saying that people who are not of color don't need that sort of help, but because it's not a level playing field, I think that even more so, that people of color need that kind of mentorship. [medical faculty]

Inadequate mentoring was also linked to job satisfaction, as described by Professors Cleary and King:

PROFESSOR CLEARY: I think what would improve my job satisfaction is having a senior level researcher nearby who could be my mentor and advocate for me. That would be very helpful. That's at the empty side, I'm going to have to develop. [pharmacy faculty]

PROFESSOR KING: I feel like if I had more mentorship in my field . . . It's unsustainable.

INTERVIEWER: What kind of mentoring have you received at your school?

PROFESSOR KING: Not much. Mostly I try to interact with people at other institutions where I've been. If I have questions, need support, asking about advancement, things like that, I talk with previous mentors that I had at other institutions . . . It [lack of mentorship at this institution] affects my satisfaction. [medical faculty]

Participants with inadequate mentoring were frequently not promoted to higher academic ranks, or if they were promoted, experienced a delayed trajectory, as described by Professor Rodriguez:

I just didn't have a mentor . . . I just did everything on my own and probably could have done things much more easily had I known what I was supposed to do. So going back twenty years, I felt stressed out a lot of the time . . . After being here for several years I felt I had to move, and I moved. So I went from assistant professor to associate professor, and my promotion came because

I moved to another school. So I actually got my promotion somewhere else, and I came back to this place fifteen years later as a professor. So I made my rounds and I traveled the circuit, but no one really guided me. [medical faculty]

The importance of mentorship for advancement and retention were also described by Professors Garcia and Hope:

PROFESSOR GARCIA: I have no guidance whatsoever with respect to promotion. And I think that's why there are so few of us ethnic minorities in academia, because there's no mentorship whatsoever with promotion. I don't know what research to do. I don't know how to apply for grants. I don't know how to write a manuscript, . . . let alone get it published or write a grant. I have no mentorship on how to be promoted. And at five years, if I cannot be promoted from assistant to associate professor, they let us go. It is a lot of pressure. And that's why there are less and less and less ethnic minorities going into academics: . . . the lack of mentorship. Most people that do go into [academic medicine] don't last very long. Retention is a huge problem. There's no mentorship. No incentive to stay. [medical faculty]

PROFESSOR HOPE: The problem . . . we've had at our school is that, yes, we may get an African American faculty [member], but they don't stay . . . They're here two or three years and they're gone. So it's not just getting them here, but keeping them here that's the problem, and a lot of that has to do with the kind of mentoring that they receive. The mentoring is absolutely inadequate. There was one faculty member that we talked to . . . and he had not received any mentoring at all. And so, as he was getting toward tenure promotion decision, somebody realized, "Wait. Nobody ever talked to him about it." And so, one of the other African American faculty members found this out, and called a group meeting of African American faculty—and there aren't that many. I think we're probably ten on the whole campus, maybe a few more. But we all got together with this gentleman and tried to figure out, "What do we do now?" I mean, "You've been here long enough that it's not . . ." And so he left, but he just didn't get any mentoring at all in his department. They just didn't do it. [dental faculty]

Despite the importance of mentorship, many participants did not have strong mentors at their institutions. Professors Garcia and Rodriguez described their belief that receiving quality mentorship was based on luck:

PROFESSOR GARCIA: I think there was luck of mentorship, and it's been like a slight frustration of mine . . . Career mentoring has been a little bit tough. [medical faculty]

PROFESSOR RODRIGUEZ: You have to be in the right place at the right time. I had a mentor and I learned a few things from him, but I didn't learn much in terms of how to get funded and being recognized. I could have done so much more with a good mentor, and I just didn't have that opportunity. [medical faculty]

Participant concerns that mentorship was to some degree a matter of luck speak to the need for a systematic approach to meet the mentoring needs of all faculty. The luck of mentorship depended on a number of factors, such as the number of senior mentors available at an institution, availability of mentors in a shared research area, interpersonal fit, presence of discrimination, and as Professor Rodriguez said, being in the right place at the right time. Participants' stories reflect the importance of mentorship for faculty satisfaction, success, and retention. Mentorship may be even more vital to the success of faculty of color in exclusionary climates.

Sources of Mentorship

Participants sought mentorship from individual and institutional sources. Individual sources of faculty mentorship were those not created by institutions and included educational and accidental mentors. Institutional sources were supervisors and mentoring programs.

INDIVIDUAL SOURCES OF MENTORSHIP

Educational mentors who recognized the value of "grow your own" approaches to fostering racial and ethnic diversity used their influence to help participants get positions at their institutions after completing graduate or postgraduate training and continued to offer mentorship as participants transitioned to the faculty role. Although most participants did not become faculty at the institutions where they completed graduate or postgraduate training, many continued to receive mentorship from past educational mentors when they went to work at other institutions. Finally, some participants were also helped by accidental mentorship, receiving guidance by happenstance.

Mentors who recognized the value of the "grow your own" strategy understood the value of diversity and equity for excellence, were aware of racism and exclusion at their institutions, and helped mentees navigate the institutional landscape. Because they were at the same institutions, these mentors were able to more directly affect participants' careers, offering wisdom, guidance, protection, and advocacy and opening doors that might otherwise be closed. Professor Davis described her mentoring experience:

PROFESSOR DAVIS: I actually joined the faculty [at] the same place where I was a fellow. My primary mentor was instrumental in [my] being offered a position here ... He's a relatively big kahuna here, and he pointed out that we had some people who were finishing faculty fellowships who would be ideal junior faculty candidates and were from URM groups ... And I'm one of two URMs in my section ... When a new person comes in they kind of look at the entire complement of faculty and put everybody in a box who's going to be promoted who's not ... and I am a minority and also a woman as well, and those things are in the room and I know that ... [but] I have this connection to my mentor, who's very big in the school of medicine, and that looms large over these conversations as well.

INTERVIEWER: How would you describe your mentoring relationship?

PROFESSOR DAVIS: He's lots of different kinds of mentors. So he's really a godfather kind of mentor. He is the mentor on my training grant, the last author on my papers, somebody who reads my papers and comments on them, reads my grants and comments on them, those kinds of basic mentoring things. But he's also mostly this sort of overseeing kind of mentor, so he's really my advocate here at this university, and also tries to promote me outside of the university to get my name and work out there ... He doesn't do the same research that I do. I have a lot of mentors who are sort of more content mentors around my research. But he's sort of my career godfather kind of mentor ... [I confide in him] to make sure I haven't missed something important, so for example he will tell me who I should go and have a conversation with, who things need to be right with ... He's my advocate, so if anybody's going to be saying anything about me, he's got to know the substance of it so that he can do whatever he does on my behalf . . . He advises me to take a business attitude about things; it's not personal. He says, "Don't worry about those kinds of shenanigans . . . Go do this, do that, make sure that you are protecting your flank and don't think any more about it." . . . I can bring problems to him and he can keep his ear to the ground about me.

INTERVIEWER: When you say "godfather," what do you mean?

PROFESSOR DAVIS: I mean by that somebody who is watching out for you, who puts the right word in, who lets you know the scuttlebutt as it's importantly related to you, who's going to make sure that you have a chance at an opportunity that [he] hears about, that you might not otherwise ever have gotten, who even outside the institution is going to put a word in somebody's ear about you when it seems appropriate. So I mean more broad strokes rather than the nitty-gritty of reading my work and making sure my research looks exactly the way it should, although a godfather does those things, too. [medical faculty]

Like Professor Davis, Professor Flores's mentors used their influence to help him obtain a faculty position and access opportunities. Professor Flores, having completed medical school and a fellowship at the same institution, had more than one mentor:

The program director on the educational side . . . created a position for me to go into after graduating from my fellowship into faculty . . . [He] was instrumental in creating a job for me, and he helped oversee a little of both. I also had a couple of other mentors that helped with the nonclinical side of it. That was during the first year of becoming a faculty member. I felt that the same people I had known since medical school were still there, particularly those program directors in internal medicine. I had developed a reasonable relationship with the Chief of Medicine. After I did my internal medicine residency, I was selected to be a Chief Resident, so going back after residency, I did two years in my cardiology fellowship, and the Chief of Medicine meets with the Chief Resident pretty much every week . . . So I think that was key . . . not very many people were able to meet with the Chief of Medicine every week for a year . . . I was able to develop a stronger and special relationship with him, and it has really borne fruit even to this point, where I feel I have a lot of support from him and the Chief of Cardiology as well. Over the course of my fellowship, I was not a typical person in that I didn't follow one of the usual research tracks, so with his support they were able to make kind of a special path for me where I would be a physician educator, which is unusual for our cardiology division and our cardiology training program. So I think what was key [was] to have the mentors that I had early on for medical school and then have opportunities where I was able to capitalize on being mentored by people who had particular influence within the department or the division. [medical faculty]

Other examples of postgraduate training mentors providing faculty mentorship at the same institution were provided by Professors Larson and Kapoor:

PROFESSOR LARSON: I ended up staying here for the duration of my training . . . I've had two mentors . . . So the mentoring . . . was really strong; they were looking out for me as far as you need to work on establishing your own area of research, but they still involved me in some collaborative work that we did. They also were helpful in guiding me through what portions of service I needed to be involved in and steering me clear of committees that would ta[ke] too much time and helping guide me toward committees that would be appropriate for my position at that time. Then [they] counsel[ed] me through what types of national organization involvement I should be in. How much teaching should I do and all that kind of stuff. They were very helpful. So my support system here has been fantastic actually. [pharmacy faculty]

PROFESSOR KAPOOR: [My postdoctoral mentor] believed in training, tremendous training . . . He was a Distinguished Investigator for several years and so had seen all kinds of people from all nations, gender, and color . . . I told him from the very beginning, "This is what I want to do." And his focus was really getting me there. He was amazing in the opportunities he opened up the door for me . . . He told me this is what you have to do, this is where you have to go to pursue something . . . When I had trouble with a person in the grants office giving me so many roadblocks, he used to say, "Well, you know you're different, so there are going to be times like this and you have to get past them and not be bogged down by them." And he continues to be my mentor. He's part of my junior faculty mentoring committee. [pharmacy faculty]

Mentors who were committed to increasing racial and ethnic faculty diversity used a "grow your own" strategy. They had established relationships with mentees as students and were committed to their long-term success in the faculty role. They understood the importance of diversity and equity for excellence and the need to counteract exclusionary processes by using their influence to give mentees as many advantages as possible. As Professors Davis's and Flores's stories show, these mentors did not necessarily share a research area with mentees. Professor Davis's mentor, whom she described as a "godfather," transcended the delimited roles of a research or teaching mentor, ensuring these needs were met by others in the organization.

EDUCATIONAL MENTORS AT OTHER INSTITUTIONS

Although most participants did not assume faculty positions at institutions where they were educated, many continued to rely on mentors from their educational programs for guidance. Professors Noble, Swan, and Morgan described these continuing relationships:

PROFESSOR NOBLE: I had people that I have built relationships with before I joined this school. I talk with them all the time. I still have mentors from my undergrad [program] and I call them. They give me great advice. [pharmacy faculty]

PROFESSOR SWAN: My dissertation cochair . . . is now an associate dean . . . and she's remained my mentor and she's an African American female. So I see her as someone I [want to] emulate. She's been very productive; she's been very successful . . . She has been someone who has helped me out tremendously. [pharmacy faculty]

PROFESSOR MORGAN: I did my fellowship at Southern University, so it was kind of a natural thing for me to have [him] continue to mentor me even after I left there . . . My specialty was something that [he] could help me . . . get expertise in. [medical faculty]

Students and postgraduate trainees of color often report a lack of access to mentoring in health professions education and color-blind mentoring relationships that reinforce racial inequities (272–277). The findings of this study speak to the importance of educational mentors for students and postgraduate trainees of color, not only for recruitment and retention in the present, but also for the satisfaction and success of future faculty.

ACCIDENTAL MENTORS

Some participants described accidental mentoring as vital to their development. Accidental mentoring was usually a one-time event, occurring as the result of happenstance when someone unexpectedly offered help or advice. Accidental mentoring came from a variety of people, including staff, colleagues, and interested observers. Professor Jones provided an example of accidental mentorship offered by a staff person:

> I did go for promotion; however, the process was very interesting in the sense that . . . I didn't know how to prepare a dossier for promotion. I was fortunate in that one of the administrative staff, when I got my little packet together she looked at it and she came back to me because she was collecting them and pulling them together and she said, "This isn't going to work. Did anyone tell you how to do this?" And I said "no." She said, . . . "I'll tell you what, don't tell anyone, but I'm going to give you a copy of a good one. Now look at that and that's what you need to do." And that's how I learned. Because she went out of her way to show me. [medical faculty]

Professor Murphy received accidental mentoring from two different physicians, both of whom were instrumental in influencing her choice of medical specialty:

> When I was going into medicine, I was really trying to decide between OB [obstetrics] and ophthalmology . . . [but] since you're a black person in medical school, they're always trying to get you to go into primary care . . . Actually it was one of my Jewish colleagues who said his father had been an ophthalmologist, and he was going to be one . . . He said, "Do you want to have my slides?" and I said, "Sure." He was giving a talk on diabetes; I found it to be absolutely fascinating. I mean I would have never been in ophthalmology otherwise. I got involved; I went to do my elective . . . and . . . while I was there, they hired a black female glaucoma person. I was in the library and she came and tapped me on the shoulder and said, "What are you doing here?" I said "doing research," and she said, "I'm going to call my friend who is doing important research and see if you can go there for a few weeks and really get some stuff together that might help you." I was like, "Wow." I mean she picked up that phone and within the next week I flew out to work with that researcher. I got three papers out of that. I still talk to the lady even today . . . I got into ophthalmology and that was one person, sort of making a difference in having those connections . . . It's that one person . . . even when I got into ophthalmology she was saying, "What do you want to do now?" I said, "I think I want to do cornea." She said,

"Glaucoma needs you." I said, "Really?" . . . and then I found that I really loved it for many reasons. [medical faculty]

Happenstance encounters, short-term, and ad hoc mentoring helped build professional skills and in some cases led to pivotal career changes. Participants' openness to learning from a variety of people fostered this unexpected support.

Institutional Sources

Health professions education institutions employ faculty in a variety of roles, with titles such as clinical and research professor, clinical educator, and scientist. The extent to which faculty can successfully pursue the career most congruent with their talents and aspirations is highly influenced by the support they receive from supervisors and leaders, as well as the availability of mentoring programs.

SUPERVISORS AS MENTORS

The granting of release time from teaching to focus on scholarship was vital for participants. Supervisors were responsible for overseeing activities that led to tenure or renewal of multiyear contracts. Hence, mentorship was inherent in the role of supervisor. As experienced faculty members with institutional authority, supervisors were positioned to offer mentorship, which simultaneously communicated a message of institutional support. Professor Howard's supervisor mentored him through the promotion and tenure process:

> He served as the division director at that time, [and he] just took a personal interest in seeing me promoted and tenured . . . He just took it upon [him]self to help me along and did a great job in that . . . extremely helpful. [pharmacy faculty]

Professors Curtis and Davis received mentorship from their supervisors in the areas of grantsmanship, clinical practice, and teaching:

PROFESSOR CURTIS: I applied for my first grant and I got a lot of help . . . My mentor happened to be chair of the department and I also work with him in clinic . . . The doors are open at all times. It's been unreal . . . and . . . [I] don't have this ridiculous workload. [medical faculty]

PROFESSOR DAVIS: I was very pleasantly surprised that the chairman of the department came and worked with me when I was doing consultation liaison.

When I first started I was getting really bad feedback from residents. They thought that I wasn't teaching, and there were all sorts of issues I couldn't understand, and I just felt really badly about it. What was very nice was he said, "You know this happens to a lot of faculty. Let's work together for a couple of weeks, and I bet we can work this out." So he just would come over and watch with the residents and give some feedback, and the feedback I got from residents was a lot better. So that was a very nice thing for him to say, "Hmmm, this is a problem; let's see if we can fix it." And it was fixed, and I thought that was very nice. [medical faculty]

In addition to providing mentorship in common areas of concern, some supervisors also protected participants against racism, as described by Professor Morgan:

My boss was very interested in having a diverse faculty . . . I had a bad run-in with the neurosurgery chair . . . He complained to my boss about me. Luckily my boss was on my side. He said, "Dr. Morgan, I know this is kind of a racist guy." But every time I had an interaction with this neurosurgery chair he complained about it, and my boss would get an e-mail, "Dr. Morgan didn't do this, didn't do that." And then my boss would call me, and I'd say to my boss, "I did it," and he'd say, "I know you did" . . . I tell you, if my boss hadn't protected me from that neurosurgeon and I had left, I would have told everybody, "Until that neurosurgeon dies, you're not safe." Because that neurosurgeon didn't like black people, he just didn't. And he was out to get me and I didn't do anything. I'm just showing up for work and you're after me because I'm black. So if I had not lasted at this university and somebody had called me and said, "Would you go to that university?" "No, no. Not until, you know, some of these folks have move[d] on." [medical faculty]

Participants who experienced racism but were not supported by their supervisors became disillusioned, often warning other faculty of color against coming to their institutions. These participants were more likely to leave their institutions or academe altogether.

MENTORING FOR LEADERSHIP

A study of twenty-six US medical schools found URMs were more likely to report having leadership aspirations than other faculty groups. Despite their interest in leadership, URMs also rated their institutions lower on relationship trust, inclusion and connection, equity, and institutional efforts to improve diversity (266). Furthermore, Mainah and Perkins's study of black women leaders found many "faced pressure to ignore their identity, beliefs, cultural competencies, and values to fit into a white male prototype in order to succeed" (278) p.10. By virtue of their positions, leaders have the power to remedy this situation. Leaders can counteract exclusionary processes that keep faculty of color out of leadership by purposefully grooming and hiring faculty of color for leadership roles and opening up a space that allows diverse values and perspectives to flourish. Professors Pryor, Ahmed, and Howard described their experiences of being mentored into leadership:

PROFESSOR PRYOR: [My supervisor has] allowed me to be very flexible in my schedule, my work. She's recommended me for things. When I did the interim director position, she came to me. She sat me down. She said, "I think it would be a great career move for you. If you don't like it, we're going to hold a job for you here." She has always been extremely supportive and helpful in kind of mentoring and guiding me in this institution. [nursing faculty]

PROFESSOR AHMED: When I started at my current position I didn't have any administrative experience. I think that the Associate Dean really took me under her wing. She helped me with what I needed to know and who I needed to [know], and the ins and outs of who [was] on our side in the office and who was not, and the politics in the office as well. I can say that she really supported me and mentored me in my current role and helped me along the way. If I was stuck in any way in terms of support or sending [me] to professional development that I needed, and if I needed to attend any meetings or if I needed to do anything, she was always there for me. [pharmacy faculty]

PROFESSOR HOWARD: My present department chair has worked a lot with me, and he's the person that actually recommended that I go into the leadership program. So he and I worked a lot together, especially during that year. He [my chair] really works hard with his faculty in regard to improving our skill sets and helping us to grow as leaders. [pharmacy faculty]

Although mentorship for leadership was greatly appreciated, some participants expressed concern about a glass ceiling. This suggested that participants faced challenges moving into higher leadership roles. A glass ceiling is an unseen barrier that keeps women and people of color from rising to the upper levels of leadership, regardless of their qualifications or achievements (279). Professors Walters and Chen explained:

PROFESSOR WALTERS: Depending on how high up you are ascending in your career—there [are also] going to be ... unspoken things [like], "Well, maybe we really don't want this." [medical faculty]

PROFESSOR CHEN: My first day here ... a senior faculty member said, "I'm going to mentor you." And he did. And he's now the chair of the department ... He's kind of washed his hands of me ... now that I'm trying to advance on the administrative pathway ... I feel like, "Well, couldn't you guys just try to go to bat for me a little bit?" ... So he's been great, but to certain limits. Same with my dean ... He's been great, but to a certain limit ... They want to promote me and see me succeed, but they want to keep me here under this glass ceiling. [pharmacy faculty]

Who is selected for leadership positions says a great deal about what groups are being taken seriously in health professions education. When racial and ethnic diversity in leadership is lacking, signals are sent about the lack of possibilities, recognition, and appreciation of talent in people from these groups. In contrast, the presence of a racially and ethnically diverse leadership creates a sense of opportunity and offers role models for everyone at the institution. Moreover, an ethnically and racially diverse leadership is essential to avoid homogeneity of decision making, which limits openness to new ideas and ignores approaches to education and health care that are most beneficial to a pluralistic society (4). Although information on racial and ethnic diversity in faculty and students is not uniformly accessible across the professions, in general it is more readily available to the public than leadership data. The AAMC and American Association of Colleges of Pharmacy (AACP) include demographic data for deans and other leadership positions in their annual faculty surveys, which are available to members and can be purchased by the public (20, 280); I found no AACN or AACP data on the racial and ethnic composition of academic leadership freely available to the public or published in the literature. Moreover, the AAMC does not provide faculty at member schools, or the public, information about the racial and ethnic composition of deans and associate deans at medical schools. Nor does the American Dental Education Association (ADEA) regularly report such information to faculty at member schools or the public, although a profile of dental school deans can be found in the literature approximately every ten years, and a profile of department chairs was recently published (281–283). I was unable to determine if medical and dental school deans and academic health center provosts and presidents receive this information separately. In my communications with AAMC I was told the only way to get current data on the racial and ethnic composition of deans and associate deans in US medical schools is to request a special analysis for a fee of at least $1,000. Dr. Kristin Lutz, who asked the ADEA for data on the racial and ethnic composition of deans and associate deans in US dental schools on my behalf, was given the same response.

The data I was able to glean suggest that faculty of color in health professions education are severely underrepresented in leadership relative to their proportion of the US population. Census data from 2015 reported that non-Hispanic whites comprised only 61.6 percent of Americans (75). In contrast, the AACN faculty survey reported that 88.7 percent of nursing school deans are white (280). The AACN faculty survey uses the term "dean" to refer to chief executive officer of a nursing school as well as persons with institutionally determined titles such as director, chair, head, and coordinator. Moreover, Yu and colleagues' retrospective analysis of AAMP data on faculty at US medical schools from 1997 to 2008 found that, averaged over the twelve years, whites accounted for 91.28 percent of deans (16). Medical school chairs also lack racial and ethnic diversity, and change is slow. Rayburn and colleagues' analysis of AAMP data on first-time chairs found that whites went from 91 percent in 1978 to 85 percent in 2007, only a 6 percent decrease over twenty-nine years (284). Pharmacy schools' leadership fares minimally better than that of nursing and medicine. The 2016 AACP faculty survey reported that 81.4 percent of deans and 85 percent of associate deans were white. Finally, a 2014 survey of US dental schools that included Puerto Rico found 88 percent of deans were white (282). Although the number of women dental school deans had doubled between 2002 and 2014, the proportion of white deans had decreased by only 1 percent (281, 282). Similarly, a survey of US and Canadian dental school chairs conducted from 2013 to 2014 found 89.4 percent were white (283).

Racial and ethnic diversity in health professions education leadership is abysmal, and change has been minimal given the increased diversity of the general population. For those who are committed to excellence and equity, such an impoverished leadership can only be seen as a state of emergency. Racially and ethnically diverse social identities influence perspectives and concerns that are not introduced by homogeneous leadership groups and promote stronger ties to underserved communities. Moreover, racial and ethnic diversity in leadership represents values concerning power sharing and equity. Hence, racial and ethnic diversity is a requirement for excellence and equity in leadership. Institutions that simultaneously describe themselves as open and committed to diversity, while failing to improve the face of leadership, can only be seen as disingenuous (239). Genuine commitment requires accountability. Thus, leadership data should be analyzed and tracked annually and the results be made available to the public across the professions. Furthermore, because faculty of color are severely underrepresented in the health professions relative to the general population, benchmarking leadership relative to faculty is not an acceptable standard. Such an approach would only serve to reify inequities.

MENTORING PROGRAMS

A systematic review of the literature on development and mentoring programs for faculty of color found that such programs increase retention, productivity, and promotion (161). Most published data on faculty mentoring in health professions education come from medicine, and several schools have described examples of promising mentoring programs (61, 285–287). Despite the existence of such programs, in an environmental scan of 124 US medical schools, Adanga and colleagues found only 22 percent offered mentoring programs for faculty of color (288).

Only three of the one hundred participants in this study reported accessing a faculty mentoring program. Some participants from medicine said mentoring programs were available to women but not to faculty of color at their institutions. Of the three programs accessed by participants, only one focused on the needs of faculty of color. Professor Dickerson described her experience:

> I joined a faculty advancement and mentorship program for minority faculty in the first few years that I was a faculty member. As part of being in the program I had to identify one mentor in my department and one outside of my department to work on a particular research project and just general mentorship kinds of things . . . [T]he person who was my mentor was in my department [and] was simply awesome and stayed my mentor after the program was over . . . His people were from India . . . When he accepted me as his mentee he said, "I will be your mentor as long as I am here. It is not just for this program" . . . and he was great. When he ended up leaving the institution, I think I went

into a depression . . . I mean I cried . . . He was really a good mentor . . . He was my mentor when I moved from being an assistant to an associate professor many years ago . . . [Since then] I haven't had anybody who has accepted that mentoring role. [medical faculty]

Recognizing the benefits mentoring programs have to offer faculty of color, participants in administrative and faculty service roles were involved in addressing this concern at their institutions. Professors Smith and Adams described their work:

PROFESSOR SMITH: I think there are some unique aspects for faculty of color compared to majority faculty that [are] important to understand . . . Understanding what opportunities are available is a very important aspect. That's the mentoring program that we're developing for the center; that's one of the things we're trying to do is provide ways in which junior faculty can match up with senior level faculty and basically learn about what experiences or what opportunities are available. [medical faculty]

PROFESSOR ADAMS: It doesn't take a rocket scientist to know that mentorship is a very critical component . . . In . . . the Minority Faculty Affairs Committee, we recognize that mentorship is a key area, so we actually have a couple subcommittees . . . and there's another subcommittee that's devoted just to mentoring. [medical faculty]

Professor Adams went on to talk about the critical nature of successful mentoring programs for faculty of color and the need for institutional commitment:

[The Minority Faculty Affairs Committee has] identified mentorship as being a huge deficit, but we have no clue how to really go about doing it. I've talked to people at other institutions to try and get an idea, but most of these are very labor-intensive programs, [and] you have people who are dedicated (i.e., paid to do just that). We don't have that sort of leverage here. And they totally get it . . . I have some of the most fascinating conversations. It's a meeting . . . where you have invested interests of the leadership to mentor those beneath, so every time I run into one of these guys who are in the leadership, they look at me and say, "What are you doing? How successful have you been? What are you working on? How can I help you?" All the things that you wish . . . somebody . . . was sitting right there at your home institution [providing you with]. [medical faculty]

Professor Adams's description of leaders who "get it" and the investment of resources their institutions provided to support faculty mentoring captures some of the ingredients needed for successful programs. Her receipt of mentorship from leaders not at her institution reflected their commitment to mentoring, and her desire for such mentorship at her own institution speaks to the importance of dedicated institutional mentors for faculty satisfaction and success.

Mentoring Needs of Faculty of Color

Faculty of color are a diverse group whose mentoring needs and preferences are heterogeneous. Professor Rutledge described the importance of tailoring mentorship for each mentee:

> Mentorship does need to be tailored to the individual involved. Certain faculty of color probably need some elements of support that . . . nonminority faculty don't, but everyone needs [mentoring] . . . I think mentorship is a process of data collection and thoughtfully spending time with people and figuring what to do and figuring out what their needs are. Because everyone is going to have something . . . I think this is something that the mentor needs to probe regardless of that person's background. I think it needs to be addressed with women faculty. I think it needs to be probed with faculty who are of lesbian, gay, bisexual, transgender, whatever, and ethnic and racial minorities. What's going on with this . . . Let's talk about this. Where is it surfacing? And I think particularly junior faculty need to feel like they have the full support of the institution behind them. And I think there is often a reticence [from] people during the first five years of their faculty appointment to bring concerns forward. [medical faculty]

Differences to be considered when individualizing mentorship for a faculty member include the influence of their various social identities, cultural background, life history, values, family obligations, strengths, career goals, and prior academic experience (289).

Despite the diversity of the sample, many participants described mentoring needs specific to faculty of color in two areas: relating to and validating experience and navigating exclusionary climates. Participants shared with us the racial, ethnic, gender, and sometimes religious backgrounds of their mentors, allowing us to analyze the importance of these social characteristics in their mentoring relationships. Mentors who were able to meet the unique needs of faculty of color were often from the same racial or ethnic background and sometimes a racial or ethnic minority of a different background. Fewer participants described white mentors who met these needs.

Relating to and Validating Experience

Making an authentic connection with another person means understanding, empathizing, and being able to see the world through his or her eyes. White privilege and the dominance of Eurocentric norms in society create different standpoints from which to view reality for whites than for people of color. This makes it less likely that a white mentor will relate to and validate the experiences of faculty of color. Professors Corbin and Noble talked about the importance of having a mentor who can understand your experiences:

PROFESSOR CORBIN: Generally, the life experiences of minority faculty are quite different. So I do think there are some unique aspects for minority faculty that require some very specific mentoring . . . when you're working with other faculty who are so different from you and don't really understand your perspective. It's nice to work with people who do understand how you feel and where you come from. There's a great deal of satisfaction when you're struggling in certain areas, and here's someone you can talk to and bounce these ideas and feelings off, and they can relate to what you're feeling and what you've experienced. I think that's really important. Old white men cannot necessarily relate to those experiences. [medical faculty]

PROFESSOR NOBLE: I think that if you have a mentor [who] can sort of relate or understand and hear out your issues, it's very, very helpful. Even now, as I think about it, when I had a lot of my problems I would call a faculty [member] of color to discuss what was going on. Even one of my mentors is Asian, and I call her all the time. She's a senior faculty member and I talk to her all the time and it's really, really helpful . . . Right now we don't have senior faculty members who are minorities. [pharmacy faculty]

Professor Flores, who appreciated and benefited from having multiple white mentors in senior administrative roles, described the added benefits of receiving mentorship from faculty of like background:

I think that there is definitely something unique about the mentoring needs of faculty of color . . . I think for someone like myself, it's nice to hear what other faculty members have gone through . . . It's kind of a little bit of showing someone the ropes, knowing that they've been through a similar experience as you have, even down to the lifestyle issues. It's like I know you couldn't afford to move to the suburbs, either, but these are the things you can do, and it's okay not to live in whatever town. So I think that's very helpful, and for me . . . he doesn't have to be the sole mentor, but I think there should be someone that can identify in some way with the faculty member and say, "I've been through the same thing," especially on committees, getting pulled everywhere, being the limited resource, and feeling guilty for not do[ing] this or the other thing. The other thing is to also focus a little bit selfishly on your career to make sure you are acknowledged for what you do. I know there's nothing like living it. I know my mentors who aren't minorities can identify, but there's just something about knowing the feelings that you have are not just you alone, and others have gone through the same deal. [medical faculty]

Professor Flores talked about the importance of having a mentor who has been through the same thing because there is "nothing like living it" and how having such a mentor forestalls feelings of isolation. Similarly, Professor Garcia described how a mentor of like background put her at ease, allowing her to be herself in ways she felt uncomfortable doing with others:

I think because I grew up in a low socioeconomic setting . . . I'm not used to . . . being in conversation with people that are VIPs . . . Not VIPs—I don't know [what] the right word is—the people above me, basically. And so I don't fall into conversation as easily with, for example, my bosses. My mentor, although his title was much higher than my boss'[s], I could fall into conversation with him easily because we talked a lot about the same things. We talked about the same booze, the same celebrations, family issues, things like that. And sometimes I feel—and I know this is silly—but sometimes I feel a little ghetto in how I speak, carry myself, or things that I do, when I hang out with my colleagues. And so I tend to hide a little bit of my culture or who I am with them. And with Dr. Pérez, it was just so easy because I could totally be myself even though he was Vice Provost and all these things. [medical faculty]

A personal connection between mentor and mentee, appreciation of "the other as a whole person," trust, open communication, confidentiality, and a safe environment are characteristics of successful mentoring relationships (290) p.75. Participants did not object to being mentored by white faculty, although some did express a preference for mentorship by someone of like background. Regardless of preference, the vast majority recognized the value of faculty of color as sources of emotional support. Because there are few senior faculty of color in health professions education, particularly URM faculty, they may be stretched thin by the number of junior faculty and students of color seeking mentorship. This group is deserving of recognition and reward for the unique skills it brings to mentoring (289). Such recognition and reward is essential to equity and diversity in health professions institutions and our ability to diversify the professions.

Navigating Exclusionary Climates

Many participants expressed a desire for mentoring that would help them successfully navigate exclusionary climates. As Professor Swan stated, "Faculty of color need to know how to deal with being a minority in a majority academic situation, because it's very different at times" [pharmacy faculty]. Professor Green described the need for faculty of color to receive "extra tips" to be successful:

When there are not many of us above us in terms of . . . associates . . . and professors, . . . how many we do we see at this institution that look like us? Without that, we lose that hope where there are unique things that we need to do. How do you protect yourself? . . . Even . . . senior faculties to partner with, who . . . has our best interest[s] at heart? . . . I'm a little bit concerned about it. The institution doesn't have a good track record of minorities here. I think it takes a little longer for us to get where we're going . . . Knowing that we will . . . oftentimes have to be . . . extra good . . . We do need those little tips. [pharmacy faculty]

Professor Dickerson described some of the unique guidance faculty of color may need:

I think faculty of color need to have a mentor who can recognize that the fact that [he or she is] mentoring a faculty [member] of color can be a big deal—that the person who's the mentor needs to be able to have an objective assessment of how the color issue plays into that mentee's career and in [his or her] life. It could be a person that's not of color. But [he or she] should be able to say, "Okay, this is what the landscape is here at your institution. And when we go over here your color's going to matter. When we go over here, your color's not going to matter. But what we're going to do is this so that you are going to be able to progress no matter what." [medical faculty]

Professors Howard, Davis, and Swift provided examples of mentoring as a source of guidance and support in exclusionary climates:

PROFESSOR HOWARD: There are probably a number of hurdles that faculty of color have to cross that others would not. I . . . mean sometimes there is the feeling that you're not quite sure whether or not your evaluation, or the way people assess you or feel about you, has anything to do with race or ethnicity. Or if this is their pure assessment or evaluation of who you are as an individual. I mean [there's] always the possibility that someone's opinion of you is colored by that, and I think you have to kind of work through that. I mean how do you handle a situation in which you think someone may be biased in some way or someone may be misunderstanding something that you're trying to say or do because of differences in cultural beliefs and cultural behavior? So I think helping someone to kind of navigate those waters is very important. [pharmacy faculty]

PROFESSOR DAVIS: I think there [are] unique mentoring needs for . . . minorities . . . Minorities can use mentorship specifically around the area of the kinds of responsibilities that we take on because we are minorities and how to navigate that. When [do] you say, "Yes"? How do you decide "Yes" or "No"? Where do you draw the line thinking about how to leverage the kinds of things that you are doing toward recognition, which is another thing we don't get? . . . How to be in the right position to have a really solid impact? . . . Like I said, it's invisible how racism is playing behind the curtain when you are junior [faculty]. And senior people would have a lot more insight into that, so if you had that kind of mentoring, to say, "No, no, no, you need to go and do this because that's where things can get hairy . . . Don't deal directly with that person. Let me worry about that." Or, "Let your other mentor worry about that. You go deal with these people." Just having that knowledge could be incredibly beneficial. [medical faculty]

PROFESSOR SWIFT: I feel like my race plays a part in how . . . I present things . . . I'll give you a perfect example. I had a run-in with administration regarding how I handled a situation in my class. When I went to administration, I asked them the first time and they told me to handle it the way that I felt was appropriate. I handled it, and they didn't like it. When we had our back and forth, I felt like before I even walked in, he [the administrator] was potentially already on guard about how he thought I was going to react to it, meaning being very emotional, high strung, and the angry black woman . . . When I didn't do that, it kind of took him [a]back a little bit because I knew that's what he was expecting me to do. He knew I was very angry. I was very angry about what [had] happened. I felt that's what he expected me to do. He was really ready for a fight, I think. I was like, really? . . . Because for that particular administrator I think because I am woman and a minority he felt like I shouldn't have questioned him . . . I can't say that race wasn't an issue, because I've had other faculty members talk to him that weren't minority and had the same disagreement, but his reaction toward me was totally different compared to how he approached them . . . He was more like scolding me. I was like, really?

INTERVIEWER: Scolding. How do you cope with that?

PROFESSOR SWIFT: I vent to someone who I think would understand. Then I ask what could I have done differently? What could I have done to not—I don't want to be wrong. Once again, there's not anything I can prove. It's the feeling from discussion that I had and with other faculty members that look like me, and their interactions with this particular administrator . . . So I guess I should have asked before I went into the office. I should have asked, how do you handle him? . . . Like I said you can't prove it. It's not anything that I can do . . . You can take him to human resources, but it's just one of those things where you shake your head and try to not feel so bad when I walk out of the office . . . He would never admit the racism. A lot of the stuff you can't prove. People aren't going to come out and say this stuff most of the time. They're smart enough to know better than to come out and say stuff. A lot of it is very covert . . . I usually vent . . . I also usually ask if I'm being too sensitive, because that's also the other issue from the other side that people think you're too sensitive . . . Usually I ask my mentor because she's like an old rock and has been here for a long time . . . I will say that definitely there have been things that I talked to her about that if she wasn't a faculty [member] of color I don't know if I would've been comfortable enough talking to her about it. I would've thought

[she] wouldn't necessarily understand the way I feel, that I feel about a certain situation. I felt really comfortable after my interview with the administrator. I felt really comfortable talking to her very candidly about it and how I felt. I'm not sure if she wasn't a minority if I would've brought it to her that way. I doubt that I would have. [pharmacy faculty]

Other unique mentoring needs were related to teaching and practice. Professor Ibori talked about race in the classroom:

Essentially, what happens . . . and especially if it's the first year that you've come into a professional division, you go into that class, you have students there who have never had a person of color stand in front of them as a teacher before. And so, there's that kind of mentoring on, "How do you command a class being an African American, standing in front of eighty mostly white people?" Maybe you have two or three nonwhite [students] in that group . . . There are all kinds of mentoring that has to do with how you conduct yourself . . . in a predominantly white community, how do you conduct yourself as a faculty member? [pharmacy faculty]

Professor Hayes described the importance of having mentors available who are connected to underserved communities:

INTERVIEWER: Would you say that you would have wanted to have an African American mentor?

PROFESSOR HAYES: Yes . . . I moved into an area that I'm not from. So giving me perspective on the setting and what my patients are coming from. And our patients are largely African American, so having an understanding of their health needs, the general social and economic circumstances of the area, having more insight into those areas. [medical faculty]

Relating to and validating experience were critical aspects of the mentoring role, and mentees were more likely to receive this help from mentors who understood the minority experience in health professions education. Participants described senior faculty of color as having many years of experience and important insight about how to strategically maneuver and adapt in health professions academe even in exclusionary climates. Yet in addition to being knowledgeable and experienced, the most effective mentors are also visible and powerful in their institutions and professions. Few participants described mentors of color who possessed this kind of institutional power.

Summary and Recommendations

Barriers to quality mentoring create an opportunity gap for faculty of color. The mentoring needs of the majority of participants were not fully met; some participants had difficulty finding mentors, and others experienced discrimination from assigned mentors. Many participants reported a desire for mentorship that included understanding and validation of personal experiences related to gender, race, and ethnicity, as well as guidance on how to navigate and succeed in exclusionary climates. Participants with inadequate institutional mentorship were dissatisfied with their jobs and more likely to leave their positions. In contrast, participants who received mentorship from educational mentors who helped them transition into the faculty role at the same institutions where they were educated, and supervisors, were highly appreciative and felt more positive about their institutions. This was particularly true for participants whose supervisors helped mentor them into leadership.

Leaders have a responsibility to attend to the mentorship needs of the faculty they are supervising. This requires an understanding of exclusion and control processes and a willingness to protect and support faculty of color when needed. Leaders should also work to increase racial and ethnic diversity by purposefully identifying, mentoring, and hiring faculty of color into leadership positions (291–294) and fostering a "grow your own" approach to filling the pipeline with well-mentored, advanced graduate students and postdoctoral trainees (295–298). Leaders can "grow their own" racially and ethnically diverse faculty, particularly URM faculty, by fostering this practice at their institutions and by offering incentives (299). Faculty development programs to increase the pool of qualified mentors that include competencies for working effectively with students and junior faculty of color are needed to support "grow your own" efforts. Quality of mentorship should be considered in faculty evaluation, promotion, and recognition (289).

Comprehensive and well-developed mentoring programs for faculty of color can increase the number of URM faculty and improve faculty satisfaction (161). However, Guevara and colleagues' study of faculty development programs in medicine found that only intensive and mature programs are effective in improving future minority faculty representation (300). These findings point to the importance of long-term investment and commitment to the development and sustainability of mentoring programs. Every program should include training and competency expectations for mentors involved in the program as well as both formative and summative evaluations of mentor-mentee relationships and program components (65, 285). Cross-race mentoring competencies include cultural humility and an interest in understanding how culture influences mentor-mentee relationships; the ability to establish trust; acknowledgment of the influence of racial dynamics on mentor-mentee relationships; discussion of the operations of institutional power and identification of potential landmines; monitoring for visibility and risk specific to faculty of color; advocacy and support for the voices of mentees in institutions; and good communication skills (301–303).

Best practices for mentoring faculty of color identified in the literature include one-on-one mentoring with an experienced investigator, group-based skill-building seminars, access to pilot grants, and support for conducting pilot studies (60). Other literature documents the importance of having a constellation of mentors to increase faculty satisfaction and success (252, 257, 289). In addition, some authors have recommended alternative mentoring models for faculty of color. Characteristics of these models include an emphasis on cultural and social networks, collaborative relationships, interprofessional and interinstitutional collaborations, and community connections (62, 65, 251, 304). E-networking and peer mentoring have also been cited as useful resources that may be used to supplement institutional mentoring (289). Hence, there is a need to provide resources, plan carefully, and be willing to think outside the box when developing mentorship programs for faculty of color. Making sure that faculty of color have strong mentoring is one of the most powerful actions institutions can take to ensure the retention, satisfaction, and success of this group. Visionary and bold leadership with an explicit commitment to the development of faculty of color is required to take the steps necessary to ensure the mentoring needs of this important group are met (240, 295, 305).

CHAPTER FOUR

Strategies for Thriving
in Health Professions Academe

The plain truth is that we are living in a white man's world, so we might as well learn to make the best of it. Regardless of your field of interest, if you are an African-American or any under-represented minority you needn't take on other people's expectations of you, nor let other people set your goals. You can decide for yourself what *you* want and then work hard to make it happen. Find realistic ways to turn the negatives into positives, and work to lift yourself and those around you along the way.

Donald Wilson (306) p.vii

When I retire from the academy, I want to exit the way I entered—authentic. That is, I want to look like someone I know.

marbly and colleagues (307) p.60.

People enter academia hoping for long and satisfying careers. Yet many faculty experience burnout, and some leave academia altogether. Why do some faculty do well and others poorly? How might this phenomenon be qualitatively different for faculty of color? Participants' stories reflect different levels of satisfaction and success, providing some answers to these questions. Some participants were frustrated with their careers and faced challenges to progression. Such dissatisfaction occurred most often when participants' core values and work were devalued by their institutions. Participants who worked in inclusive climates, received recognition for their work, and enacted strategies for success were most likely to thrive. I call these two groups survivors and thrivers. Many participants experienced both struggle and accomplishment, moving back and forth between surviving and thriving. This chapter describes participants' strategies for thriving, which I labeled having a vision, knowing the game, living your values, seeking and managing opportunities, and coping with everyday racism.

Having a Vision

In his book *Wilson's Way: Win, Don't Whine*, Donald E. Wilson, MD, the first black person to become a dean at a medical school, said, "Great accomplishments don't happen by accident. Knowing where you want to go is always the starting point for any future success" (306) p.201. He referred to this as "having a vision." Engaging in self-reflection about core beliefs and values and what one hopes to achieve is essential to developing a career vision (238). Thriving participants focused on their strengths and natural talents to build motivation and worked to cultivate a positive attitude in the service of their vision. Professor Hope, a full professor who was active across the missions, is a robust example of a thriving participant. He stayed at the same dental school for his entire career, which he began with a vision and strong awareness of his needs and goals:

> I had pretty strong ideas—I knew I didn't want to go into community-based practice. I knew I'd be bored; I would not see the kinds of kids that I would see at a university health center. Number two, the guy I was going to who was running the program, Dave Richardson, was a renowned educator researcher, and I had heard really good things about this guy . . . And I knew from the interview that Dave was not a micromanager and that definitely was not what I wanted. I really wanted to have a free hand and kind of manifest my views of what should happen, because after finishing my residency program I could see there was a huge problem in what I didn't see in dental school. So I came here and—the hospital wasn't even—it was just a hole in the ground when I got here. That was good because I wanted to be the person who could make the rules, not have to fit into a set of rules . . . I had pretty strong ideas about what needed to be done in dental education, so I figured this was the place. [dental faculty]

Professor Hope thought carefully about what he wanted in a faculty position and gathered information about his prospective supervisor and institution. He displayed a high level of awareness about his own needs and found an institution that matched them, including supervisory style, availability of mentorship, and opportunity to impact educational programs. This laid the foundation for later success. In contrast, Professor Adams, who lacked a career vision when beginning her faculty role, described in hindsight the importance of knowing your academic focus and the need for mentorship:

I got here directly out of scholarship training . . . Initially when I got here my goal was to be clinically competent and make sure that I have a good strong clinical foundation, prior to really concentrating on any research efforts. So I did that first, passing my boards and getting comfortable in the operating room. And then the second year I tried to figure out what my research area was going to be, and I did not come in with kind of a preconceived notion of what I wanted to really study or anything. And so I think I spent a great deal of time that was wasted flitting about here and there and talking with various people but not really taking time to focus. One thing I wish I would've had would have been someone or some influence from above that could of directed me a little bit better . . . I think ideally most people should come in with a strong strategic plan for their academic career already, then they should come in with that being acknowledged and then with their division chief or whomever saying, "Listen, I have these things going on, I don't have any time to do them, but I think that they could be good, and at least while you're trying to figure out what you want to do, why don't you try working on these things so you're at least being productive during this time period[?]" And that's what I wish I had, and I haven't had it. [medical faculty]

Professor Adams emphasized the importance of having a "strategic plan," which is consistent with having a focused area of scholarship as part of a career vision. Having a vision also facilitated participants' ability to select institutions that matched their career goals. Professor Rangan described his experience:

I really like teaching, so that's the basis of m[y] going into faculty. I started applying for jobs, and I was looking mainly for small pharmacy schools, not really big state schools, because I don't want the burden of research to be something that will stop me from continuing my job. So I was looking for small pharmacy schools where teaching is more prominent and my income is based on teaching rather than getting grants. That's why I chose this school, which is a small, nonprofit pharmacy school that basically does dental, nursing, and pharmacy. [pharmacy faculty]

Professor Rangan enjoyed teaching and wanted to avoid the pressure to bring in research funding common at research-intensive universities. This awareness led him to seek a position at a small teaching institution where he was extremely satisfied. In contrast, Professor Iglesias envisioned a research career:

When I joined the combined PhD/perio track I knew that research was going to be a priority for me . . . I had been lucky enough to publish, getting my name out there and network[ing], which was essential in the job-seeking process: meet with people, talk with people, and let them know what you really want and what you really expect to be doing while you are a faculty member . . . And I was fortunate enough here to receive protected time . . . People have been extremely helpful, open, willing to collaborate. [dental faculty]

Selecting the best institutional match, professionally and socially, was an important step for participants' career journeys. Having a vision enabled participants to mindfully select institutions where their career goals could reach fruition.

Having and sustaining a career vision required that participants focus on their strengths to create a sense of empowerment about their career paths. Professor Morgan started his career believing in himself:

I do take a little bit of pride because I did take a bit of risk. My favorite story is when I left for my fellowship and I did a year or two as a faculty member, and John, who is African American, . . . was neurosurgery chair, and as soon as he heard I was going to this university he came to my office, almost running to my office, and he said, "What are you doing?" and I said, "I'm going to Southern University. I went there to graduate. I'm from that area." And he said, "That university is white by design, and they don't want you there." And it kind of frightened me a little bit, because when I got to this university I was thinking, "John was right." I'm looking around and nobody looks like me, but you have to have somebody go first, and I think because I was maybe one of the first folks to go in and say, "I'm going to be successful here." It then brought in other folks, so that the playing field is totally different now. [medical faculty]

Professor Morgan told himself, "I am going to be successful here," and with the help of a supportive supervisor and mentor, he was eventually able to change the cultural landscape of his department. Professor Blakeley spoke about the importance of fostering a positive self-image to combat negative messages:

I think for us we have to—and it's not being narcissistic—but we have to love ourselves. And we have to be confident and competent. And not only competent but confident in our ability, and know that we bring something positive to the environment that we're in. [nursing faculty] (308) p.140

In turn, self-confidence and self-worth provided a foundation for a positive outlook to support one's career vision, as described by Professor Hope:

You say, "Hello" to twenty people in a day, and they say, "Hello" back, some of them may not, but that's not your problem. That's not your fault. The fact is you should not do things because of what you think people are going to do in return, but it should be a core for you about how you carry yourself . . . and being positive . . . If you want anything in life you have to work for it. Ain't nobody going to give it to you, nor should they. And you should share your good fortune with people because you are going to feel good. And I guess that is what it is for me. [dental faculty]

Assuming an attitude of success, competence, and confidence and nurturing a positive self-image and outlook about one's career were important thriving strategies. Integrating resilience as part of personal identity, which has been recognized as important for faculty of color (309), was also evident in participants' narratives. Making a conscious effort to focus on strengths was particularly critical for participants who faced negative messages (310, 311). A strengths perspective assumes "that every person has inherent strengths that can be drawn upon to help them improve the quality of their life and further, that in even the most desolate environments resources can be found. Therefore it becomes imperative . . . to recognize, celebrate, and build on . . . unique strengths and abilities" for success (312) p.12. Consistent with this view, participants who emphasized and capitalized on their strengths were most successful in realizing their career visions.

Knowing the Game

Thriving participants understood the rules of the game in academe. The rules of the game have been referred to in the literature as "learning to play the game," and rules that are not overt as "unwritten rules of the game" (313, 314). Rockquemore and Laszloffy used the term "rules of engagement" to refer to the written and unwritten rules of an institution, including the "race rules." Race rules are unwritten and include various forms of unequal treatment (197). Written rules of the game are official and can be accessed in policy documents such as those for promotion, tenure, and merit. Faculty of color need to know what is valued and discern and negotiate the power structure at their institutions to make informed career decisions (149). Examples of unwritten rules of the game relevant to promotion, tenure, and merit include what areas of scholarship are considered worthwhile, which journals fall within the realm of acceptability, and how much scholarship is enough to meet a standard (313, 315). Various emphases on the missions of teaching, practice, service, and research exist across time and institutions. Moreover, leaders may change unwritten rules to fit professional and personal biases (149). Unwritten rules may also govern unspoken expectations about office hours, demeanor, and dress. Sources of information about rules include faculty policies, trusted peers and mentors, and quiet observation. In a study of the success strategies of tenured black women faculty, a participant recommended:

> Know the rules of the game that you have chosen to enter and play the game by the rules. If you want to succeed in this system, you have to abide by the rules whether you agree with them or not. Don't enter the game and then try to change the rules, unless there is enough support behind you to do so. Know the rules and play the game by the rules. That's the way the system is, rightly or wrongly. (316) p.76

Consistent with this view, Professor Achebe provided an example of learning unwritten rules to be successful:

PROFESSOR ACHEBE: You learn about what are the most critical indexes and push hard on those. My insight from all those experiences would just be that you need to find out what the rules are. What are the rules? What does your university value? Is it more teaching, more service, or more work; what exactly are going to be the indexes by which you will be judged . . . And you've got to focus on those indexes, and you've got to learn that we are in an age now [when] this thing called the Internet, which is a very beautiful thing . . . You can collaborate and you can find mentors, collaborators that are on a different coast or anywhere and those can help you . . . For example, let's say you're in an institution where they're focused on getting grants. Okay, and . . . at the end of the year, at the end of four years, at the end of seven years, there will be key evaluations where grants play a role. Then ... go ahead, head on, and try to find who can help you ... and it doesn't have to be people at your university. You can try to find mentors and collaborators all over America that can be of help.

INTERVIEWER: So Professor Achebe, when you're talking about finding out what the rules are, do you think that the rules are always explicit, or are there some rules that aren't so explicit?

PROFESSOR ACHEBE: The rules are never explicit. [pharmacy faculty]

A previous quote from Professor Achebe (in chapter 1) illustrated how the rules were interpreted differently for him than for white faculty, providing an example of race rules. Similarly, Professor Drake described how promotion and tenure criteria were interpreted unevenly at her institution:

I have always known that the rules were different. The rules in terms of success. The rules in terms of productivity. The rules in terms of getting promoted and tenure. They are different for people of color. They just are. But I didn't really see it until now. Really see it ... I've been told I have to have a second R01—nobody here has a second R01 at the associate level, nobody. Very few even have one R01. But the rules for me, I need to have five papers a year ... But the majority [of] faculty, they only have to have two papers a year. And when I say, "I was told I have to have five," they say, "Oh well, you misunderstood." And I say, "No, I heard it from more than one person, that is what was communicated to me from more than one senior faculty member that sits on the APT committee." So anyway that is fine, because I know that as an African American if I get a second R01 and if I have five papers a year, I can go anyplace in the country I want to ... I think what people respect is productivity. And I just recently got published in a prestigious journal, and I can really tell the difference in how they treat me now. [nursing faculty]

Professor Drake's response to uneven interpretation of the rules at her institution was to increase her productivity and use her success to her advantage, increasing her marketability as a faculty member. While uneven interpretation of the rules of the game in academia is unjust, faculty of color need to know when this is happening to make informed decisions about application for promotion and tenure. Professor Hope described his experience with the promotion process:

I was promoted here just like anybody else when [the] time came that I was eligible to be promoted. I never had a setback. My chair was really very brilliant. He knew the game, and he told me exactly what I had to do. And he said, "Until you do it you won't be prepared, and I won't put you up because I don't want any excuses that you didn't get past the committee." So when I was ready, I guess if I got turned down it could not have been because I wasn't academically—my credentials, whatever the evaluation system was, it was not going to be because I wasn't qualified. [dental faculty]

Professor Hope made sure that he clearly met or perhaps exceeded all the promotion and tenure criteria when he went up for review to ensure that if he was denied it would be clear it was not due to a lack of achievement. As a faculty member of color, Professor Hope could not afford to be average. In a chapter describing success strategies for faculty of color, Adams wrote:

Many faculty of color have been instructed to always do their best and be better than the rest. While excellence is demanded of you, mediocrity is accepted for others. Do not get frustrated; just accept the situation and adjust. (317) p.39

Consistent with Adam's statement, none of the participants described receiving the benefit of the doubt in promotion decisions.

Lack of interest in promotion of faculty of color was part of the race rules at some institutions. Professor Griffin learned what was expected for promotion late in the game:

I was very naïve in that I thought, "Oh well, I'll just come here and I will teach medical students and work with the residents, blah, blah, blah." But there's a whole other thing—you are trying to figure out ways of okay, how can I get what I ultimately want? Otherwise, they're happy to keep you in the assistant professor position because you are the worker bee. They're happy, everybody's happy to keep you kind of where you are, and if you are not being very intentional about what you are doing and it is not having a purpose, then you ultimately won't ever get promoted . . . You end up spinning your wheels . . . Like you've been doing it ten years and you think you're doing everything you're supposed to be doing, and then you look up and they're like, "No, we can't promote you yet because of this, because you haven't done this" . . . and I think that happens to minority faculty. No matter how much work you've put into it, I think for the most part they'll let you spin your wheels if you aren't intentional about things. [medical faculty]

At first, Professor Griffin was naïve. As she gained experience in academe, she learned the race rules of the game, gaining sophistication. Because she developed this awareness later in her career, her advancement was delayed.

Knowing the rules of the game, and playing it to one's advantage, increased the likelihood of participants' career success as traditionally defined in academe, despite the injustice often inherent in the system. Some participants who chose to pursue work that was not valued by their institutions were able to forge a personal definition of success when they saw through unwritten rules. In such cases, participants understood lack of recognition for their accomplishments was not a personal failure, but rather failure on the part of universities to affirm the choices and successes of faculty of color (226, 315). Professor Rivera rejected the unwritten rules of the game:

We recently had a faculty recognition award that was given to a white faculty member who is a good scholar but is not so great in other areas—very little teaching and nothing in community or diversity. But the selection criteria for the award included all of it, so the written and unwritten rules were very different. [T]here are faculty of color here who are much more deserving of the award . . . When white faculty who have never lifted a finger to promote diversity are rewarded, that sends a really negative message to faculty and students of color and our community . . . I think for me, I have chosen to invest a lot of my time serving the Latino community—I'm not really focusing on prestige. I would say I am a well-rounded scholar, but I can see that the unwritten rules here are not for me . . . Sometimes I think, "What if I had taken that other career path, just really focusing on my self-interest?" If I had that other road—of really try[ing] to promote myself—then I would have truly failed, because I would have had to sell my soul. So in one sense it feels defeating not to be recognized, but I can also evaluate my own career in light of my values and know I've done right. [medical faculty]

Speaking to the need to find sustenance in institutions that failed to recognize the contributions of faculty of color, Bonner shared age-old wisdom from Archie Dorsey, a church musician: "This joy that I have, the world didn't give it to me—the world didn't give it and the world can't take it away" (196) p.127.

This refrain provides context for the actions of participants who chose to define their successes based on personal values that transcended oppressive academic contexts.

Living Your Values

Thriving participants were able to align their personal values with their professional roles. This has been described in the literature as being true to oneself or situating "your voice through your content, pedagogy and your scholarship" (318) p.144. This finding is consistent with Mainah's study of black women leaders in academia who defined success in accordance with their personal values and found meaning and purpose in what they did, in the relationships they had with the people they served, and in serving a goal that was bigger than themselves (292). For participants in this study whose scholarship was grounded in social justice frameworks, this could be challenging in the context of the health sciences, where the dominance of empiricism circumscribes inquiry (4, 319, 320). Social justice scholarship focuses on promoting a society that balances benefits and burdens among people, promoting full participation and equitable living in a justly ordered society (321). Participants at institutions that supported or at least respected their values were more likely to be satisfied at their institutions and in many cases to receive support needed for advancement. Professor Meriwether received support that helped launch his career:

> I came up with the idea of working with African American men. And I'll tell you the former dean . . . she did not completely understand, but she was good enough to say, "Okay, let's see where this is going." And I think that was the start of my career . . . She was open enough to recognize my area and could really push me in that area of knowledge . . . and I was recognized. I was given an award for my work in the community with African Americans at the university level. [nursing faculty]

Professor Meriwether's dean provided him with protected time to pursue his area of interest, leading to a fruitful program of research. Even though his dean did not necessarily understand the work Professor Meriwether proposed, she supported it, indicating a respect for the value of his research. Similarly, Professor Cleary experienced her school as supportive of her research on Native American health. Professor Cleary's institution was in the process of building a center in her research area and recruiting other faculty of color to add synergy:

> The support that I get to do my research. That always stands out—from my associate dean and definitely the dean of our college—is significant and supportive of my work. So that definitely stands out. It is nice to be in an area [where] what I'm doing is deemed important by them. [pharmacy faculty]

The importance of being valued and receiving institutional recognition for participants' satisfaction was described by Professor Baboor:

> I'm living the dream . . . I just couldn't be happier. I'm in the best possible place . . . It's amazing. Not only being supported here, but I am also appreciated here. Which I think is very important for development of any individual, professionally or otherwise, is that any significant contribution that you make is appreciated and that makes a huge difference. It's kind of a motivator. So I do have a good support system and good people who are constantly integrating and appreciating all the work that I put in. [pharmacy faculty]

Although institutional recognition and support was important, participants' ability to integrate their personal values in their work was critical to their satisfaction. Professor Yazzie integrated her Native American cultural values into her scholarship and teaching, infusing meaning across the various dimensions of her faculty role.

> And we looked at Native values, and part of the Native American is living—well, for Cherokees, is living the white path, staying on the white path, following the white path. Which means following and being a good person and not doing harm to another person. These are just basic values in Native American culture, remembering that what goes around comes around. And how each person does that, you kind of have to figure that out on your own. I was lucky. I had people who helped me, and one of the ways I did it was through my research, through writing, through presentations—living it. My office is filled with Indian character and influence . . . I do a lecture on burns and I talk about Indian culture. I look up examples. And not only does that allow me to express myself as a Native person, but it also teaches the students how to

look holistically at their patient, even if we're talking about shock and what do with it. [nursing faculty] (308) p.140

Professor Pope, whose position focused on diversity in a school of medicine, described the sense of satisfaction he derived from his work and its connection to his values:

It is going to take a whole lot of change to increase the number of black physicians if you are looking at the numbers. But I have decided to be satisfied in my time trying to get as many as I can into the profession. I can't deal with what's happening at other medical schools or other institutions, but I can try to make a difference here. When I first came here, our percentage was 3. Now our percentage is 22. And I am not going to be satisfied until it is 25. And so if I just keep pushing the envelope here in my corner of the world, and if there are other people out there who will push it in their corner of the world, we might be able to do something. [medical faculty]

Professor Pope spoke with a sense of mission. He was committed to increasing the number of black physicians. Not only was it his job, but he conveyed a sense that the greater number of black students who graduated during his tenure was very meaningful to him. His personal values and professional role were perfectly aligned.

Seeking and Managing Opportunities

Thriving participants were proactive in seeking collaborations, networking, showcasing their work, and engaging with professional organizations. Cultivating relationships with mentors and leaders and developing a supportive network were also crucial thriving strategies.

BEING PROACTIVE

By proactively seeking, creating, and responding to opportunities to advance their careers, thriving participants earned the respect of others at their institutions and took the steps needed to enact their career visions. Professor Jennings described positive changes in his career that occurred after he made an effort to be proactive in seeking out opportunities:

I think the biggest thing is just feeling alone and not necessarily having the support to succeed. I felt like I had two strikes against me. I'm the only African American faculty [member] at my school of pharmacy, ... plus I was the one who did not have a previous connection with any other faculty here. So because of that it definitely was difficult. Things have definitely changed now, and it's because I've become very proactive. I've sought opportunities to network with other faculty of color on the main campus. I've sought out opportunities to get involved in diversity leadership and fellowship that I'm currently in now, and it's opened up many doors. When I was initially here, there was just no exposure that I received. And I don't know if that was intentional or not, but now that exposure ... over the last year or so—I've become very proactive in seeking that exposure, networking, finding ways to propel my career and just to grow professionally ... We provide a yearly dean's report. This goes out to the community, it goes out statewide, just to show and to recognize the faculty and students. And I was never in there ... When I started to really realize that, I felt like, well, I can't blame others. I've just got to be proactive and I've got to do some extra things to expose myself versus feeling like others should expose me. Because I saw that other faculty members were clearly being exposed and showcased, but I had to seek out ways that I could as well. [pharmacy faculty]

Despite feeling isolated and alone, Professor Jennings displayed a sense of empowerment in his decision making and the will to create his own path. Rather than focus on what was beyond his control, he decided to seek opportunities to network and showcase his work, both important elements of academic success. Similarly, Professor Sewell was able to achieve the status of department chair despite a lack of mentorship. He forged his own path, finding opportunities by "inviting" himself to the table:

Very seldom have I ever had anybody who wakes up [in] the morning and says, "What can I do to make sure that Dr. Sewell has another opportunity to succeed? Hey, Dr. Sewell I got this opportunity, I need you to call so and so at Hopkins, there is a specific opportunity for you to collaborate on this project. I think you are the perfect person. Let me know what I need to do to create headway for you if there's any problems." That has hardly ever happened. So you develop a skill set of finding opportunities, and I oftentimes ask myself, invite myself to the table, and a lot of times people say, "Sure." [medical faculty]

Professor Wakefield attributed 90 percent of her success to "inviting herself to the table":

I started networking to see who was doing research in the area I was interested in and to see if I could write with them. I knew Dr. Michelle Castle from my risk management days . . . And I happened to see her at the hospital one day and she said, "Oh, how are you doing?" And I said, "You know, I'm fine. I'm back at a historically black university, but I'm having trouble finding a mission." She said, "Oh, let me put you in touch with a Dr. Harper at NIMH. She does research in your area . . . and she has a focus on African Americans even though she's white." So I made an appointment and went over and talked to her, and we talked about the ways we could collaborate. And while we were talking, she said, "Oh, do you know Van Withers at your university?" And I said, "I haven't met him yet, but our chair has been encouraging me to contact him." Well, Van Withers is the director of research for the medical school. So that next week, I actually met with Van Withers, and he has a writing group, and he's had several grants, and he invited me to participate with his group. So for a year I was going to their meetings, and they were reviewing their grant and their cases, and that was good. And I met a doctor who was interested in doing research, . . . but she wasn't really committed. So I spent some time writing a grant with her, and in the meantime, I discovered the nurses who did research in my area. And one of the people was Lillian Hughes Sawyer at a state university. And I was looking for somebody who might be able to add me on as a minority supplement. So I contacted her, and she was interested in communicating with me and assisting me. She invited me up [to] her campus to meet her. I e-mailed her for a whole year before I even met her. And I've published a continuing education with her and coauthored another article with her. She also has included me in the activities she does with her graduate students. So I've presented at conferences, and she has helped make things happen. In the meantime, Van Withers is still mentoring me, and I'm working on a grant with him . . . focused on faculty in medical schools. Van said, "Don't worry about it. We will get you a faculty appointment [in the medical school] if you need that to qualify." . . . I think time has helped—I knew what I needed, and I knew that I couldn't wait for it to happen. I would say probably 90 percent of my success has been related to my reaching out. My philosophy is if I am not invited to the table, I will ask for an invitation. [nursing faculty]

Other examples of being proactive included taking advantage of opportunities to showcase one's work and being involved with professional organizations, as described by Professors Yazzie and Morgan:

PROFESSOR YAZZIE: Every so often, they would have a speaker . . . to get some faculty to talk about their research . . . and . . . the associate dean for research heard me talking about how . . . you have to take Native American ideas and translate them into researchable concepts. And it's almost like speaking, you have to learn to speak and think in a different language. You have to learn to speak Indian research and you have to learn to speak mainstream research. And I was talking about how I'd like to develop or write something about what words are appropriate . . . in Native research and Indian research . . . She asked me to present that. So I did—and this was something that a lot of people never came to, this little seminar . . . and the room was packed. [nursing faculty] (308) p.138

PROFESSOR MORGAN: Well . . . my mentor . . . sort of said, "You've got to come if you're going to be a player." And I don't like that term, "player," necessarily, but he said, "If you're going to be an influential person in—again, my cooperative group—you've got to come." So it wasn't too long after I actually got involved in a cooperative group that I was . . . a person they would look to ask questions. [medical faculty] (143) p.8

CHOOSING OPPORTUNITIES.

Thriving participants selected career opportunities that would propel their careers forward but also provide a sense of satisfaction. Professor Bell chose to take on the role of center director at his school, recognizing the opportunities it would afford him:

Being the co-director of our center here, I think adds to what I do—it has been elevated across the institution. So I'm in my role as a center director, a member of our faculty executive committee, which only opens to department chairs that are directors and institute directors . . . This position [provides] the support . . . to pursue my research areas of interest in high level discussions here at the medical center. [medical faculty]

Professor Bell's work as a center director dovetailed with his research and his personal values. He found the work both meaningful and fruitful. Professor

Drake provided an example of choosing opportunities on a smaller scale. She chose the journals she published in carefully:

> There was a lot of pressure for me to hurry up and get these papers out. And I didn't because I wanted to wait so I could publish in top journals. So I got a lot of criticism for that. "Hurry, hurry, hurry. Get the papers out." And I kind of said, "Okay, okay, okay," and I didn't do anything but wait. I'm happy [with the result]. [nursing faculty]

Learning how to balance service and scholarship was also part of choosing opportunities wisely. Faculty of color are often asked to serve on more diversity-related committees and mentor more students of color than white faculty, resulting in a heavier service burden (311, 322). Professor Adams described her experience of being subject to this burden:

> The whole minority tax and being on every committee that has to deal with diversity in some way. I mean I'm on the women's committee, I'm on the diversity committee, and I'm on this committee of minority faculty affairs. I'm asked to be on panels all the doggone time. And . . . my instinct is not to say no, because they are important things and geez, if we can't be there and represent, well then it's never going to happen. And if I don't sit on that student panel then the students will never see someone who looks like them or will never aspire to be where I am, and then you have more issues and the isolation is perpetuated, so I think many of us feel a social obligation to do it when asked. I may not necessarily seek it out. When someone is asking you, you feel a little bit special because someone asked you. But then you also feel like "gosh, if I don't do it, who is going to do it?" Or the next person who is going to do it probably won't do as good a job as I tend to do, so therefore I should, and therefore your calendar gets filled with all these commitments and whatnot, which are otherwise not promotion-generating activities, and so you fall into that trap. You're not productive but you're busy. But in all the wrong ways. [medical faculty]

Professor Adams was doing important diversity and equity work, but it was not recognized by her institution, a common experience for faculty of color (48, 226). Similarly, Professor Cleary expressed concern about the amount of service she was doing:

INTERVIEWER: You feel like you're being called on to do more service because of your ethnicity?

PROFESSOR CLEARY: Yes, definitely. I do feel like I'm being called on more. On [the] one hand, I feel like it's valuable and it could be positive. So I'll accept different positions. On the other hand, I keep remembering, well, I was supposed to have two years free to publish and get caught up . . . So it's a double-edged sword. On [the] one hand, I want to be included and I'm glad they respect me and value my opinion. On the other hand, there are complications I've been suffering.

INTERVIEWER: Yeah. Trying to find that balance?

PROFESSOR CLEARY: Yes, exactly. It's pretty difficult. [pharmacy faculty]

As Professors Adams's and Cleary's quotes show, learning how to balance one's desire to be involved in meaningful service activities with the need to select career-promoting service activities could be challenging for junior faculty. The literature documents this dilemma; it is important for faculty of color to avoid service overload but also to stay true to themselves by giving back. Bonner described this difficulty:

From colleagues who are external to the black faculty experience, "Just tell them you are not available" is commonly advanced as the panacea perceived to cure all ills. Yet, it's that feeling of being conflicted caused by the head's stern admonishment to protect yourself from time-consuming tasks like mentoring, and the heart's wise counsel to support them, that causes the faculty member of color the most angst. (196) p.125

The help of a good mentor was essential to participants successfully working through this dilemma. Professor Singleton described the critical role of mentors in helping guide these decisions:

Faculty of color may not have the mentorship . . . You don't have the mentorship, so you may not have a person say to you, "Don't you dare get on another committee" . . . I did that when I worked at another school, and I was really overextended. I was doing too much stuff and not dealing with some of the key things I should have been dealing with. I know even here, there's a young woman who's not here now. She started out here and she went up for promotion and I think didn't get it . . . I think she got shafted. She didn't have the guidance. I think she was the only one in her department, she was young, inexperienced, and no one was giving her the guidance that she needed to be a faculty member. She was trying to do too much. I believe for her to be engaged in so much service, we did her a disservice. [nursing faculty]

As Professor Singleton described, when junior faculty members did not receive mentoring to help them prioritize service activities, they could fail to achieve promotion and become dissatisfied. Professor Hope was an example of a successful faculty member who engaged in service but knew how to reduce service activities when they interfered with his productivity:

When we had a little bit of a puff, explosion of people of color here, it was because I would be going out to the health profession society meeting, conferences, medicine and dentistry, all these things. And when a student came up of color, and I'd be at the table of this university, I would threaten them that if we give them an interview, they had better show up. And so we had a little run of students. But then what happened, I got so busy that I couldn't represent the school anymore. I just couldn't do it. [dental faculty]

Professor Hope was able to effectively manage his career by balancing service and scholarly obligations, recognizing the importance of letting some things go to achieve his academic goals. Although he stopped recruiting students of color for a time, Professor Hope's commitment to nourishing the pipeline remained. Later he continued his efforts to engage students of color, integrating these efforts with his clinical work:

My clinical program is being used by this high school. And I came to talk to the people about it. I said, "Look, one thing I want to do out of this with you guys, I want to make a pipeline from this high school to my dental school. I don't know how we are going to do it, but I want you to start." Now we have the students that have been doing it for about four years. Once a year they'll bring a busload of kids out to the dental school, and we have them here for half a day. We give them a tour. And finally, one woman said, "You know what? I think I want to be a dentist." So we watched her through college, and she applied and she's here now. And she's been here three months. I said, "Angela, one thing you are going to do while you are here, you are going to be our face back [at] your school, because I want to create a pipeline—because they don't want to talk to me, your students. They want to talk to you because you came from there. So we are going to start this thing where you are going to give a PowerPoint presentation at your school. And I am going to be right there . . . And we are going to start this thing . . . I think African American students respond to—how can I say—we have to be tribal if that's a word? It's not enough to throw a bunch of pamphlets out there. You are going to kind of press the flesh, okay?" Whereas if the kids see her they say, "Oh, okay. We can do this." And maybe it will be just one. I don't care. But as long as I am here, I am going to keep on Angela to try to visit her school once a year. And then maybe we will get another kid next year or maybe in two years. And we are going to keep this thing going . . . [W]e have to dig a tunnel that goes from our door to their door. [dental faculty]

Professor Hope's ability to integrate his personal values across the missions provided a stellar example of how thriving participants were able to balance service and scholarship to meet their career goals while staying true to themselves.

SEEKING MENTORSHIP

The breadth and depth of findings on mentorship woven throughout this book reflect its vital nature. Defining mentor/mentee role expectations and goals, planning frequency of contact, establishing confidentiality and relationship boundaries, and periodic evaluation of mentoring relationships have been identified as useful strategies to promote successful mentoring relationships (289). Here I describe thriving participants' strategies for cultivating and making good use of nurturing, guiding, and protective mentoring relationships. Professor Sanchez described the guidance she sought from her mentor:

I'll ask her [mentor] questions on how to do things in the classroom, how to handle different things in the classroom . . . She also helps when it comes to surveys and scholarship. So we talk about research. We actually are almost in the same field of research, so we both do breast cancer research, [and] we talk about that as well. We talk about research; we talk about how we can work together to get some things done in the lab. We talk about admissions. We are both in admissions, so then with this whole diversity thing, it is like we also talk about that: What can we do to increase our diversity here? [pharmacy faculty]

Professor Sanchez's mentor was assigned to her when she started her faculty position. Other participants had to find their own mentors. Professor Ames described how she sought out mentorship:

I personally sought out a lot of things. When I first started, I signed up for a bunch of [listervs] . . . That's how I even found out about the mentoring program that I've been in, and what was even better, it offered financial support . . . That's part of the biggest key is when you come to a new campus or are taking on a new role that you have to be proactive. [dental faculty]

The mentoring program Professor Ames described was campus-wide. She took advantage of this program in a way that fit her needs:

Thankfully, the campus as a whole—not necessarily the school of dentistry but the campus—does have some programs that provide mentoring, so I actually have just finished up a yearlong mentoring program where I was paired up. I applied for this particular program, and I received a mentor, and I was very specific that I wanted a mentor not in my school just because I wanted a different perspective. Which has been extremely helpful because I had a mentor who has a nursing background but who . . . has a technology background as well, which for me is great because she has the nursing background. She understood what I did for health care because I have a background in informatics as well. It just ended up being for me the best of both worlds . . . And it was funny, when they were pairing me up, they said there were people in dentistry who want to be mentors, and I said, "No." I want someone who has gone through the promotion process for the entire campus who can look at what I am doing objectively and say, "Yes, no, you shouldn't do that or don't take that on, that's too much." [dental faculty]

In addition to faculty mentoring, Professor Ames also sought out peer mentoring and helped to create a peer-mentoring group:

We actually just started a peer-mentoring group. We used to call it the Junior Faculty Club, and we're like, "We are not going to be junior faculty forever." So it changed to peer mentoring. [dental faculty]

Similarly, Professor Cleary was proactive in establishing mentoring relationships:

We actually don't have a formal mentoring committee process yet. We're developing one for our college. So I developed one, I guess, personally formally. I've contacted the people and asked if they would serve on my committee. They all agreed. So I have members selected. [pharmacy faculty]

Professor Hope described the importance of connecting with people and being open to new relationships to cultivate mentorship:

> I've had incredible mentors. I definitely feel that it takes a village in the world to be in the world . . . If you feel alone that's really terrible, because all you have to do is just open yourself up and you will be connected to other people, because that's what we want to do no matter how we behave. We want to be interconnected to each other. So I've always felt that there were people around me that if I just—as my mom used to say, especially if you just pay attention you will connect to people. If you just open your eyes and just let yourself—let the sunlight hit you, you're going to find people who, for some reason, make a difference for you. [dental faculty]

SEEKING SUPPORTS

Thriving participants developed supportive networks through relationships with colleagues, family, and friends. These relationships provided a place where participants could be themselves, let their guard down, and check things out. In her personal essay on promotion and tenure, Turner eloquently described the importance of having such supports:

> It is important to have a small but strong personal support system that can validate your experiences. Loneliness is discouraging in itself; but when it is combined with self-doubt (Am I good enough?) and the constant need to negotiate one's reality (Am I being left out or am I imagining it?), the burden can become heavy indeed. (323) p.134

Professor Adams described how her faculty support group helped her process covert racism:

> That whole concept of the microaggression . . . What do you . . . do with all of that? . . . The majority of us don't sit around all day trying to be . . . that introspective and . . . trying to deal with all that on . . . a minute-to-minute basis. But it is real, it does exist, and it's something that's very difficult to quantify, and it's very difficult to convey to someone who has an otherwise experience . . . And even if you could convey it, to have the security that in doing so, that you haven't otherwise ostracized yourself or given the impression that you are . . . weak, or you're unworthy in some other way, is a . . . heavy burden. So . . . where's the repository for all that? And I guess our group [of junior faculty

of color] is a repository. Because . . . you tell it to people who, who get it, who know no further explanation is required. [medical faculty] (143) p.8

Professor Belmont sought support from colleagues to help him deal with the effects of racist messages on his psyche:

This percentage of people who will never come back to me and say, "Congratulations for your publications, congratulations for getting into this journal, congratulations for your paper being cited in this article." I had one paper that had a worldwide press release done on it by the journal . . . and this person had nothing to say. And that was okay because I thought, "You know what? It does not matter, it doesn't take away from the fact that it was done." . . . I don't walk around with that same fear, that same lack of confidence. That's gone. It's just gone. And I don't think it would be had I not worked through all of this stuff and had I not got the support that I did, and I had a lot of support. I had a lot of people that I turned to for help who sat me down and helped me work through all of this; most of them are white, but they helped me understand what was going on and more important they validated my experiences not being something that I made up in my head. [nursing faculty]

Despite facing significant exclusion and control earlier in his career, Professor Belmont was able to thrive, reflecting a growing awareness of his own needs and of the rules of the game in health professions academe. Finding sources of validation and support, including support from white colleagues, was a vital component of that journey. Professor Belmont's connection with white faculty is consistent with Edwards, Bryant, and Clark's description of fostering mutual engagement and empathy within and across racial lines:

You know when that connection has occurred, because someone takes the time to listen to your thoughts, share your excitement, to give you an extra pat on the back and to offer a helping hand when you get stuck. When someone "has your back" and you have theirs, you are mutually engaged . . . "mutual empathy is the unsung human gift" . . . the creation of mutuality involves a leveling of the playing field. (324) p.42.

Connecting with others who "have your back" is also consistent with Stanley's recommendation that faculty of color identify allies (59). Powerfully, Alfred's findings suggest: "Try to find somebody who will help you. They may not look like you expect them to look. It may not be the sister; it may not be the brother; it may be a white person; it may be a white man" (316) p.77. Finding sources of validation, from any supportive source, was vital for participants who experienced exclusion and control in the workplace in addition to the usual daily stressors of the faculty role.

Coping with Everyday Racism

Participants encountered racism, sexism, and other "isms" in their everyday interactions as faculty members. Awareness of and preparedness for racism and other "isms" allowed participants to identify, interpret, and thoughtfully select responses congruent with a specific situation, an institutional context, personal values, and priorities.

CHOOSE A RESPONSE

Professor Swan described the need for faculty of color to decide how they are going to respond to racism and other "isms":

> If you are a minority, you have to make a conscious decision on whether you are going to allow a majority group to use that in defining you. I say don't assume just become someone's part of a majority group that [he or she has] a certain belief. I would say to try to become integrated into the organization and figure out the culture and try to be part of the group. If you experience some overt racism or classism or whatever, then you make your conscious decision [about] how to deal with it. [pharmacy faculty]

Similarly, Professor Hope described how he dealt with racism:

> Not that I found any problem, but I could see very clearly that people behaved and their attitudes . . . You could tell they did not grow up in a big city. I admit my parents raised me, I guess, to see that if you think there's a wolf behind the door, there probably is. But if you just knock the door down, there may not be a wolf there, or if there is, [it's] probably not going to bug you. So my attitude has always been, I don't see a problem until there's a problem. I was pretty much for quite a while probably the only doc of color—physician or dentist of color in the health sciences center. I don't think I saw that as an obstacle. It was just kind of the background in a way because I just had my agenda. And if

you were cool then you were cool with me. And if you're not, then as long as you're not standing in my way, I [have] no problem with you. [dental faculty]

Professor Hope showed a remarkable level of positivity about every aspect of life and viewed himself as a very fortunate human being. This was evident when he said, "How can you not choose to try to feel good about the world and yourself?" Inherent in this outlook, he tended not to focus on covert racism, although he was aware of its existence. He chose not to focus on racism unless it posed a clear obstacle:

My parents raised me to say, "If you take care of your business and you're courteous and you're respectful of people, no matter how they might first start looking at you. If you just mind your business and take care of your business and get your stuff done and you're respectful, usually you'll begin to separate the contenders from the pretenders." I mean, unless you are going to stand in front of me with a brick in your hand, I really don't have any time for you. I'm not paying any attention. I'm just too busy . . . Unless someone is going to stop you, why get yourself distracted from where you're going? . . . So I can't tell you if there was anything [subtle or covert] here in my way. I really can't tell you if there was or wasn't. [dental faculty]

Professor Singleton's threshold for responding to racism was also primarily at the overt level of observable behavior:

I can't change people. I can't do anything about what people feel, but I think in a work environment we can do something about how people act . . . Maybe when I was a lot younger I would say well, we have to change people. [nursing faculty]

For Professors Swan, Hope, and Singleton, only overt racism warranted a response. In contrast, Professor Said expressed concern about covert racism:

INTERVIEWER: Have you ever reflected on how to respond to racism?
PROFESSOR SAID: Yes, I have thought about it, but only sporadically and in the moment. I have not sat down and identified any well-thought-out strategy . . . I have not really done anything to respond to racism targeting me personally because I have not felt empowered. I would have had to lodge a formal complaint . . . to get any action . . . and there is a lot of fallout that comes with doing something like that. On the other hand, I feel a sense of responsibility to respond to the covert racism that is so prevalent here because I am con-

cerned it affects how we are educating students . . . Mostly when I respond to something like that [covert racism], it will be in the classroom when a white student uses coded language. Sometimes I will also address racism in faculty meetings but . . . not as much there. I have a better relationship with students, and I provide them with the tools to understand racism as part of their education—they are kind of a captive audience and that makes a difference . . . I feel like I have a responsibility to respond to racism in the environment, but I just feel so powerless. I often bring up equity, and most of the faculty have racist assumptions that filter how they see equity—they are wearing blinders. They don't see past their privilege. So they don't listen, or they roll their eyes. Leadership only gives lip service to equity, and that is upsetting, and it makes me want to disengage. If I was more thoughtful about what is realistic, I would probably be better off. [nursing faculty]

Professor Said's concern is consistent with the higher education literature, which has documented covert racism as a pervasive problem (48, 199, 325). Yet the subtle nature of covert racism makes it difficult to address at the individual level. Although findings on the influence of exclusionary climates suggest that addressing covert racism and its negative effects is critical, each person must carefully consider what he or she can take on individually rather than collectively. Recognizing that individual responses to covert racism are inherently challenging may help faculty of color let go of feeling personally responsible to address such acts on their own. In sum, it is important to recognize there is no one "right" way for an individual faculty member of color to respond to racism in academe; this decision differs from one person to another. The key for thriving is to thoughtfully choose a response. Reflecting on current habits and associated results can inform decision making and future choices

STRATEGIC ENGAGEMENT

Choosing your battles was an important strategy for dealing with racism and other complex, sometimes hidden challenges in academe. Using this approach required awareness of personal values, institutional climate, and a given situation in order to assess the likelihood that actions would be effective. Considering the immediate and longer-term gains or losses that actions would likely bring to one's career and life overall were valuable strategies (197). This kind of informed approach is consistent with findings reported by Alfred:

When it comes time to challenge the system you have to know your stuff; you just have to be rational. You have to know exactly what you want; you have to give them help on how they can get there, but don't just protest on foolish stuff. I think there are ways to challenge, and I don't think a loud voice or accusations are the way to do it. (316) p.76

Professor Singleton described this skill:

I think you learn to pick your battles . . . Over time I have found that I'm not a quiet person anymore. I'm not like I was when I started out as a doctoral student. I think part of it is aging. You figure you know what is important and you know what isn't important . . . I just feel freer to say the things I need to say. I think that is a privilege of getting older and wiser. I feel that way too. Some things I don't make a comment on but at some point you say, "Look." You speak your mind, and it's always a little bit of a surprise when I say something. [nursing faculty]

When thriving participants chose to respond to racism, they used a strategic, often measured response. Professor Singleton did not speak up every time an issue arose. She saved her comments for when she felt most compelled to speak or act and when action would be most effective. This approach lent her credibility. Professor Rhodes, an experienced faculty member, also chose her battles as part of her work with students of color:

Working a lot with students, working with student scholarships and stuff like that . . . A lot of things we have learned over the years is that you have to pick your battles, decide where you want to go, to put your emphasis. In other words, you don't just fight everything. [nursing faculty]

Professor Belmont, describing himself later in his career, used this same language.

There are things that happen every now and again that I go, "Yeah, that happens." I recognize it for what it is. And I pick and choose my battles. And I have won most of them, but I pick and choose them very carefully. [nursing faculty]

Professors Singleton, Rhodes, and Belmont learned to choose their battles as they gained experience as faculty members, while other faculty like Professor

Hope used this strategy from the beginning of their careers. Thus, while some may learn this strategy over time, there is no reason a faculty member cannot use it from day one. Importantly, choosing one's battles is not a euphemism for becoming a doormat. Rather, it means asking the questions, "Does it really matter? and Will my insights change another's opinion?" before choosing to act (326) p.243.

An example of carefully deciding how to strategically respond to a control process, using, was provided by Professor Morgan. He was invited to be in a cooperative group and was the only black person in the group. Initially this tokenism bothered him, but as he thought the situation through, he decided to use it to his advantage:

> "I think you white folks [in the cooperative group] think that you're doing okay because I'm in the room. We've got diversity; look at Professor Morgan over there, he's happy." And I almost decided not to continue . . . I felt like I am being used. But you've got to be in the room even if it means they are using you to some level . . . I do have enough influence that I can tell people, "Look, there's some minority or underserved that aren't being asked," and they respect me enough to listen to it and try to address me. And I am thinking, "Okay, so maybe I'm in the room because I am black, but I am actually pushing these white folks because I am black." And I am okay with that. [medical faculty]

Professor Morgan made a conscious choice to "use the users" as a way of responding strategically to tokenism. Recognizing that he was being used, he decided to employ the platform to his advantage, pushing a diversity and equity agenda that was consistent with his values. Hu-DeHart used the term "surplus visibility" to describe how institutions thrust faculty of color into the limelight to demonstrate a commitment to diversity (327) p.34. Consistent with Professor Morgan's actions, Hu-DeHart recommended faculty "use the space created by this surplus visibility to turn the spotlight back on the institution itself" (327) p.34, starting in one's department and continuing on to higher administration.

STRATEGIC DISENGAGEMENT

Strategic disengagement was the act of carefully and purposefully disconnecting from interpersonal or group activities in order to maintain well-being in the face of exclusion and control. This decision ultimately supported career satisfaction and success because it promoted smoother functioning in the workplace and reduced stress. Professor Adams described how she purposefully distanced herself from some colleagues to avoid experiencing invalidation in trivial situations:

PROFESSOR ADAMS: Another example is some of the research that I was doing [with] . . . one of our fellows . . . looking at racial segregation . . . I showed some of that research to my chair and other people and they're like, "Oh, this is happening stuff, you've got to present this and have this be . . . a grand rounds." I don't really want to present it as a grand rounds. I don't really want that to be my . . . flag to carry, and my introduction to the rest of the faculty. They see that here I am—one of two African Americans—and I happen to be doing research on . . . disparities . . . I'm interested in it, obviously, but I don't really want it to be my claim to fame, so to speak . . . And so I've shied away from it . . . and . . . avoid some of those conversations with people because I don't really want to hear what their reactions are going to be. Because if it's anything other than what I want to hear, then . . . that may color my further interactions with that person.

INTERVIEWER: And . . . your hesitance to present that research, is that because you're worried about being typecast? Or is it because you're worried how people are going to react and you know the work that you're going to have to do—emotionally and intellectually—to respond?

PROFESSOR ADAMS: It is . . . equally distributed between my fear of being typecast and the diversity token. And . . . having to deal with the explanations and platitudes and further questions, etc., that are going to come about . . . Inevitably, I know the conversation's going to land up in a place that I'll probably disagree with . . . that person's thoughts, and I really don't want to know what [his or her] thoughts are. Because . . . I'm going to have to then carry that and figure out how to interact with this person on a regular day-to-day basis. So, not knowing is almost better. [medical faculty] (143) p.9

Professor Adams avoided unimportant conversations that could sour her relationships with peers. This was a strategic form of avoidance that promoted her well-being and ability to deal effectively with colleagues on a daily basis.

Recommendations for Thriving: Assessment and Action

Thriving for faculty of color in health professions academe is personally defined and reflects each person's unique values and goals. Hence, personal expectations for satisfaction and success do not always coincide with external standards. Taking ownership of a personal definition of thriving is an ongoing process as one changes and grows in response to life's vicissitudes and opportunities. There are two overarching thriving strategies. The first is conducting a thorough assessment, and the second is developing and implementing an action plan.

Writing about women faculty of color, Monture emphasized the importance of awareness and recommended three actions: (1) understand who you are, (2) understand where you are, and (3) understand that your experience is knowledge (315). Understanding who you are requires affirmation of your identity and struggle, as well as connection to culture and community (315). Understanding where you are dictates an awareness of institutional climate. Understanding that your experience is knowledge means seeing, validating, and gaining wisdom from your experiences as a person of color (328) and willingness to share opportunities with other scholars in ways that affirm race, ethnicity, and gender (315). Hence, awareness is foundational to self-agency because it provides a basis for informed decision making.

Participants' ability to integrate deeply held personal values in their work was critical to their satisfaction; the institutional support and recognition they received for this work was also important. Because a successful interaction between an institution and faculty member promotes thriving, self-awareness and awareness of one's institution are vital (197). The "Diversity and Equity Climate Stages Rubric" in table 4 may be used as a guide to institutional climate assessment. This rubric points out key elements that faculty can assess using information such as institutional policies; racial and ethnic composition of the faculty and student bodies, higher faculty ranks, and leadership; history of racially and ethnically diverse faculty retention; data on URM student admissions, graduation, and resident match; the presence and effectiveness of diversity programs including mentorship for racially and ethnically diverse faculty and students; handling of critical incidents involving faculty and students of color; formal and informal satisfaction data from faculty and students of color; and so forth. Other data can be obtained through quiet observation and conversations with faculty and students of color. Synthesis of this information will provide an overall picture of institutional climate and its written, unwritten, and race rules.

Self-assessment focuses on personal values, career goals, and patterns of behavior with associated results. Ideally, personal values drive one's career goals and behavior. The best examples of this are faculty whose teaching, research, practice, and service are integrated around a focus that matters to them and who are able to achieve their career goals because they have learned how to navigate academia with sophistication (191). Reflecting on one's values and their fit with long-term career goals is part of this process. Reflecting on one's beliefs about how to appropriately respond to covert or overt racism encountered in academia is also critical. Tools for this reflective process include reading a wide array of relevant literature (e.g., on strength assessments, career planning, information about the faculty role, racism in the workplace); quiet observation; journaling (329); and conversations with family, friends, mentors, and colleagues to gather information and clarify ideas (330). Faculty of color should also carefully study decisions and behavior made in past situations to expose patterns and identify new approaches to managing situations if appropriate. Synthesis of this information will provide insight into short- and long-term career goals and concrete strategies for navigating the minefields of exclusionary climates.

The next step is to integrate the information gained from institutional and self-assessments to create an action plan. The action plan includes three components: core values, short- and long-term goals, and behavioral strategies. Core values are at the top of the plan because they are the foundation for other components. Short- and long-term career goals should have an estimated timeline and include specific activities for achieving goals (197, 331). These activities might include cultivating and accessing mentors; developing collaborations; developing new skills such as improving communication, writing ability, or public speaking; writing papers or research proposals; service work; and developing a robust support network (197). The behavioral component of the plan should list and describe strategies for decision making and behaviors faculty want to cultivate, such as being proactive, positive thinking, self-affirmation, and choosing your battles (326). The assessment and action planning process should be revisited and revised on an ongoing basis. Such steps provide a framework for systematically developing the conscious decision making that is the hallmark of thriving faculty of color.

CHAPTER FIVE

Working toward Equity

I tell my students that "When you get those good jobs that you have been
so brilliantly trained for, just remember that your real job if you are free
is to free somebody else, if you have power then your job is to empower
somebody else. This is not just a grab-bag candy game."

Toni Morrison (332)

Although faculty of all races and ethnicities have contributed to efforts to achieve equity, faculty of color bear a disproportionate burden of this work. The term "minority tax" has been coined to describe these extra responsibilities (333). Although this work often has great meaning for faculty of color, it leaves far less time to produce what is most valued by academic institutions for promotion: grants, patents, and academic publications and presentations. Although institutions rely heavily on faculty of color to support their diversity and equity initiatives, few recognize or reward the work required to make progress toward equity (48, 226).

Most participants were involved in diversity and equity efforts of some kind, often feeling a sense of responsibility to do this work. This chapter makes explicit the taken-for-granted, unrewarded, and hidden work many participants took on and the unique contributions participants made to diversity and equity. Through their presence, hard work, and dedication, participants made contributions to their institutions and communities that are deserving of recognition. I describe these contributions in the following categories: mentoring people of color, diversity-related teaching and service, and promoting health equity through research and practice.

Mentoring People of Color

The previous chapter focused on faculty mentorship and described some of the unique contributions faculty of color make to mentoring their junior colleagues.

In this section I focus primarily on mentoring students of color, although minor reference to junior faculty is also made. Commitment to and passion for the success of students of color was a common theme among participants, who recognized that many students of color face disadvantages in an educational system designed for middle- and upper-middle-class whites.

Many participants were able to mentor students and junior peers of color in ways particularly important for these groups. Role models are living proof of the possibility of success. Sharing and emotional connection are also important for development of successful mentor-mentee relationships. Because of their life histories, participants were able to relate to many of the experiences of students and junior faculty of color, offering a safe place to share personal stories. Participants were able to help mentees successfully navigate exclusionary climates, offering guidance and advocacy. Finally, participants nourished the pipeline, working to increase racial and ethnic diversity in the health-care workforce.

SUCCESSFUL ROLE MODELS

Role models send powerful messages about what is possible. According to Zirkel, "Young people learn the racial and gendered structuring of the culture in which they live by noting the race and gender of adults in different professional positions. The presence or absence of like others in different social positions implicitly conveys information to young people about the possibilities for their future" (334) p.357. Institutions lacking visibly diverse faculty and leaders send hidden, invalidating, demeaning, and hurtful messages to students and faculty of color. As Sue explained, "From the perspective of students and faculty of color the absence of administrators of color sends a series of loud and clear messages: 1. 'You and your kind are not welcome here.' 2. 'If you choose to come to campus you will not feel comfortable here.' 3. 'If you choose to stay, there is only so far you can advance. You may not graduate . . . or get tenured/promoted'" (335) p.26. Proactively grooming faculty of color for future institutional leadership and hiring outside candidates of color for leadership roles are essential measures for addressing these negative environmental messages.

Professors Rice and Woods described the discouraging impact that lack of institutional role models can have on students and faculty of color:

PROFESSOR RICE: I think that for the majority [of students], they see things whether they're walking in the hallway and they see all the previous presidents and they have these huge oil paintings on the wall or a bust and everyone is an old white man. So therefore if I was a white male I would say, "Yeah, I mean look at these halls and everything. One day I'll be on these walls too." Well, I don't see anyone that looks like me on an oil painting. [medical faculty]

PROFESSOR WOODS: Of the pharmacy faculty who are non-tenure track, most of them are females . . . And I do have a sense that the odds are stacked against me. I do notice who are the tenure track and tenured faculty . . . They're mostly Caucasians. Those are two areas where I don't fit . . . and so it's definitely something I am aware of . . . I'm looking to see, well, who are the ones who have made it through, and I know that they don't look like me. And so I wonder what's happened to the other ones that didn't make it to that level and maybe moved on. What did they look like? And I wonder, why is that the case? [pharmacy faculty]

The exclusionary messages some institutions send may generate feelings of discomfort, anger, and anxiety in faculty and students of color (325, 336). In contrast, a successful role model can help students visualize future success. Sharing her own student experience, Professor Swift described how a role model of like background was both inspiring and reassuring to her as a student:

Thinking back to myself as a student, I think it was more of an unconscious thing, but you see this person and at least the person looks like you, so you think that [he or she] could at least relate to you . . . One of my main mentors that I had before I got into pharmacy school was a black lady in Tuskegee, Alabama, working at a VA, and I was just like "this lady is superwoman." And so when you see that person you can almost see yourself. It's almost like a reflection of yourself, and it's like if she can do it, I have to believe now that I think I can do it . . . It's just that reinforcement that it's okay and it has been done and it can be done. [pharmacy faculty]

Professors Zeno and Garcia also recognized the value of visible role models:

PROFESSOR ZENO: [Students] definitely see me as a role model, and that's something that I see as very important because I want those students to get in their heads that . . . someone who looks like them can make it big. [pharmacy faculty]

PROFESSOR GARCIA: I think it's nice for all students of all colors to see me, a Hispanic physician. They get a sense of my background and culture and appreciation for having someone that knows the language and understands the culture . . . From a teaching perspective, I think the residents need to see attending physician role models of color . . . especially like students applying for medical school and residents, they need to know they can get there, that despite cultural barriers . . . they will eventually get there. [medical faculty]

Identification with a faculty role model was not always based on racial or ethnic background. Professor Sanchez spoke of his value as a role model for students with English as a second language:

I make a point of telling them . . . that I grew up in Puerto Rico . . . I think especially for some of the Asian students, if they're first generation or something they're like, "Oh see, there's people here whose first language isn't English, they're doing well and they teach and they do all these things, so it's possible." I've heard that from a couple of students in my years here. I think some of them perceive me to be an immigrant. They kind of relate to me in that way. [pharmacy faculty]

Professor Ortiz described how her presence motivated students:

When my students find out I am Puerto Rican—especially my Hispanic students [who] want to do well to impress me more . . . I see it in them. And when they make a mistake, they are like, "Sorry." They will apologize to me, whereas with the other faculty it will be like, "Whatever." But with me they don't want to let me down. [dental faculty]

Although there is an abundance of white role models in health professions education, there are far fewer options for people of color. Because of the critical importance of role models for visualizing what is possible, the presence of visibly racially and ethnically diverse faculty now is essential to greater diversity in the future. As Professor Bailey said, "I think that just the very fact that I'm here where I'm visible makes a difference" [medical faculty].

SHARING AND VALIDATING PERSONAL EXPERIENCE

Understanding what it is like to be treated as a member of the out-group provided a basis for connection between participants and students of color. Professors Hazelwood and Meriwether described how their life experiences informed their mentoring relationships with students of color:

Professor Hazelwood: I bring an understanding of what it's like . . . to be a minority student, because I think when you look at having gone to school in a white institution in the early [1980s,] it wasn't easy. When you walked into school people automatically thought you weren't going to make it through the first semester . . . So I bring that perspective, that struggle. What it means to struggle. I think I bring the perspective of an African American . . . We understand the struggles an individual has to go through. So I think we can put ourselves out there a lot more, available to students and want everyone to succeed. [nursing faculty]

PROFESSOR MERIWETHER: I think as faculty of color we tend to . . . extend that nurturing to no matter what student . . . but I feel more of a need with the African American students . . . The white kids . . . don't always have to remember what color they are before they can do anything . . . I know the black experience in a predominantly white school because I lived that experience. [nursing faculty]

Some participants described students of color as being closer and more comfortable with them than with white faculty, as explained by Professors Zeno and Kendall:

PROFESSOR ZENO: The tendency is for the students of color to definitely relate to me and the other faculty of color more personally. They definitely seek us out more . . . They see us as faculty they can connect and share with and they feel comfortable. [pharmacy faculty]

PROFESSOR KENDALL: I've had students tell me . . . certain stories or they'll tell me something thing and they'll say, "Well, I'm comfortable saying certain things to you because you're like me." [pharmacy faculty]

Although many participants mentor students of the same race/ethnicity, many were also sought out by students of color of other races and ethnicities. These relationships were also formed to some degree based on a shared understanding of what it is like to be different. Professors Ahmed and Sanchez described their ability to relate to students of color across racial and ethnic lines:

PROFESSOR AHMED: I think that because of my background, it's very different than everyone else's. So I think for me I feel that I'm the only one of the Middle Eastern or one of two . . . I think with the students on that scale they can relate to me. I just think that I offer a different eye or different view. [pharmacy faculty]

PROFESSOR SANCHEZ: The students who aren't born and raised white, I think I relate more with them . . . I think they consider me ethnic for lack of a better word . . . I think they gravitate toward me because they perceive me to be different from the norm and perhaps then they think [I'm] more open-minded or broader or whatever . . . I think they can tell, "Oh, there's someone who's different here." [pharmacy faculty]

Participants successfully provided mentorship to students of all races and ethnicities; however, they were able to offer unique support to students of color both within and across racial and ethnic groups. Having someone to connect with who understands where you are coming from, and with whom you can share, is powerful. Many students of color in predominantly white health professions schools experience marginalization and covert racism (337–341). Some may be mistrustful of the environments they find themselves in. For these students, connecting with a faculty member of color can be a lifeline.

NAVIGATING THROUGH EXCLUSIONARY CLIMATES

Participants in exclusionary climates helped students of color progress through their programs, offering critical guidance and advocacy. Professor Pope, an assistant dean for diversity, described his commitment to shepherding students of color through medical school from start to finish:

What I tell students . . . this analogy—since it's Black History Month, I used this just the other day because I had attended . . . a little presentation—someone was doing a presentation on Harriet Tubman. And Harriet Tubman was talking about how she'd led people on the Underground Railroad to freedom, and her train never went off the track, and she never lost a person. I'm your male Harriet Tubman here at the school of medicine. I know how to get you through. I know how to get you to the Promised Land that you say you want. You want to become a physician. I know the pitfalls. I know the people to avoid. I know how much you need to study, and I will lead you if you come here and if you listen to me. Now, I understand Harriet Tubman would shoot you, if you didn't listen to her. Well, I'm doing none of that, but I tell the students—I almost guarantee them—if you follow my lead, I will get you the MD degree. These students have come here simply because of the support system that they perceive in me and my office. Because I've never lost a student . . . That's what I tell them. [medical faculty] (143) p.10.

Similarly, Professor Ross coached her students on how to manage being treated differently:

You see a student who is a strong student, but for some reason [she has] fallen off track. You say, "Sally, why don't you come to the office?" And then [she comes] in and you shut the door. "What's going on with you? Do you need me to call somebody for you?" . . . And you appeal to people because you are—you may be of a similar culture and so I reflect back to them what they will find as minority nurses. I reflect to them how you manage yourself, carry yourself. You may be confident, you are confident, but you are still going to be second-guessed on how you are going to handle this and especially in this program where the nurses have experience. They say, "Dr. Ross, you are so correct" . . . And I talk to them in a realistic manner so that when they go out, when they interview . . . when they interact with physicians, this is how you carry yourself. And so they come back and report that this incident happened or this event happened, and so it increases their image of me as a credible administrator. I'm just not a hide-behind-the-door or book administrator. They know what I am speaking of, and I speak about patients and examples of patients and I share . . . Because we [faculty of color] want to make sure they succeed and succeed at a higher level, but it's the nuances of the profession that other people don't understand that we face and we try to translate to them: this is what you are going to face. This is what you have to do. [nursing faculty]

Many students of color sought guidance from participants on how to handle racially charged incidents. Professor Swift's office was "home base" for many of the black women who were students in her program:

I will say that I do feel like a lot of the African American female students tend to come by my office and . . . they all kind of congregate . . . They come to me with things like career questions and some personal things. I feel like it's because I'm black . . . even if things happen in the classroom and it's not even my class. They'll come and want to ask for my advice. This is what happens, and even racial things that they feel have happened to them, or there was a huge Facebook incident with a minority student and a European American student. They stopped by my office to ask me what should they do. [pharmacy faculty]

Professors Meriwether and Said both worked in exclusionary climates. Their knowledge of the racial landscape at their institutions allowed them to support students' progress despite obstacles and hidden traps:

PROFESSOR MERIWETHER: I remember one student who came to my office . . .
I said, "I know you want to go in there but you want to go the instructor [to
protest]" . . . but I said, "Mike, the one way that you can really hurt them is to
walk across that stage and graduate . . . because if you walk down there and
you say something disrespectful, they will get you out of here." And I said,
"You will have paid out all of this money and [have] no degree." I said, "But
when you walk across that stage on graduation day and they hand you your
diploma, there is nothing they can do about that." I said, "You stand there and
you smile and you take it . . . and when you get your license that's the time to
come back and confront us" [nursing faculty] (342) p.158.

PROFESSOR SAID: I recently had a student of color who was looking to round out
her committee. And we were looking for a dissertation committee member
with specific expertise. The student suggested Dr. Smith, whom I know and
have worked with in the past. I have seen Dr. Smith railroad two black students
out of this school . . . So I told my student that I believe Dr. Smith is a racist
and that I am worried she will try to sabotage your education if she joins the
committee. I said, "No I can't live with [the] possibility of that happening
knowing what I know now. Let's find someone else." [nursing faculty]

Participants also advocated for students who were being discriminated
against. A common example of discrimination occurs when white students
are afforded opportunities and/or given the benefit of the doubt, while students
of color in similar situations do not receive these benefits. Professor Kirkpatrick
described how she protected a black student who had been targeted for dismissal,
ultimately allowing the student to graduate:

PROFESSOR KIRKPATRICK: There was one black student . . . they [other faculty
members] essentially tried to do her in. And if I had not been there . . . she
would not have gotten out of that program, because they were ready to kill
her. So I had to kind of intervene to keep her from going under.

INTERVIEWER: And it wasn't because of her inability or that she lacked the ability?
It was just the way in which they treated her?

PROFESSOR KIRKPATRICK: She had some issues with writing . . . but that you can
overcome with work and good editing. This woman . . . she knew the literature
in her field in a way that I had rarely had a student know their clinical literature.
And she had done very good work and . . . had received funding. And they still
ran her out. When she came back—there's a black man that was a student ad-

visor who came to me and said, "Would you be willing to take her on to keep her from going back to these women?" and I said "Yes," because I had known her from before. And . . . when she came back, they were trying to get her again. To really finish her off and . . . she had a time getting out of there. It took her a long time to get out of that program. She was finally able to get finished . . . There were pockets of it, of racism in various programs. [nursing faculty]

Similarly, Professor Hazelwood advocated for a black student in crisis and after ascertaining the problem referred him to emergency student support programs:

I had one young man . . . he came to me one time because his mother—he was depending on his mother to help with rent on the apartment he was sharing. Her phone had become disconnected. He couldn't get in contact with her, and I kept saying, "Why does he look so dazed when I'm seeing him in the hallway?" I finally brought him in the office and I said, "Can you share with me. Where are you? What's going on?" He said, "Dr. Hazelwood . . . I don't have money to pay my rent, I'm worried about whether they're going to evict me, I don't even have money for food." He . . . was having these headaches. I said, "This is stress"; he said, "It probably is." I said, "What are you eating?" He said "I buy . . . those cups of noodles that you put water in"—they're loaded with sodium and MSG and everything else. And he was having an MSG reaction with the headaches and so forth . . . I put him in touch with counseling service and also with student affairs in order for him to get emergency financial aid . . . And then he finally was able to get in touch with his mother and she reconnected, but this was a very unstable family situation. He was the first generation to graduate from college. And . . . you want . . . [students] to be successful . . . The white instructors were saying he may be on drugs and wondering if he was going to become hostile in the classroom . . . There's still racial undertones at this school. There's no question about it. [nursing faculty] (342) p.158

Faculty also advocated on behalf of groups of students. Professor Belmont suspected discriminatory grading practices were affecting black students in a course taught by another faculty member. He advocated for the entire class and took the problem to administration:

I told her [the dean] that I thought there was something odd going on with this group of students and I wanted to do an experiment to see whether or not

. . . these students were being singled out. So she agreed. She called the course faculty member, and she agreed. What we did was . . . we agreed to take the names off of the papers and we would just grade them and then we met. All the African American students that [the course instructor] didn't realize . . . that . . . she had . . . She gave them A pluses on their paper; one of them got a B plus. And when it was over, the dean comes in and says, "Well, we have the grades. We have some Cs . . . Ds, Fs. We have some As, Bs," and so on . . . And she [the faculty member] said . . . "Well, I'm sure it's the students of color who fell into those areas . . . the Fs and Ds." And the dean said, "As a matter of fact they didn't. You graded them and gave them A pluses on their papers." And she [the faculty member] said, "That can't be." And [the dean] said, "Yes," and she showed her their names and so forth. So we exposed her that she was singling out these African American students for no other reason than the color of their skin. So it was a thing that really affected me there in a profound way. I thought, here I am working with colleagues who at one point will be reviewing my track [record] for promotion and tenure and who are flunking these African American students, and she was getting so much support for doing so by other folks. That was pretty scary for me at that time to witness that going on. [nursing faculty] (308) p.135

These findings suggest that participants were vital resources for students of color, who sometimes needed guidance and advocacy in exclusionary school climates. Awareness of the institutional landscape allowed participants to help students of color consider what strategies were most likely to help them successfully graduate. A willingness to advocate for students, while sometimes placing participants in vulnerable positions, speaks to the dedication of this group to student success.

NOURISHING THE PIPELINE

Several participants nourished the pipeline of students of color through mentorship and outreach activities with middle school, high school, and undergraduate students, and by engaging with students in their programs to support retention. Professors Murphy and Jones mentored youth in their communities:

PROFESSOR MURPHY: I have always felt being an African American physician . . . that I want younger kids to be able to look up and say, "Wow, I can be a doctor; I can be the specialist; I don't have to be the person who's transporting the people." We know that it is important for young people to have successful role models who are like them. [medical faculty]

PROFESSOR JONES: I get a lot of African American students who come in telling me their stories, and some of the students can be high school students, because I am trying to mentor them. They will call me to mentor them because I'm the African American in the health sciences that they see and [I] will spend time talking with them. And so because I do a lot in the community, people know me for the most part and they find me to be approachable, so they will want their kids to come and talk ... I try to be available ... There are students in the community who will periodically come and show up and they want to go into medicine; we'll sit and talk about what they're doing, and they say, "Okay, I'm going to do this," and I'll come back and I might not see them again for a year. And then they will show back up, and I'm thinking I thought you changed your mind. "Oh well, I'm doing this or that but yeah I'm still around." "Well okay." I just sort of accept them and try to give them direction. But part of it is just thinking about the community and how people do things, but at the same time, letting them know that this worked for me, but it's not going to work for the people that you're trying to sell your application to. So you can be late [turning in your application] if you want to, but they're not going to accept it. And we actually did what we call an education fair aimed at the students, and [I got] some of the students I am mentoring ... to participate, to educate the other students, [who] were mostly some undergrad, some high school, and even middle school kids that we're telling if you want to go to the next level, this is how you have to think about it. And so the mentoring is formal and informal. [medical faculty]

Similarly, Professor Zeno reached out to undergraduate students as a means of recruiting URM students to his pharmacy program:

I think that culturally the fact that I'm not only faculty of color in terms of my skin being dark, but me being Hispanic, like maybe Puerto Rican goes beyond me being black. That brings a different perspective ... Because I try to get involved in other things beyond what happens in my college. I [got] involved in the cultural festival at the university that took place last week, and so I was involved with that not only with our graduate pharmacy students but [also] undergraduate students around campus. Now they know of me and of my culture, and yeah, so I feel that I am definitely making a difference. [pharmacy faculty]

As described previously, Dr. Garcia voluntarily ran a mentoring program for undergraduate students:

> I started my mentorship program . . . for students from disadvantaged backgrounds . . . for undergraduate students . . . in a health-care career at this campus because . . . they tend to get a lot of local brown kids into that university and in this mentorship program . . . we have about twenty students and I think we have twenty students in the second year as well, and basically the curriculum--these students shadow their mentor--a physician assistant twice a month for two half days about four hours each time. They also were mentored once a month by their mentor, and we have one lecture per month at the hospital, and the lecture usually integrated the general sciences with whatever they were seeing in the hospital . . . And [the mentorship program] was very successful. Oh, and on top of that, we also had a book club . . . And I found out that 100 percent of my students found a role model in life to be their mentor from the program. And I believe all but one said they wanted to work with patients from a similar background . . . So it was very, very, very successful. In that way they all wanted to stay local and go to health-care school here, so you know, potentially a way to reduce health disparities in this state. [medical faculty]

Participants also volunteered their time to supervise student associations to support and connect with students, promoting retention and graduation. Professors Woods and Swift described their work:

> PROFESSOR WOODS: I'm co-advisor for our school's student national and pharmaceutical associations . . . It's predominantly been minority students, African American students for the most part. While it's never been explicitly stated, it's just kind of been understood that it's an African American organization. So I'm one of the co-advisors. And at the meeting in February, I was the guest speaker. It was very informal, but I just told them, "Hey if you're interested in pharmacy, if you become interested in research . . . I'm here to help you guys. So ask me whatever you want. And afterward a lot of the students . . . said, "We didn't even realize what you did and how you're able to help us out. Now that we know what you do we see that you're so unique. And you can really be

helpful to us . . . pointing us in different directions and . . . especially you are a minority at the school." A lot [of] the students say, "That's cool. We're glad you are here." [pharmacy faculty]

PROFESSOR SWIFT: I am the advisor for the student pharmacy organization, which is a minority student organization. They validate me. We had a banquet a couple of weeks ago and they gave me an outstanding mentoring award. I feel like being their advisor kind of makes them also feel comfortable, once they're a member of the organization, to come talk to me about things. I had a student tell me that, "You're to be my mentor for life." [pharmacy faculty]

Participants nourished the pipeline with passionate dedication across the educational spectrum. Their connection with and commitment to their communities provided a foundation for this work.

Diversity- and Equity-Related Teaching and Service

Although the pedagogical contributions of faculty of color in health professions education have been poorly examined, studies of undergraduate education indicate that faculty diversity is a "'compelling interest' in that it enhances higher education through the benefits it brings to . . . students" (343) p.318. Similarly, many faculty of color engage in service activities that promote equity and excellence.

TEACHING

Research on undergraduate learning has found that faculty of color are more likely to use active and collaborative learning techniques, create environments that increase diverse interactions, and emphasize higher-order thinking classroom activities than white faculty (343). In addition, these pedagogical improvements are more likely to be used by faculty of all races and ethnicities on campuses where racial and ethnic faculty diversity approaches that of the general population than by faculty on less diverse campuses. Moreover, frequent interactions with racially and ethnically diverse faculty are associated with considerable growth in leadership skills, psychological well-being, intellectual engagement, and intercultural effectiveness across student groups (344). Interactions with faculty of color also have a significant positive influence on the academic performance of students of color (345). Participants made unique contributions teaching in the areas of cultural humility, social determinants of health, and health equity.

Professor Bailey described her unique positioning for making such contributions:

> We have diversity in the patient population . . . Cultural competency is something that I provide because I can empathize with patients of color and the way they approach things. I have an appreciation for the cultural differences or approach to care; I can relate . . . So I bring those unique abilities. They say only the person wearing the shoe knows how it fits. So if you're not of color, you don't know what it means to . . . live in a racist environment. And as a patient, you look for the best care . . . At the same time, you want people to respect you for who you are and not treat you like trash. I think working with the residents, I can help them begin to ask questions that maybe they wouldn't think of when they are talking with patients and trying to understand some of the problems that the patients may have . . . There are times when maybe I can raise issues and say, "Well, think about what it would be like if you worried that your child might get hurt going to school because there's so much crime." Those are things that maybe they've never experienced . . . I also think that it's a good thing both for the patients and for the residents to actually see that someone who looks like me is a physician, not just coming and saying, "Help me." [medical faculty]

Many participants were highly invested in improving access to and quality of care for underserved communities. These faculty were proactive in assuring students' clinical rotations included minority and medically underserved populations. Both Professors Singh and Singleton made minority and medically underserved populations central to their clinical teaching:

PROFESSOR SINGH: The whole caring for the underserved population and what it takes and how important it is, is my contribution to the college. And with it comes the cultural competence: What does it take to serve this culturally diverse group of individuals with different health literacy skills? We started clinical sites based on that. I have two students who were selected as fellows from foundations that focus on public health and health care for . . . underserved populations. So they're both in the underserved group, and one of them said he wasn't even sure he wanted to be in pharmacy school until he heard me talk about all of these opportunities with the underserved during one of the school convocations. And now he's gone so far deep into it he wants to make this his life. So I think I have opened a lot of students' eyes to [serving underserved communities]. About the importance of this . . . I think my contribution is I've opened their eyes and helped them see where their contribution will be. [pharmacy faculty]

PROFESSOR SINGLETON: I think because I'm focusing so much on community and I'm teaching community . . . and I feel that we need to provide services to our community . . . I feel a commitment to that. I think everybody knows I'm committed to that, because I just push the issue on it. I'm hoping that has impacted the people feeling like they need to be providing health services to the people that actually need them. Everybody needs health services; I shouldn't say it like that. We really, really, really do need those. To get into those communities and try to make a difference—that is kind of the key part. [nursing faculty] (342) p.161

There is evidence to suggest that curricular content on diverse populations prepares students for clinical practice with minority and medically underserved communities (346). Yet several studies have documented significant decreases in commitment to caring for medically underserved populations occurring between enrollment and graduation in medical and dental students (347–350). Underrepresentation of faculty of color in total numbers, the higher ranks, and leadership likely contributes to this problem, leaving health professionals unprepared to address inequities in the nation's health.

SERVICE

Baez's study of academic service by faculty of color found that participants differentiated between general and race-related service (351). General service included community, institutional, and professional activities that all faculty members are expected to perform, but that had little direct connection to race, ethnicity, diversity, or social justice. The latter category included any community, institutional, or professional activity perceived by the faculty members as benefiting the health of minority and medically underserved communities. Professor Ibori explained his sense of responsibility to address diversity and equity at his school through service:

I say to myself, "What if there were no senior professors of color at this college? Are there going to be things that don't get brought up?" Or not even that, but more than that is, "Are there things that don't come up because there's no African American faculty?" One of the things that I always bring up is that we have a class of eighty to one hundred students and out of those every year [we admit] people of color—maybe five, if you're lucky, maybe fewer—out of a class of one hundred. So the question has to come down to recruitment, retention, that sort of thing. And so that comes up constantly, and so it's looked at. But I suspect if there wasn't a person of color, of someone who was more aware of these things, it probably would come up periodically, but it would be on the back burner.

Although participants described a variety of race-related service, the most commonly mentioned was serving on school admissions committees. Some participants expressed concerns about admissions criteria that prioritize grades and standardized test scores. This practice has been termed "testocratic merit" by Guinier. According to Guinier, "Testocratic merit makes the assumption that test scores are the best evidence of applicants' worth, without paying much attention to the environments in which one finds those individuals. It thereby ignores several built-in biases that privileges those who are already quite advantaged" (189) p.x.

Consistent with this view, Professor Murphy expressed concerns about medical schools' admission practices:

I think personally that one just has to relook at the whole way that we even pick people to go into medicine, and I mean there's nothing—I don't know even if we have anything that says just because you get good grades in school or the highest grades, if that makes you a really good doctor . . . So I hope it is really looked at, and I mean you can have a passionate person who is dedicated who is maybe smart in a lot of other ways but maybe not smart enough to get a 90 on a [test] score . . . I think we have to look at where a person . . . comes from, obviously you have to have a minimum of something, but also what [her] passion, what [she is] committed to, how strong [she] might have worked to get to a particular point. And really figure out what [her] qualities are . . . I think we need to look beyond numbers and GPAs and consider other qualities that we're looking for in students. Our medical school year after year has magically 20 percent of students who are minorities; well, why couldn't it magically be 25 or 30 percent or other things? It's difficult because whom are you excluding, and whom are you taking spots away from? . . . I think really you could easily consider that they are taking spots away from the minority students, but just to realize that there is more to a physician than numbers. [medical faculty]

Service related to admissions was often described as important to promote equity. Professors Drake, Ainsworth, and Green described their motivation for serving on admissions committees:

PROFESSOR DRAKE: I sit on one of the admissions committees, and there have been many issues—there was an instance where they accidentally miscalculated an African American applicant's grade point average. And I brought it to their attention and they corrected it. And she was admitted. But I don't know if I had not been there that anybody would have picked that up or said anything about it. [nursing faculty]

PROFESSOR AINSWORTH: I sit on a number of committees like the admissions committee, and I interview students, and I decide who gets in. I put in a request some years ago, if there is any student of color who comes to apply to this school—they usually undergo three interviews—I said, "I want to be one of those interviewers." So far the office of admissions has done that. Whenever those students come before the admissions committee, everybody wants to know, "Professor Ainsworth, what do you think?" [medical faculty]

PROFESSOR GREEN: We had a highly qualified applicant who was an African American male, and he asked about the schools' resources for students in need of academic support during his interview. Because of that question a white colleague said the student would fail academically and he should not be admitted. That question killed the student, and that would not have happened if he had been a white student . . . I always ask about the diversity of the incoming class, and I am told at the meeting [that] they don't know because the students start next week. Last time I asked one of my colleagues [she] said, "She asks that every year," which I felt was a racist comment. They don't check on the racial and ethnic diversity of the student body so they don't look bad. If I wasn't here, there wouldn't be anybody to contest these practices. [pharmacy faculty]

Concern about admissions standards and practices for students of color was common among participants, reflecting recognition of the lack of URMs in the study body and health-care workforce. Although it is widely considered legitimate to offer preferential college admission to veterans, athletes, and children of alumnae, many do not support affirmative action practices for URMS who face systematic discrimination (4, 352); this view is reflected in increasingly restrictive judicial decisions on race-conscious college admissions over the past twenty years and the decision by eight states to ban this practice (353). Despite this trend and ongoing legal challenges to race-conscious admissions nationally, the constitutionality of considering race and ethnicity in the selection of students was upheld on June 23, 2016, in the US Supreme Court ruling in *Fisher v. University of Texas* (354).

Recognizing the importance of racial and ethnic diversity for the health professions and potential for negative bias during the admissions process, the AACN, AAMC, AACP, and ADEA have urged use of holistic admissions processes (355–358). Further, the AAMC and AACP have published guidelines recommending that admissions committee membership include faculty of color (355, 356). The holistic admissions process goes beyond the narrow lens of test scores to consider other qualities candidates bring to the health professions. Price and colleagues described holistic admissions thus:

> Decisions based on a comprehensive evaluation that balances the quantitative and qualitative qualities of a candidate. It refutes the practice of overreliance on standardized tests by detailing the whole-file review process to measure merit and professional promise. Also described is a range of noncognitive variables (e.g., leadership, ability to sustain academic achievement with competing priorities, volunteerism, communication, social background, and disadvantaged status). (359) p.S87

A national study of 228 health professions schools found that dentistry schools reported the highest rates of holistic admissions practices, at 93 percent, and nursing schools the lowest, at 47 percent (360). The number of holistic review elements used by schools was also significant. Whereas 81 percent of schools that used many holistic review elements reported increased diverse student enrollment (diversity was broadly defined), 60 percent of schools that used few elements reported increases (360). Other authors have documented increases in URM student enrollment following implementation of holistic admissions processes (361, 362). Participants contributed to holistic review, in the sense that they were able to identify the strengths students of color could bring to their future roles as health professionals. Further, participants understood academic criteria offered a narrow lens through which to view candidates, who must be prepared for complex social roles in health care; they also guarded against bias on admissions committees. Thus, despite being overextended, most participants found meaning in serving on admissions committees, which for some offered an opportunity to promote change. At the same time, participants frequently described lack of institutional recognition or reward for this important work as a source of dissatisfaction. These findings suggest a mismatch between academic reward structures and national priorities to graduate a racially and ethnically diverse health-care workforce to achieve health equity.

Addressing Health Equity through Practice and Research

Health professionals of color are more likely than whites to provide care to minorities and the medically underserved (45, 363, 364). Participants shared not only the importance of being there, but also connecting with and caring about patients, many of whom rarely see a clinician who looks like them. Many participants described the pleasure patients expressed when they saw them, as well as the difference their common racial and ethnic backgrounds made in their care. Professor Jones described her commitment to providing care to underserved communities that was based on her personal values:

> Somebody has to provide the care. Because growing up I wouldn't have, none of us would have made it, if we didn't have the support of our own community doing . . . the health care, because we didn't have access to doctors. There were a couple of black docs in a nearby town that we could go to, but we all lived in the country. And people didn't have money, so our health care was literally practiced out of the church, and my grandmother and other older women, on Sunday when we'd go to church because it was an all-day event, they would go from whatever vehicles people came in and be it a horse and buggy or car or truck or whatever and find out how families were, find out if somebody didn't come, who saw them. Because we didn't have any telephones, we didn't have any electricity. You rode past somebody; usually you'd stop to check on them. And so it was a big community thing. And so we looked out for each other

and we supported each other. And I feel that . . . given what I know based on my history and the support I have received from those people who believed in me, that I do believe I have a duty, a responsibility to help the next people come along. [medical faculty]

Professor Bailey described black patients' appreciation for having a physician of like background:

There [are] very few African American female doctors, and my patients that happen to be African American, they love, love, love, love that they see me. And they feel as though I can relate to them more and understand them more . . . How do I explain this? Like I said, my patients who can relate to me and they feel like they can relate to me more than they can relate to anyone else. If I can make that special connection to help them understand their diagnosis, their disease, recovery, then I've made a difference . . . I have patients who, they're like, "Oh, I'm so glad that I have you" because they're coming and they want to talk about their experiences, their problems, and they feel very comfortable being able to talk to someone who looks like them and knows some of the things that they've been through; they haven't just read about it in a book. That's a constant thing that I see . . . I feel like if I were in their place, it would [be] awfully comfortable to have somebody whom I didn't have to re-explain everything to. I mean there are a lot of cultural things that you can just sort of say without having to explain it to someone. [medical faculty]

Dr. Garcia described her dedication to her patients and differences in the care she provided to Latino/a patients compared to her colleagues:

Well at our hospital rehab, we have a very large undocumented population that seek medical care here. And we have a large number of patients [who] have kidney disease and need dialysis, but because they're undocumented they don't have the access to routine dialysis, which is three times a week. The undocumented population comes here whenever . . . usually once a week. And the number of patients with renal disease that come here once a week [for] dialysis is growing such [that] we have about close to fifty now. And all of their stories are just so sad; they just have such sad stories; many of them are parents to toddlers, many of them were the only working parent. Many stories of abused, I mean it's just so sad. I empathize with this population a lot, and I feel awful for them. I pay for many of their medications because they don't have money. I think at times I feel isolated and different from everyone else because I empathize with them, and my colleagues are annoyed by them. And that's what I find a little hurtful and makes me feel kind of awkward and different. They are annoyed because they are here every week, and it adds a lot of workload every week. Yeah, and I really loved seeing them, I've gotten to know their families . . . There are four of them that I pay for their medication every week. And it's just different, like I see these very sad stories and I think that my colleagues see them as just people they have to admit, people they have to work on. I mean to them it's just work; to me it's a life, that life. [medical faculty]

The contrast between Dr. Garcia's approach to her patients and that of her colleagues rings true. Clinicians are busier and busier these days, making it easy to see patients, particularly those with complex needs, as just more work to be done. No doubt faculty of color are not immune to this pitfall. However, participants' stories suggest that many felt a special connection to the minority and medically underserved patients in their communities and that this connection had meaning for the care provided as well as for that modeled to students.

In addition to practicing with minority and medically underserved communities, many participants engaged in research in support of health equity. Professor Meriwether's research with black men in prison provided an example of work with an underserved and vulnerable population:

I always used to think, . . . why am I doing this type of work with African American men besides the fact that I'm an African-American male? But now that I'm in psychiatry, I do forensic psychiatry, so I work in the jail. All of that research that I've done understanding health dangers and how black men think really helps me in the jail. And when these men come in my office and they say certain things, I can immediately understand. And I don't identify with them, because I didn't grow up in this city. I may have grown up in the inner cities, but I didn't grow up here. I didn't grow up in the same environment that they did, but I understand what they're saying. [nursing faculty]

Professor Smith described her work with American Indian tribes:

Being an American Indian, I help research that aspect, which was lacking on our campus. I think even in colleges where there were not people who had looked into community-based participatory research, [they] are now working with the tribes. [medical faculty]

Professor Morgan made an effort to support recruitment of black subjects into clinical trials:

> I can tell you that [I am] the number one recruiter of African American patients to clinical trials here. And it's not magic. I think it's just people who look at me, trust me, and I think I try to do a good job of being honest about things. And I also worry that it might . . . be that some of the non–African American folks can't speak to those folks. It worries me. I can tell you yes, I think African American patients who see me do feel like there's some connection with me. [medical faculty]

Many participants made important contributions to health equity research and practice. Although the work that is part of an independent funded program of research is no doubt recognized, other work worthy of recognition is often hidden, such as Professor Garcia's seeing extra patients and paying for their medications and Dr. Morgan's helping colleagues with research recruitment.

Summary and Recommendations

The US population has become increasingly diverse, and as a result of the Affordable Care Act of 2010, 20 million formerly uninsured Americans now have health care (365). The need for health professions education to graduate clinicians capable of providing equitable, high-quality, culturally sensitive care to all patients continues to be urgent. However, making changes to the way we educate clinicians "will not be developed just by calling on the traditional players" (366) p.1487. Rather, engagement with a diverse array of perspectives, expertise, and life experiences is essential to innovation. Thus, diversity and equity in health professions education is integral to the achievement of excellence (366, 367).

Notwithstanding the need for diversity and equity in higher education to achieve national priorities, the work of faculty of color is undervalued. In a mixed methods study using data from a nationally representative sample of faculty and in-depth interviews with forty women faculty of color, Castro found that despite discourses in support of diversity and the presence of faculty of color, the boundaries of professionalism have remained rigid and unchanged from previous eras when only white males were found at universities. Although diversity and equity work in the forms of teaching, research, and service were integral to the professional identities of participants, their work was "systematically undervalued and denied legitimacy within the academic rewards system" (36) p.140. Hence, institutions incorporated faculty of color to satisfy the rhetoric of diversity, while structurally denying them legitimacy as scholars and educators due to the fixed and immutable norms of professionalism (36). This disadvantage is compounded by the minority tax, which results in faculty of color having less time to engage in pursuits that are more valued by institutions (333). Yet to teach, model, and achieve national goals for educational and health equity, health professions education must change.

Touting the importance of educational and health equity while simultaneously devaluing the time required to address this important goal is not only dishonest; it also reinforces inequities. Institutions that value educational and health equity must reject the status quo, expanding narrow definitions of merit and prioritizing work that improves education and health in the underrepresented, poor, and underserved. This will require encouraging expanded forms of knowledge generation, such as social justice frameworks and community-based participatory research, use of innovative pedagogies, and involvement in community-based service and practice. Broadening conceptions of merit means recognizing that such work is certainly as valuable as, and in many cases is of greater value than, producing an academic publication. A meaningful commitment to addressing educational and health equity would also help eliminate the minority tax that unjustly affects faculty of color (351).

Participants were able to powerfully influence the lives of students, other faculty, and their schools and communities in profound ways. Although it is known that faculty of color play a critical role in mentoring students and junior peers of color, what has not been well understood is the unique nature of this mentoring and the expert knowledge of exclusionary climates in health professions academe that faculty of color bring to the mentoring role. Moreover, the influence faculty of color have on health professions schools and in their communities is strong because it is often based on personal connection and moral commitment. In light of the often taken-for-granted and behind-the-scenes work that faculty of color engage in, making their strengths and contributions explicit is critical to our ability to appreciate, support, and aid them in this work. In addition, understanding the contributions of faculty of color sheds light on the nature of the work that all faculty must learn to do.

CHAPTER SIX

Group Differences

Institutionalized rejection of difference is an absolute necessity
in a profit economy which needs outsiders as surplus people.
As members of such an economy, we have *all* been programmed to
respond to the human difference between us with fear and loathing and
to handle that difference in one of three ways: ignore it, and if that is
not possible, copy it if we think it is dominant, or destroy it if we think
it is subordinate. But we have no patterns for relating across our human
differences as equals. As a result, those differences have been misnamed
and misused in the service of separation and confusion.

Audre Lorde (2) p.115

Beloved community is formed not by the eradication of difference
but by its affirmation, by each of us claiming the identities and cultural
legacies that shape who we are and how we live in the world.

bell hooks (368) p.265

Whiteness is a set of unearned privileges disguised behind structures of silence, obfuscation, and denial in Western societies (369). Because people of color in the United States live outside the boundaries of whiteness, they have many experiences in common. For example, rejection of Donald Trump's candidacy for president by a large majority of racial and ethnic minority voters in the 2016 election reflects common concerns about white supremacy. At the same time, people of color are an extremely diverse group. The use of in-depth interviews in this study provided the opportunity to gain a deep understanding of the contexts and conditions shaping participants' experiences and to identify patterns both within and across social groups. This chapter describes group differences based on gender, class, foreign-born status, and race/ethnicity. Although data from participants from historically black colleges and universities are included in other chapters, the experience of working at these institutions is included in this chapter. Thus, the last group difference I describe is institution type, specifically historically black colleges and universities.

Gender

In medicine 44 percent of assistant professors and 21 percent of full professors are women. Among full-time pharmacy faculty, women make up 61 percent of assistant professors and 30 percent of full professors (19, 20). In contrast, the total number of women faculty in nursing and dentistry is 94 percent and 31 percent respectively (18, 370).

Sixty percent of the sample were women, including seven Asian, forty black, seven Latina, four Middle Eastern, and two Native American women. That 60 percent breaks down into 23 percent from nursing, 16 percent from pharmacy, 16 percent from medicine, and 5 percent from dentistry. The small number of women dental faculty in the sample did not allow an assessment of gender-specific patterns in dentistry.

Women participants' experiences were shaped by representation of women among the faculty in the higher ranks and in leadership at their institutions. Women in medicine were more likely to report having their personal appearance scrutinized and their clinical judgment questioned by male colleagues than women in other professions. Consistent with the literature documenting a glass ceiling in medicine for women (371), there was a clear pattern that being a woman was a disadvantage in male-dominated fields, particularly in specialties such as surgery. Professor Rivera described this imbalance of power:

> We had a female chair who had some challenging personality traits. I'm not going to pretend that there was nothing. But the backlash, and this is in pediatrics, where now it would be slightly more than 50 percent of pediatricians are women, the backlash from the senior men in the department, the hostility toward her, was amazing, amazing. So there, it's still an old boys' club . . . There are a significant [number] of women sort of floating up to the top, but the men are still really holding the purse strings, which is really the critical thing. So you may have a lot of women surrounding the dean, but the dean's a man, always has been a man . . . And so the women have not got a hold of those divisions yet here. But they're at least at the, sitting at the table. So . . .

there are women sitting at that top table, but they're not the most powerful people in the room. [medical faculty]

The backlash against a "difficult" woman and lack of recognition of women's contributions, though reported less often, were also present in pharmacy. Professor Chen described her experience:

They [men] don't expect they need to listen to you . . . I know the women here on campus feel like we're not really heard. If we say something, it's somebody else's idea. It's not our idea. Or if we are assertive or express concern about something, then we're just being a bitch. And in that respect . . . I think there is sort of a stereotype—at least initially—about how they expect you to behave . . . I think they are especially . . . less receptive to people who are outspoken or pushy, particularly from an Asian woman, whom they expect to be submissive. [pharmacy faculty]

Dominant cultural norms that devalue women's abilities and police their behavior to promote conformity with gender stereotypes create roadblocks for women. Gendered/raced stereotypes further restrict women's behavior. Whereas Asian women described being stereotyped as submissive, black women feared being stereotyped as loud and angry. Either way, an assertive woman risked triggering a backlash. Professor Griffin provided an example of how raced/gendered stereotypes were used as a means of controlling women's behavior:

My girlfriend, a person of color, is a surgeon, and we hung out . . . I had more in common with her . . . which is kind of interesting, because . . . certain people say, "Oh well, that person is a hard ass" . . . like that person is not nice. And I'd go, "Oh, she's fine with me." I think it's how they perceive her because, okay she's tough on her job, she does her job, but does that make her a bad person? I've had nothing but positive interaction with her, and if we disagree about a case, well we just disagree. But I think it's perceived differently. Right now she's doing transplants . . . I think in her mind she has to be assertive. I mean you can't go into the operating room and not have some level of confidence about yourself. Because she's confident, some people take that as being cocky. I had the same experience when I did my residency at another university. There was one particular cardiology fellow who would get the same kind of treatment from some of the residents. They'd be like, "Oh, I don't want to talk to her." And I'm like, "I don't have any problems with her." And she was a person of color ... Maybe to them she came across as being a little bit too aggressive or trying to, and I'm like, "She's doing her job." We have more white males than we do anything else. I don't know what the whole big deal is but ... I've noticed that more so with the white males toward other African American[s] ... they'll just, they'll make that type of comment. It'll be like the angry black woman type of thing. [medical faculty]

Professor Swift described how the angry black woman stereotype affected her ability to speak:

As an African American, one thing you don't want to be characterized [as] is the angry black woman, which is the typical stereotype of my culture. I have to be really careful when I object or have an opinion about something. I feel like if my voice goes up maybe an octave or so in a faculty meeting, that people are a little—I have to make sure that I say it with the least amount of emotion ... possible, because I feel like it might be construed the wrong way. [pharmacy faculty]

In the female-dominated profession of nursing, the policing of women's gendered behavior in nursing schools was not reported as a concern, although gender inequity at the larger university level affected them just the same. Nursing is unique in that it views white men as a minority group because they are numerically underrepresented in the profession. Nursing schools pursue men, mostly white men, as students, faculty, and leaders. Reasons commonly given for pursuit of men include gender inclusivity and the belief that having a greater number of men in the profession will elevate status and pay (372).

Several authors have identified prejudice against men in nursing as a significant problem. In a review of gender discrimination in nursing, Kouta and Kaite stated, "Men entering the nursing profession encounter barriers that limit their choice of specialty and risk being labeled and stereotyped" (373) p.59. Given the existence of patriarchal gender-role socialization and the fact that nursing has long been seen as "women's work," it is not surprising that prejudicial attitudes toward men in nursing have been reported. In contrast, men are paid significantly more than women in nursing, and there is evidence to suggest they are overrepresented in leadership roles, the opposite pattern of what one would expect to see in an oppressed group. Hence, reports of prejudice against men in nursing paint an incomplete picture.

Sexism is an institutionalized and systemic form of oppression that privileges men over women in society. A system of oppression is the combination of power and prejudice, and men are systemically privileged throughout all sectors of society. Thus, while some women are prejudiced against men in nursing, such prejudice will not result in structural disadvantages for men, because women lack systemic societal power. Hence, as Smith described, "A man's experience in a traditionally woman's field is asymmetrical to that of a woman in a man's field" (4) p.36. In her study of men in female-dominated professions including nursing, Williams explained that men "take their power with them wherever they go" (374) p.260. As described above, examples of men's privilege can be found in salary studies. Muench and colleagues compared the salaries of 87,903 men and women registered nurses over a period of 11.4 years. The authors found men's salaries were significantly higher than women's for every year during that time period; they estimated an overall adjusted earnings difference of $5,148 (375). Similarly, Westphal's study of nurse leaders in US hospitals from 1992 to 2008 found the average salary for men was $5,443 greater than women's, despite greater proportions of men having less education and on average being younger than women. In addition, men were overrepresented in leadership relative to their percentage in nursing overall by 2 percent (376). Salary survey findings are consistent with the literature documenting a glass escalator effect in nursing and other female-dominated professions. The glass escalator effect refers to systematic advantages such as higher pay and rapid promotion, enjoyed by men in female-dominated professions (374, 377–381). Professor Said described her concerns about a glass escalator for white men in nursing:

> In nursing men are considered a minority, but almost all the men in the pro-
> fession are white, which means they are at the top of the food chain in the
> world, in the government, at the NIH, and [in] the university leadership. And
> white men at my school are treated like they are golden. They make more
> money than everyone else even at the lower ranks. They are overrepresented
> in administration. Nursing is a white man's heaven. [nursing faculty]

Although Professor Said's concern suggests that white men benefit from their gender in nursing, this study clearly indicates that black men do not. Black male nursing faculty were among those with the most negative experiences in the nursing sample. These findings are consistent with Wingfield's study of men's experiences with women's work. Wingfield found that race and gender intersect to determine which men will ride the glass escalator, stating that the advantage received by men "appears to be unequivocally true only if the men in question are white" (381) p.23. Consistent with the findings from this study, black men in nursing did not experience the advantages of white males, instead facing barriers to satisfaction and success, including a chilly climate and bias in promotion and tenure.

Class

Most participants reported coming from working-class or middle-class families. Participants from working-class families were more uncomfortable sharing information about their personal lives with colleagues than those from privileged backgrounds. Professor Howard described how her class background affected her experience as a student and faculty member:

I come from a very working-class background. My mother's a licensed vocational nurse and my father . . . never really kept one steady job. I came from a rural southern state, and it wouldn't have been any different for me, but luckily . . . I got a chance to go to a high school for science and math . . . And so it kind of put me in an environment where I was among people of different classes and . . . So I didn't feel as socially awkward as I think I would have if I didn't have that experience going into college. And so went into college—I went to a private school. I still felt some awkwardness, but I felt more comfortable with groups of people of different social classes. I would find myself not necessarily talking about where I came from as much. And so that was one of the difficult things, because other students would talk about some things that were going on in their lives and their families and . . . I felt kind of awkward not being able to share those things. My brother is still trying to find himself, as my mother calls it . . . sometimes in and out of jail . . . And my father is constantly unemployed, and so it is just a different type of experience. So when I got into pharmacy school, it was different at a historically black college . . . I met some people who had similar backgrounds to myself . . . There were a lot of students who . . . had varying backgrounds . . . I found a little group who had a similar background to me . . . At times, even here, I kind of still find myself with a little bit more social awkwardness . . . because my family . . . is still working class. Even I think possibly lower than working class at this point . . . And then . . .

my colleagues, when we're talking about things their family is giving them or having these trips or doing those type of things—so I will say, it's very difficult at times. [pharmacy faculty]

Similarly, Professor Garcia described the effects of class on her relationships with peers:

Because of my class background I just don't fall into conversation as easily . . . I feel like there is more of a hierarchy with people from different ethnic backgrounds, socioeconomic backgrounds, that have the same titles I do. And as far as falling into conversation easily, what I mean is, my colleagues will sometimes sit down and talk about the trips their parents took them on when they were little, something like that. Like "Europe, blah, blah, blah." And I just feel a little bit different. I didn't get to do things like that. And even now, I contribute to my mom's mortgage every month, and I contribute to my dad's therapy or other things. And I have school loans. They don't. Different worries, different things, I guess . . . They're just different. [medical faculty]

In contrast, participants from middle- and upper-middle-class backgrounds described this as a cultural advantage. Reflecting the intersection of race, class, and gender, Professor Dickerson described how her middle-class background helped her deflect the angry black woman stereotype:

The fact that I grew up in kind of a middle-class setting contributes to me not being an angry black woman, which I think helps things go better. I'm not perceived as a person who is always pulling out race, even though I'm on the Multicultural Affairs Committee . . . I'm not an angry black woman. If they're going to listen to anybody, perhaps they'll listen to me if I can find a way to get this working in different parts of the school. [medical faculty]

Professor Davis, who came from an upper-class background, talked about the link between poverty and educational disadvantage:

There still is a lot of inequality when it comes to the schooling system. I really still do feel if you're not born into at least—not like privileged, like super-rich, but privileged enough to go to the good schools and make the right connections—that you really are kind of crippled when it comes to trying to get on that path . . . If it's a private school, I mean obviously, you're paying and you're getting a good education. Out there the public schools are so poor that the only way you're going to get a good public school is if you're living in a rich area. I still think that that's a problem. [medical faculty]

At the same time that Professor Davis expressed concern about educational inequities, she also felt the need to differentiate herself from poor blacks when she experienced racism in academe. Here she described her response to discriminatory treatment during a job interview:

She [faculty interviewer] insulted me by just assuming that I was from a poor background and that I was just like all the other blacks. And I explained to her that I come from an affluent family, you know private school all the way. [medical faculty]

The racialization of Professor Davis on the part of her job interviewer assumed a working-class background based on race. Professor Davis felt the need to distance herself from poor blacks in response to the stigma associated with this background. She went on to describe negative perceptions of young minorities living in poverty, suggesting her own identification with a middle- and upper-middle-class bias:

When I talk to a lot of young people I say "Hey, what do you want to do when you grow up?" And it's always, "Oh I want to play ball. Oh, I can sing" . . . If I get lucky I'll find somebody who says [he or she wants] to be a nurse. And I say well, did you ever want to be a doctor? . . . And a lot of times these young people will say, "Well, it just doesn't take as long as medical school" . . . I just notice they sound like they're lazy . . . It's sad, but . . . a large majority of many minorities when they see how successful we've become as recording artists and sports stars and so forth—heck, why go for anything else? . . . And . . . in the lower income areas I've heard that and seen that, and it's really unfortunate. [medical faculty]

Although Professor Davis's class status was unclear to those unfamiliar with her, once that status was established at an institution, her privileged upbringing allowed her to fit in more comfortably with similarly privileged colleagues than did faculty of color from working-class backgrounds.

Foreign-Born Status

The 1965 Immigration and Nationality Act made significant changes to US immigration policy by sweeping away a long-standing national origins quota system that favored immigrants from Europe and replaced it with one that emphasized skilled labor. More than fifty years after passage of the landmark law, nearly fifty-nine million immigrants have come to the United States, reshaping the racial and ethnic composition of the country. Consistent with these changes, the migration of health professionals in search of a better standard of living, access to advanced education and technology, and greater political stability has changed the face of health professions education (382).

DEMOGRAPHICS

For the past half-century modern-era immigrants and their descendants have accounted for 55 percent of the nation's population growth and have reshaped its racial and ethnic composition (383). The attitudes of US adults toward immigrants vary depending on immigrants' origin. A recent national survey found attitudes are on average more positive toward Europeans and Asians, neutral toward Africans, and negative toward Latinos and Middle Easterners. Middle Eastern immigrants were viewed more negatively than any other group (383).

Each year the United States invites thousands of immigrants with professional skills to work in this country, including academicians and health professionals (384, 385). Academic employment of foreign-born, US-trained science and engineering doctorate holders has increased continuously since the 1970s, at a rate that has exceeded the growth in academic employment of US-born science and engineering doctorate holders. As a result, the foreign-born share of the total academic employment of US science and engineering doctorate holders increased from 12 percent in 1973 to about 26 percent in 2010 (386). In 2010 the foreign born accounted for 27 percent of physicians and 22 percent of nurses in the US health-care workforce (387). International medical school graduates make important contributions to the US health-care system; they are more likely than US-born graduates to work in primary care and to provide care to medically underserved populations (388, 389). Despite the importance of foreign-born faculty and their large numbers, many educational associations in health professions education do not publish data on foreign-born faculty, and none differentiate foreign-born and US-born URM representation. This lack of information poses challenges to assessing the proportion of URM faculty who are US born.

Twenty-four percent of the sample were foreign born, primarily from India. The remainder of the foreign-born sample came from other parts of Asia, Africa, the Caribbean, South America, and Mexico. Most foreign-born participants reported positive experiences, particularly Asians. Black and Middle Eastern immigrant faculty were more likely to report negative experiences.

THE EXPERIENCES OF FOREIGN-BORN FACULTY OF COLOR

The characteristics of having English as a second language and being a foreign-born person of color were intersecting exclusionary social positions. Faculty from Asia, Africa, and the Middle East frequently talked about the stigma of speaking with an accent. In addition, foreign-born faculty across the professions seeking resident status described barriers to career success. Finally, some participants suggested that faculty from countries with educational systems different from the West and who had not previously taught at a US institution would benefit from additional supports to ease their transition into the faculty role.

Speaking English as a second language and being foreign born were associated with experiences of discrimination and xenophobia. Professor Rodriguez perceived a preference for US medical graduates as a form of overt discrimination:

PROFESSOR RODRIGUEZ: Ranking agencies and reputation and a lot of prestige [are] given to how many US graduates a program has as opposed to having foreigners, so that is an incentive for programs to try to fill their ranks with US graduates. So ACGME [Accreditation Council for Graduate Medical Education] and the residents and review committee in other accrediting agencies are looking at the proportion of US graduates. That is basically pushing training programs to try to fill their openings with US graduates, which tend to be 80 percent white.

INTERVIEWER: Why is that distinction made?

PROFESSOR RODRIGUEZ: Because of discrimination . . . There's always been open discrimination against foreign medical graduates. Now things are changing, and the only reason [is that] there are not enough US graduates to fill all the openings, so they are forced to take foreign medical graduates . . . It's part of the whole equation. Because most foreign medical graduates are not white folks. They are minorities. Either from Africa or from South America, from

Asia. There [are] actually data from the American Board of Internal Medicine that foreign medical graduates perform better, with more sophistication than, us graduates. But I can tell you that as a resident I was discriminated [against], being a foreign medical graduate, but that's not race related as opposed to being foreign born. I'm foreign born, and I'm still being discriminated [against] . . . to some degree. You don't really see it, right. But you sense it sometimes. [medical faculty]

Similarly, Professor Gupta connected his schools' avoidance of international hires with racial/ethnic discrimination:

Racism, there are some issues . . . Sometimes our school does not want to have any race other than white unless they are bound to . . . For my position, for example, it was open for more than two years. And they are not hiring because they are not getting the type of people they expect . . . I applied here a year ago . . . They didn't even consider my application because at that time I didn't have a green card . . . He [search committee chair] was telling me, "Even though your cv was the best . . . we have a policy that we cannot talk about—our dean would not want anybody without [a] green card." . . . Other schools in the whole university have no problem with that, but the pharmacy school was like, "Okay, we'll not have anybody without a green card." . . . Very, very hard attitude toward people because they are not white. I serve on a lot of committees, and they don't want to interview international candidates. And I was really angry. I said, "How do you know after not even talking to them? How do you know if they are good?" . . . The attitude was like that. "Oh, they don't know anything. They cannot talk. They cannot speak. They cannot communicate. We don't even want to talk to them." . . . We had one applicant who was white American and so we didn't look at any other applicant. The committee . . . wanted to hire him. I said, "I have a problem with this guy." "Why?" I explained, "Because he . . . moved as a chair to a new school and within ten months, he was out of a job. Now he's trying to come here. Why is he out of a job? . . . Maybe he had some problem . . . We have to find it out before we do anything." Then they said "Oh, no, no, no, that is not his problem. That is the problem of the dean." I said, "How do you know?" And then I found out the dean was black. I said, "A school should not grow with a problematic dean—I don't think that is justifiable. To me, that is not the case and we should find it out." But nobody would hear me that it's not the dean's problem . . . Nobody would even hear me because he's white and the dean was black and my word has no value in fact. But after he was hired they found out all these things . . . When you are working on a committee closely, then you find . . . From the outside everything is good, nothing is wrong. But inside, there are some problems. [pharmacy faculty]

As a faculty member of color who spoke English as a second language, Professor Rangan was subjected to a humiliating requirement for speech remediation:

They were having the pharmacy accreditation site visit. And before that they asked all the faculty to be present so they can give orientation about accreditation . . . and there were a couple of faculty who were of different color and whose native language was not English . . . The management told us, "What if the accreditors think that because your native language is not English and you're teaching students and students won't understand" . . . and then that made faculty of other color, or faculty whose language is not English, a little bit uncomfortable because we all cleared our English proficiency exams even before entering into graduate school, and even after graduate school we went through a series of English proficiency exams . . . to prove that we can speak good English. Anyway, coming back to that . . . Management asked us to go through speech therapy to get our English better so they can show the accreditors that we have sent these non-native English speakers to go through speech therap[y] and now they are good. So this experience I did not like at all, and it was the same with other faculty too, they did not like it . . . I decided at that moment okay, I have to get another job. [pharmacy faculty]

Speaking with an accent was described by most participants as stigmatizing. Professors Gupta, Kone, and Hamid described how some people focused on their accents to embarrass them and exclude them from academic life:

PROFESSOR GUPTA: If the students are doing [well], they say good things. They say I am the best professor they've had in their entire life, something like that. And when the students are getting Fs or Ds they have complaints. I think that is usual. And the most [common] complaint is, "He has [an] accent." I say, "All of you have an accent. I have an accent and you have [a] different accent . . . I have [a] different accent. That's all." [pharmacy faculty]

PROFESSOR KONE: They [colleagues] try to always say, "Can you please say it again? Can you say it again?" . . . to make you embarrassed. [pharmacy faculty]

PROFESSOR HAMID: I have an accent so that sometimes . . . people try to give you the impression, "I don't understand you, what you are talking about?" . . . Sometimes people do that on purpose to embarrass you. Like my accent does not make me comfortable sometimes while talking in a meeting. [pharmacy faculty]

Professor Hamid went on to talk about how his school avoided using non-European, foreign-born faculty as representatives to market academic programs:

The school wants to show the people who do not have an accent and they are white . . . When the school does a video or any marketing the dean would choose the people who don't have an accent . . . She wants them to represent the school. [pharmacy faculty]

Foreign-born faculty without US residency faced disadvantages to career success. Professors Iglesias and Jan commented on such barriers:

PROFESSOR IGLESIAS: I still don't have a green card. And I have been applying for one, but it hasn't been successful yet. Hopefully now that the university is sponsoring me there is going to be a change to get a green card and at some point become a citizen . . . That has not been easy, and I have been spending a lot of money on it for lawyers . . . That's been a hurdle . . . The one thing that I would feel segregated by is the fact that, yeah of course, some resources are for Americans and some others are not, which to some extent I do understand, but it's really unfair to the highly trained people because, like just to name a name, the president is very adamant about it. He says, "We're training PhDs and we're not doing everything we can to keep them and generate jobs for them." And of course some people would agree and disagree with that . . . But of course it makes it more difficult; if I didn't have that barrier I would be able to apply for grants at an earlier stage of my career. [dental faculty]

PROFESSOR JANI: When you come from a foreign country you need sponsorship. So I think when I was applying for my permanent residency I was the first person in the university who was going for this, so they were not very well aware of the process. They were not initially very serious about things . . . My boss ... was like, "If you leave because of this that would be [a] shame." I think what seriously happened was that they [the university] had their own lawyer and they were not really pushy about things. They were kind of lax, but it's my will and I need to take things more serious. I would say something, and it would never go to the right person. I kind of struggled in that and for me it's very important to get permanent residency, because if I don't get that in a specified time, I'm on a work visa, I'll be kicked out of the country. I had to get that done. I think things were moving really, really slow because I couldn't communicate directly with the lawyer. It has to go through steps. I communicate to my chair, and it goes to [the] dean, and then [the] dean goes to HR. So it was going through a lot of steps and all that. Eventually when I got another job offer my boss got serious, and I was able to communicate with the lawyer and things went really fast. [pharmacy faculty]

Faculty from South Asia and the Middle East, where educational systems are different from the West, suggested orienting foreign-born faculty who had not previously taught at a US institution. Professors Hamid and Rangan described the need for such an orientation:

PROFESSOR HAMID: Normally they [foreign-born faculty of color] don't have any exposure [to] for example . . . benefits. We don't know anything about 401K . . . life insurance or disability insurance . . . and that stuff or teaching, or sometimes there's some things in my culture different from the culture here. For example, in my culture it's okay that the faculty would marry his student, but here it's forbidden . . . So I believe these things should be, more orientation . . . I believe especially in the beginning . . . there should be more orientation or different orientation programs . . . for the faculty of color, especially if they have a different culture. [pharmacy faculty]

PROFESSOR RANGAN: I [feel] with people of color who haven't been trained in this country, they go to either extreme. Some of them, they're too nice to students, and some of them are like too harsh . . . I think that's where faculty of color from different country need some kind of training on how to deal with students . . . Setting that nice balance of saying "No" but in a very nice way and saying, "Yes, but you have to do this instead." So that's something [that] I feel . . . we at least, I'm including myself in that, need to be trained [in] because that's something . . . we don't know. Because it's a tactical thing and it's a cultural thing, I feel because we grew up in a very straightforward environment, if there is something wrong we will put [that] in very harsh words and we'll be very stern and we'll be very effective, which will backfire very badly if [a] student doesn't like it, and it will spiral into a conflict. But it won't be the case if you can deal with that situation in a nice, calmer way. So I think that's where special training or special orientation is required. [pharmacy faculty]

Professors Hamid and Rangan's concerns may be addressed by publishing explicit policies and providing orientation materials and individualized mentoring. Schools and mentors need to be aware of the needs of foreign-born faculty without prior exposure to US institutions.

Foreign-born faculty of color are a large, growing, and diverse group who make substantial contributions to health professions academe. Their stories reveal experiences of exclusion in academic life rooted in the intersection of their foreign-born and racial and ethnic social positioning. Speaking English as a second language compounded their vulnerability to such exclusion. Despite these commonalities, I also identified differences in the experiences of foreign-born faculty across racial and ethnic groups.

Race/Ethnicity

ASIAN FACULTY

Demographics. Asians are the fastest growing racial group in the United States (390). In 2010 Asians (4.8 percent) and Asians in combination with one or more other races (0.9 percent) made up 5.6 percent of the US population, a 46 percent increase over ten years (391). Fifty-nine percent of the US Asian population are foreign born (390). In 2008 South Asians were the single largest group of immigrants with advanced degrees, comprising 7.8 percent of all advanced degree holders in the United States (384). In this study Asian participants made up 20 percent of the sample. Seventy percent (*n* = 14) were foreign born, mostly from India but also from China, the Philippines, and Vietnam. We also had one Asian Pacific Islander participant.

The experiences of Asian faculty. With the exception of nursing faculty, Asians are overrepresented among health professions faculty. Overrepresentation in the health professions and a large proportion of foreign-born faculty created differences in the experiences of many Asian and URM participants. People from countries with race relations that significantly differ from those in the United States do not form their racial identity in the same way as those who are US born. The desire to integrate into a new culture and lack of familiarity with the history and complexity of US structural inequalities decrease the depth of some immigrants' understanding of racism (392). This was true for some foreign-born participants, including Asians.

Overall, Asian faculty reported more positive experiences than any other racial/ethnic group. Although discrimination was a problem for many, Asian participants, particularly men, were less likely to report experiencing exclusion and control than others. In addition, Asian men immigrants were among those least likely to identify racism as a problem or to express concern about the underrepresentation of minorities in health professions academe. Professor Dee, a US-born faculty member, and Professor Tata, a foreign-born faculty member, shared such views:

INTERVIEWER: What do you think would need to happen to address the issue of underrepresentation of minority faculty?

PROFESSOR DEE: I'm not sure that students are asking to have more of a particular [type of] faculty member. It's not so much who, but how it's being done and whether the quality of the instruction is good or not good . . . Do you recruit on the basis of ethnicity even though they're not quite as qualified? Or just to fulfill that requirement of underrepresentation? Or do you recruit on the basis of qualification: How well they do their jobs? [dental faculty]

PROFESSOR TATA: I have not seen the experiences of minorities being influenced by ethnicity . . . I believe that it is just human nature that if somebody discriminates against me even based on my professional performance, in the back of my mind there is that 1 percent part thinking, is it because of my color? But I don't believe in that personally. But I have seen people say that or believe that might be the factor. I personally don't believe that, at least not with pharmacy, because I believe that doesn't exist. [pharmacy faculty]

In contrast to the views described above, many Asian participants, particularly those who were US born, described an awareness of systems of oppression and supported institutional diversity initiatives. These Asian participants worked to improve diversity and equity in the health professions and provided effective mentorship to other faculty and students of color, as described by professors Kumar and Mossman:

PROFESSOR KUMAR: My research focus is on race and ethnicity, . . . disparities in health-care delivery, and diversity in the health professions. [medical faculty]
PROFESSOR MOSSMAN: I think that I have a little bit better connection to students of color or prospective students of color than Anglo faculty. And the other thing is I've felt compelled to advocate on behalf of students of color in the workplace. Not only because of my cultural connections but also because [of] the concept of paying it back or paying it forward. [pharmacy faculty]

Due to a 55 percent increase in the number of pharmacy schools since 1987, there has been a dramatic increase in the number of international US pharmacy graduates. In 2011 international students made up 16 percent of new pharmacy doctorates and 45 percent of new pharmacy PhDs (217). Comments made about the overrepresentation of Asians, and in particular Asian Indians, occurred most frequently among pharmacy participants. Although some viewed the large influx of Asians into the professions as a positive contribution to diversity, others perceived it as a threat to opportunities for URMs. Professor Sanchez described this concern:

INTERVIEWER: Many of the people that I've talked to [who] were from India consider themselves to be minorities.
PROFESSOR SANCHEZ: Oh stop. You know how many Indian faculty members there are in the school of pharmacies all over the [United States]?
INTERVIEWER: Yes, I know they're overrepresented.
PROFESSOR SANCHEZ: They are so overrepresented. Stop, stop right now. If I were to roughly give some numbers about our faculty, here the group does clearly overrepresent our Asian Indians . . . I am one of two Latinos in the whole school of pharmacy . . . I think the concern in terms of health care and having Asians overrepresented is that when we go out into practicing roles where we're actually dealing with patients . . . I have African American friends who want an African American pediatrician for their kids . . . In areas where you have big immigrant populations, where there's an issue with language, then it would make sense to have health-care professionals who are of ethnicity, and

clearly we need to encourage Latinos and no other group. It's very difficult. I used to chair that committee here for a number of years, and it's very difficult to attract students [who] meet the criteria who are Latino who want to pursue pharmacy, or any health-care thing for that matter . . . We don't have a lot of students who are African American. We don't have a lot of students who are Hispanic. Sometimes I see someone with a Spanish last name and I get all excited and they're Filipino. We have Filipinos going into health care a lot . . . I'm like, "They're Latinos" and then I'm like, "Oh, they're Filipino" and I can tell because they look Asian . . . You still want to see Latinos. [pharmacy faculty]

Despite their overrepresentation in health professions education, Asians are a minority in the US population, and Asian faculty have reported experiences of discrimination in the higher education literature (164, 393). Asian participants in this study also experienced exclusion and control, but fewer described this experience than other groups.

BLACK FACULTY

Demographics. In 2010 blacks (13 percent) and blacks in combination with one or more other races (1 percent) made up 14 percent of the US population, a 15 percent increase over the previous decade (394). Almost 9 percent of the US black population are foreign born, a threefold increase since 1980 (383). Wealth inequality for black Americans has grown worse over the past twenty-five years, posing a challenge to opportunities for large segments of this population. In 2013 the wealth of white households was thirteen times the wealth of black households, the largest gap since 1989, a result of cruel historical and contemporary inequities (395). Foreign-born blacks ages twenty-five and older fare slightly better than those who are US born. They are more likely to have a bachelor's degree, are less likely to live in poverty, and on average have higher household incomes than those who are US born (383). Research has shown differences in racial identity between foreign-born and US-born blacks. Foreign-born blacks are more likely than US-born blacks to identify by ethnicity, and for Muslims, by religion than by race (396, 397). Differences in perceptions of discrimination among blacks based on native origin have also been documented (396).

Fifty-eight percent of participants identified as black (*n* = 56) or black in combination with another race (*n* = 2). Ten percent of black participants were foreign born (*n* = 6), including people from Africa and the Caribbean.

The experiences of black faculty. As described in chapter 1, black faculty reported the most frequent and severe exclusion and control of any group in the sample. Most black participants described the need to strategically manage racial discrimination to be successful in health professions academe, and many reported experiencing additional stress from this burden. Stereotypes of black people as intellectually inferior and violent haunted their interactions with their colleagues and students, requiring they constantly be on guard against making errors. In addition, black faculty described feeling the need to avoid appearing angry to escape being negatively labeled by supervisors and peers. Many also mentioned that students had never seen a black faculty member before, making students doubtful about their qualifications. Professors Jennings and Green described the pervasive nature of negative stereotyping affecting blacks:

PROFESSOR JENNINGS: I have my students write a reflective portfolio about what groups of people . . . they [have] been taught stereotypes about as they were growing [up]. I would say 90 percent of the students say African Americans. I have them . . . speak about some of those stereotypes, and this is in a reflective portfolio only I read, so they are free to be as honest as possible. And they say that their parents, their grandparents, talk bad about African Americans. They say that they're lazy, they're disrespectful, they're criminals, and so you should stay away from them. And then they talk about . . . their particular stereotypes and biases that they were taught by their family . . . So that for me that really explains a lot. And if I'm being taught something about people and hearing sarcastic comments about them and just negative comments, that's going to infiltrate into my mind and it's going to have an effect on my interaction with them. I'm not going to trust them, or I'm going to not feel as comfortable. [pharmacy faculty]

PROFESSOR GREEN: If it's Caucasian, it's assertive. If it's black, it's aggressive. I think I have to be much more careful how I speak, [adjust] tone so as not to get maligned. I have to monitor how much I say, when, tone, volume, posture, a lot more. I need to make sure that I'm welcoming in my posture. Not a whole lot of hand movements and all of that . . . I don't think people are intentional at all in their exclusion, but they are probably less comfortable with African Americans. [pharmacy faculty]

Professor Chang reflected on the severity of discrimination experienced by Asian and black faculty:

I don't think the stereotype of the model minority helps me as an Asian person. But I think from what I've seen of our black faculty, they have had a much more difficult time . . . And I think they had a very hard time proving their credibility here in the school. Which I think is just awful . . . Recruiting black faculty here, I would tell them to come with their eyes wide open. [pharmacy faculty]

Although exclusion and control was prominent in the stories of black faculty members overall, some participants described differences in treatment based on first-generation or foreign-born status. Black US-born faculty who did not report immigrant roots in recent generations were described as being treated more poorly than first-generation and foreign-born black faculty. Professor Green, a first-generation black faculty member, described his experience:

I felt sometimes I was treated preferentially above my minority classmates because I was of West Indian background. It's like, "Oh, you're basically not like them [African Americans]." The white students are [more] willing to accept me because I'm really West Indian than they are to accept other African Americans. You know, they have issues. "But you're not like them." So whenever I do good, I'm not like them. Isn't that weird? If you do bad, you're like them. [pharmacy faculty]

Professor Kendall described how she was treated differently than students from Africa during training:

I went to pharmacy school, at an African American school, so predominantly a historically black university. And we had classmates [who] were from Kenya, Nigeria, [and] so on and so forth. And we would go on rotation, and it would be like those students had less to prove than we did, for whatever reason. I don't understand why. It would be like maybe they're better at math. Maybe they're stronger at this or that. And then it just transitioned into residency, where my coresident was from Nigeria and we're both on the same rotation, and that individual is respected more than me. And it's not male-female. It's female-female. Because I think that does contribute to it sometimes, male-female . . . And then going further into fellowship. And I've just kind of seen that pattern over and over again. [pharmacy faculty]

Similarly, Professor Ibori described differences in the treatment of US- versus foreign-born black faculty:

I'm not really African American—I wasn't born here. I came from a different culture. I've always felt that the white faculty treat me differently from an African American who was born here . . . I feel that they tend to treat me a lot better than they would the African American faculty, in terms of mentoring, in terms of support, and resources, and so on . . . I must say, I got my pharmacy degree from . . . a historically black college and university. And I even saw among black faculty that there was this differentiation between an African and an African American . . . I think the African American faculty that I've encountered seem to have a much harder time than I do . . . Being that I'm from a different culture, I think I'm accepted a little better. There's less quote-unquote fear, if you will, of saying things around me, and so on.

INTERVIEWER: What do you think is the reason for that?

PROFESSOR IBORI: I've thought about that a lot . . . I really don't know why that is, but in terms of faculty treatment, I think it's just that there's less of what you might call a threat to the white faculty, especially the predominant faculty. Because I'm just from a different culture, I don't have any ax to grind or anything like that, so I think that's part of the reason.

INTERVIEWER: What do you mean when you say, "ax to grind"?

PROFESSOR IBORI: Well, I've been told by white faculty because they'll tell me this. They'll say, "Well, African American faculty sometimes come in, and they have a chip on their shoulder, if you will, and . . . they're not very easy to work with." . . . I've never found it to be true. That's what, sometimes, they tell me, but it's not because anyone is difficult to anyone else. I think it's just that they don't trust one another enough to be able to carry on the conversations and communications and maybe even work together. [pharmacy faculty]

In a book on faculty diversity, Moody differentiated between what she called domestic nonimmigrant groups and immigrant groups. Nonimmigrant groups are "African Americans, Mexican Americans, Puerto Rican Americans, American Indians, and Native Hawaiians" (21) p.xvii. Moody's distinction between non-immigrants and immigrants is based on a very specific view of US colonization. According to this view, not only are the foreign born defined as immigrants, but so too are their US-born offspring. As an example, Moody categorized President Obama as an immigrant. Moody justified this approach by saying, "The secret to power all [emphasis not added] . . . immigrants had and have is this: they chose of their own volition to come to this country to start a new life. They came with extravagant dreams and an abundance of hope" (p.xvii). I do not agree with Moody's monolithic characterization of immigrants, which ignores the negative effects of Western colonization on non-US soil as well as the influence of US policies on the formation of refugee populations. The current Syrian refugee crisis offers a relevant example. Syrian families, having fled violence and destruction, must now endure the burden of trauma, loss, and hate as they are forced to seek new homes in unwelcoming countries. Hence, Syrian refugees are not coming to Western countries with extravagant dreams and abundant hope, but instead with grief and horror that they must attempt to overcome in a foreign land. Although I recognize that there are cultural differences between Americans who are the offspring of immigrants and those who are not, I do not agree that people born in the United States should be described as immigrants. Categorization of US-born faculty and students as immigrants ignores the complexity of first-, second-, and third-generation experiences as well as multiracial and multiethnic identities in the United States. As an example, my nephew, son of an African American and an Arab American, is applying to medical school. It is not clear if Moody's scheme were in use whether he would be categorized as an immigrant or nonimmigrant. Despite these differences in perspective, I believe Moody raises a critical issue. Although differences among Africans, African Americans, and blacks of varying origin are tracked among applicants and enrollees in US medical schools by the AAMC (398), other health professions do not make such distinctions (71, 217, 399), and these group differences are not tracked at the faculty level either (18, 20, 72, 76). Moreover, measurement of these ethnic differences alone does not directly reflect US versus foreign-born status in these populations. This blurs the line of progress, making it impossible to hold institutions accountable for ensuring adequate opportunities for US-born URMs, particularly those who come from disadvantaged economic and educational backgrounds. Given the severe disparities in income and wealth that exist in America, US-born blacks are among those most likely to face such disadvantages. Black participants were more likely to express this concern than participants from other racial and ethnic groups. Professors Howard and Lang expressed their concerns about the lack of tracking of US-born black students:

PROFESSOR HOWARD: Many people other than African Americans don't see the difference . . . When our faculty look out and they see a class and they see people that you would consider black, they think the class is diverse, you know what I mean? They're not differentiating between the fact that this is an international student and not an African American student. So they say, "What's the problem? The class is diverse." I mean, how do you explain the fact in a way that doesn't sound biased itself and say, "No, I'm not talking about that kind of black person. I'm talking about another kind?" So it kind of puts you in a bad position too, because you could come across as looking biased, and you don't want to look as though there is a battle between the blacks, what I mean the African students versus the African American students and all that. So that's been a very difficult issue for me to approach. [pharmacy faculty]

PROFESSOR LANG: Every time [I attend] . . . our white robe ceremony . . . just trying to figure out how many African Americans there are . . . We have a lot of Africans. When I get one with an American name and she happens to be black, I'm like, "Oh, we've got an African American, very good." [pharmacy faculty]

Professor Jordan also expressed a wish to see more US-born black students:

I don't actually have any students at all that are like African American, just blacks, just from the United States. I don't have any. All the students that are here are from Africa somehow. So it's different. So when I look at my pool, I mean obviously I try to treat everybody the same, but it is a bit different. I would love to see that there are just more people like me, who were just born here and just, just a black girl, but there aren't. [pharmacy faculty]

Black faculty are among those who are most visible and subjected to stereotypes that undermine their credibility as intellectuals. Although this places black faculty in a disadvantaged position, the experiences of this diverse group are not monolithic. The findings suggest that US- versus foreign-born status is one difference in this population worthy of greater attention.

LATINO FACULTY

Demographics. Latino/as are the second fastest growing racial group in the United States (400). In 2010 people of Hispanic or Latino origin made up 16 percent of the US population, a 43 percent increase over ten years (401). As of 2014, Mexico was the single largest source country for the nation's immigrants (28 percent) (383).

There were fourteen Latino/a participants in the study. Of those, 14.3 percent (*n* = 2) were foreign born, having immigrated from Mexico and South America.

The experiences of Latino/a faculty. In general Latino/a participants were less likely than black and more likely than Asian participants to experience exclusion and control at their schools. Latino/a faculty living in areas with a higher representation of Latino/as in the population tended to have more positive experiences because their institutions were more likely to recognize the importance of admitting Latino/a students. Some commented on the burden having darker skin placed on faculty members regardless of their racial and ethnic backgrounds, and others commented on how having lighter skin allowed them to more easily blend in with the dominant group. The significance of having a clearly identifiable Spanish surname, the benefit of speaking Spanish for education and patient care, and the need to address the educational needs of undocumented Mexican immigrants were also themes uniquely described by this group.

Hispanic or Latino is the only ethnicity the US government uses as a standard category. According to this official classification scheme, Latino/as may identify as any race (402). Not recognizing the legitimacy of US government racial classifications for their own lives, in 2010 37 percent of Latino/as selected "some other race" as an option rather than selecting Asian, black, Native American, Pacific Islander, or white on the US Census (402). This uncomfortable fit reflects both the diversity and history of this group, made up mostly of indigenous-, European-, and African-origin peoples. Professor Rodriguez commented on the diversity of the Latino/a population:

> Latin Americans are not all the same. So I think Cubans are a certain group, and they behave in a certain way. Puerto Ricans are different, Dominicans are different . . . I'm Latin American and I try to interact with all of these groups in Spanish, so I have made friends over the years regardless of where they came from, the Philippines or Cuba or Nigeria or Mexico. [medical faculty]

Latino/as with lighter skin and more European features in the sample described having a greater ability to blend in with whites than those with darker skin. Professor Ortiz described her experience:

> Often people will say, "Oh, you don't even look Hispanic," because I guess I don't look it or whatever—and their idea of what a Hispanic person looks like . . . When I first started this appointment nobody knew that I was Hispanic,

and I certainly didn't bring it out in any way, shape, or form. But here quite a [bit] of our patient population is Spanish speaking . . . I have had occasion to have to speak Spanish. And that is how it came to be that people started asking me, well, "How do you speak Spanish?" And I would say, "I'm Puerto Rican," and they would just say, "Oh, I had no idea." [dental faculty]

When Latino/a faculty were not recognized as such by others, they sometimes endured derogatory comments made about Latinos in their presence, as described by Professors Alvarez and Larson:

PROFESSOR ALVAREZ: What I always found interesting was that I was always either the exception or I was always welcomed into the group . . . I do have the Latin culture in me but I guess not so much that it affects my interaction with them. And a great example that I have, this is when I was in school . . . I was working as a pharmacy technician and one of the lead techs said something along the lines of, "God forbid my daughter bring home a Hispanic guy." And I was standing right next to her and she's like, "Oh, oh, but not you, you're different." And that's how I've seen myself, especially in those situations where I may be the only Hispanic person, I may be the only person of color there. They see me in that way, but they don't see me in that way, at the same time . . . It probably has more to do with the fact that I don't have an accent, that I'm not super—I mean like I said you can look at me and probably tell that I'm Puerto Rican, but for somebody that doesn't really know, there can always be that shadow of a doubt. I think it's more of just the fact that I kind of fit in and I'm not too ethnic for them. [pharmacy faculty]

PROFESSOR LARSON: I'm [in] kind of a unique situation, I'll put it that way. My birth father was born in Puerto Rico. He and my mother were divorced when I was very young. I was born [with the last name of] Cruz. My mother remarried, and then my stepfather adopted me. So when they did that process, my name changed. If you were to look at me, most people would not guess just by visual appearance that I'm Hispanic at all. In fact, I've actually been categorized as Caucasian when they haven't asked, and someone has just filled out a form with my demographic information. So my experiences are maybe unique in the aspect [that] people may not identify me [as] being [of] Hispanic descent. They may actually identify me more as Caucasian. So the uniqueness of this is that people sometimes confide in me their beliefs about other races and ethnicities, not realizing the situation. I grew up in a state where there's a large Mexican American population. Moving to the South, there's not as many Mexican Americans. In my undergraduate years meeting some of the people that live in the rural areas in the South, they've made comments, derogatory comments about Hispanics in general; . . . I usually let them say all that they're going to say and then I announce to them that I'm Puerto Rican. Usually I watch their embarrassment afterward, or with other friends who knew that I was Puerto Rican, and then they would kind of—in one particular situation they kind of egged the person on and got him to say all sorts of stuff. Then they announced that I was Puerto Rican and actually asked me where my father was from. So in all the situations, the person who is making the derogatory comments was thoroughly embarrassed and apologetic . . . It will certainly make them think twice about what they say to people. [pharmacy faculty]

Having a Spanish surname was described by some participants as important, not only for personal identity, but also as a means to communicate their ethnic background to a larger group. This was particularly common among participants with lighter skin. Professor Sanchez described her experience, comparing herself to a lighter-skinned black friend:

Depending on where I am, if people meet me they'll say I'm Latin American or they'll say I'm Italian or they'll say I'm Spanish like they're not sure. I have an accent, and I know that, and it's not going to go away. I know that [in] the scheme of Puerto Ricans I'm on the lighter skin with dark hair. Some people think I'm European, but my last name is Spanish. The second half of my last name is hyphenated because I married a man from up here. I wasn't about to give up my Spanish last name for him because that's part of who I am. I think with my friend from another university, she is a very light black person, but you can tell she is African- American, right? For her the African American thing is more of a theme. She grew up here. I'm sure she experienced racism and discrimination more . . . than I ever did. [pharmacy faculty]

Similarly, Professor Garcia commented on the importance of keeping her Spanish surname:

PROFESSOR GARCIA: I think just the students can see my last name and know that I'm a fairly successful physician. I'm an educator, I think it's important to see that because I don't look Hispanic, I'm not dark, I'm very light complexioned, most people confuse me for white. When they hear me speak Spanish, they say like, "Oh! Where are you from?" I kept my last name for that reason. [medical faculty]

Professor Rodriguez commented on how relying on Spanish surnames as a marker of identity can both identify and exclude Latino/a faculty members:

PROFESSOR RODRIGUEZ: I attended a meeting last year sponsored by a pharmaceutical company on how to address health issues in the Latin American population, on rheumatoid arthritis for example. And they invited me and I accepted and I went and that was 100 percent addressing Hispanic health. There are people who do this full-time; I may have done it two to three times in the last ten years or twenty years. I don't push that much on my own. Unless I'm invited to participate.

INTERVIEWER: And why do you think you get invited to participate?

PROFESSOR RODRIGUEZ: Oh, because my name is clearly Hispanic so it's hard to miss that. I mean Rodriguez doesn't really sound German does it? So other Latin Americans have an Italian last name, which is part of our previous discussion, or they may be called Jose Epstein, and the last name would be Jewish or whatever, and they're actually Latin American, and they have a very heavy accent. But they're not identified as Latin Americans because their last name is not Hispanic, it's not Spanish. So they're also part of our group, but they're probably left alone—I mean unless [they] become permanent in our community they're not visualized as Hispanic because their last name doesn't sound Spanish … The US system from the government, federal government identifies Hispanics just going by their last name. So they are missing a whole fraction of people who are also Hispanic, they're also native Spanish speakers, and maybe they don't even speak English, but because their last name doesn't sound Spanish they're not included in that list of US Hispanics. [medical faculty]

Speaking Spanish and being able to connect culturally with Latino/a patients was described as an important contribution by participants. Professors Ortiz and Garcia described their contributions to patient care:

PROFESSOR ORTIZ: I was born in Puerto Rico and my first language was Spanish … Here quite a few of our patient population [are] Spanish speaking; they are low income, and a lot of Medicaid people come through. And I have had occasion to have to speak Spanish … So I do think that there's value in having Hispanic faculty for sure. [dental faculty]

PROFESSOR GARCIA: My colleagues are all really happy and proud that they have at least one Spanish-speaking physician, from my Hispanic background on the team . . . I think our hospital is lacking in Spanish-speaking faculty . . . We have like something like 350 to 400 patient beds . . . I feel like I made a difference in my patients' [lives] when they see a physician of color, and I can speak their language, and you could see a sense of relief. For the school of medicine, I think it's nice for all students of all colors to see me, you know, a Hispanic physician. They get a sense of my background and culture and appreciation for having someone that knows the language and understands the culture. [medical faculty]

Although speaking Spanish was usually described as an ability that strengthened their faculty roles, some participants did not receive appropriate credit for their work. Professor Sanchez described how her knowledge of Spanish was used by the university in a way that detrimentally affected her path toward promotion:

INTERVIEWER: You mentioned that you weren't promoted at your previous job?
PROFESSOR SANCHEZ: The guy who was the president at the time got invited to go on a trip to Cuba. They started looking through all the faculty to see if there was anyone who knows Spanish because they were getting these e-mails from Cuba in Spanish. The next thing you know, I have to talk to the president and translate all these e-mails for him. The next thing you know, I go to Cuba with the president of the university, which is a small university. We're in Cuba, which was great. I'm like, I really can't complain. I get to go to Cuba because I happen to be the only Latino in the freaking place. I could translate e-mails. The next thing you know, we started getting into other collaborations with the school of pharmacy in Peru, so I also got to go there. They gave me an extra appointment at my previous job, where I was a special assistant to [the] president there for Latino stuff. As I went up for promotion I claimed all those things that I did as special assistant to the president, a service to the institution. The dean at the time said I couldn't use those things because I was being paid an extra stipend for that . . . I really think he was just kind of looking for an excuse not to get me promoted. [pharmacy faculty]

Concerns about opportunities for undocumented youth to enter the health professions education pipeline were also uniquely mentioned by Latino/a faculty. Professor Larson described his experience:

As I'm becoming more senior in the college, . . . I would like to become involved with the admissions committee and see what's going on out there. Why there's not Hispanics who are applying. I don't know if there are blockades prior to pharmacy school that are limiting them, but if you look at the Hispanic population here, it is growing. I don't necessarily see that same growth in the college of pharmacy. So I don't know if the students aren't pursuing careers here in pharmacy in this city. I think maybe the larger number of Hispanics in this city relates to larger numbers of immigrants that are coming through. So when I see the demographics in the city, oftentimes the Hispanic people that I see and that I know are immigrants. They emigrated here from Mexico. My wife actually teaches high school in a town just south of the city. So like one of the students that we work with—he works with us in coaching soccer—is an illegal alien. Wonderful kid. Fantastic kid. Super smart, he is the kind of kid where I can see him becoming a pharmacist or health professional at some point, but his status is limiting his ability to do that. He is working now on becoming a citizen, and they have a process kind of laid out for him to do that. Before just this year, there was no process, like for his brother there was no process. So his brother took jobs that were cash jobs, construction type jobs even though he was smart enough that he should have gone to college and could have become a professional in any area that he was interested in. So that's my big concern with this city, is whether or not there's a blockade for people that are Hispanic to move up. That blockade is not there as much for the African American students. [pharmacy faculty]

Latino/a participants were dedicated to providing care to underserved patients in their communities. Some even paid for medications for patients who were unable to afford their own prescriptions. In addition, this was the only group of participants who specifically described their bilingual abilities as important skills for patient care and who were also uniquely concerned about educational opportunities for undocumented youth.

MIDDLE EASTERN FACULTY

Demographics. In 2015 a Forum on Ethnic Groups from the Middle East and North Africa was held at Census Bureau headquarters to discuss plans to test a Middle Eastern or North African category on the 2015 National Content Test (403). Topics for the forum included the collection of data using the term "Middle

Eastern or North African" or "MENA" and the Census Bureau's plans to classify and tabulate Middle Eastern and North African responses for the 2020 Census. Although people from the Middle East and North Africa are currently categorized as white by the US government, this has resulted in a large undercount, because many do not recognize this identity (404–407). Because Middle Eastern and North African Muslims are less likely to identify as white than Christians from the same regions, the undercount has worsened as immigration of Muslims to the United States has increased (408). Distrust of how the Census Bureau has and may again use information about Arab American populations in collaboration with Homeland Security also contributes to the undercount (409). Thus, current estimates of the Middle Eastern and Northern African populations in the United States are both unreliable and fragmented across multiple ethnic groups.

Middle Easterners and Northern Africans include a large foreign-born population. Immigration from 1948 to 1965 was triggered by political unrest, including the 1948 Arab-Israeli War and revolutions in Egypt and Iraq in the 1950s. Partly as a result of the restrictive US quota system, immigrants who arrived during this period were highly educated. The removal of the quota system in 1965 opened the door to a mix of people seeking family reunification, education and employment opportunities, and safety from war and persecution. Post-1965 immigrants had a similar level of education to prior immigrants but came in much greater numbers and included a higher percentage of Muslims. Between 1980 and 2010 the size of the Middle Eastern and Northern African immigrant population increased fourfold; between 2010 and 2013 immigration in this group increased a further 18 percent, to 1,017,000. As of 2013, approximately 1.02 million immigrants from the Middle East and North Africa region lived in the United States, representing 2.5 percent of the nation's 41.3 million immigrants (410). The total current population of Middle Eastern and Northern Africans is 3.7 million (411).

Although there are no data on representation of Middle Eastern and Northern African faculty in the health professions because this category is not generally counted, we did find one study reporting Middle Eastern ethnicity. A study of medical school deans at eight Ivy League schools in 2013 reported that 7 percent were Middle Eastern, providing evidence of overrepresentation of this group in medical school leadership (12). We interviewed five Middle Eastern participants. Four were Arab, one was Persian, and three were foreign born. Three of the five spontaneously reported their religious affiliation as Muslim. The small group of Middle Eastern participants experienced exclusion and control in the same ways that faculty of color from other groups did.

Experiences of Middle Eastern faculty. Themes unique to Middle Eastern participants included rejection of government classification, being mistaken for another ethnicity, post-9/11 alienation, and for Muslims, religious stereotyping.

A public opinion poll in 2015 found that only 40 percent of Americans had favorable attitudes toward Arab Americans, and only 33 percent had favorable attitudes toward Muslim Americans (412). A second poll found that 32 percent of Americans favor placing limits on the civil liberties of Muslims (413). In light of the reality of anti-Arab and anti-Muslim racism in the United States (414), the categorization of Middle Easterners as white sometimes paradoxically placed these faculty in positions of greater marginality. Professors Hassan and Said described their concerns:

PROFESSOR HASSAN: Sometimes by some of the white faculty we're considered white. We don't contribute to this diversity business that you are saying, that you want a diverse faculty. But in the meanwhile, we don't get treated as white. It's very obvious at all kinds of levels, and even walking in the street you are treated differently, and you can recognize that treatment. Even if it's subtle, you can recognize that I'm not treated as mainstream. So I'm thinking, well, I don't get thought of as white . . . Like I'm not asking for a scholarship . . . I'm not trying to use the resources and not . . . be beneficial to the country or to the state. In the meantime, again, you can see a difference in how people treat you. [nursing faculty]

PROFESSOR SAID: I am not white. That is not my culture. Also I don't get treated as white. I don't get paid the way they do, and I don't have the same workload. I don't get the same treatment. It's at work. It's on the media. It's attitudes everywhere that are very extreme and insulting and go unchecked. I always check "other," or else I leave race information blank on forms. [nursing faculty]

Middle Easterners' and Northern Africans' skin tone and appearance vary widely and include both light skin with straight hair and dark skin with Afro-textured hair. Like participants from other racial and ethnic groups, some Middle Eastern participants endured derogatory comments made about their group in their presence, as described by Professors Ahmed and Said:

PROFESSOR AHMED: I'm at somewhat [of] a disadvantage or advantage because sometimes people don't know what I am. They'll say things in front of me they probably wouldn't say in front of other people of color . . . It feels awful because then I look at this person and go, "Oh, so that's what you're really like." So kind of like getting inside knowledge on someone. [pharmacy faculty]

PROFESSOR SAID: My skin tone varies depending on the time of year, but I have an olive complexion. The university diversity office staff member thought I was Latina for years until I told her otherwise. It is common for me to be approached by people speaking Spanish. I always feel bad because I don't fit the bill. People seem disappointed . . . As an RN working in the hospital, the patients would often call me that "Indian nurse," or the "Hawaiian nurse." Pretty much every shift patients would ask me, "Where are you from?" Since I was born and raised here, this can be an annoying question. In the beginning I would just tell patients about my ethnic background, but the response was always so negative that I quickly started making up answers and that worked much better . . . I do remember once a patient making negative comments about an Arab physician who was not in the room that were pretty bad . . . I didn't say anything because it wasn't worth it. I learned a long time ago Arabs are an unpopular group, so a lot of times it is better to keep your mouth shut. [nursing faculty]

Middle Eastern faculty also described not fitting in, an experience that was intensified in the post-9/11 era. Professor Hassan described the impact on her family:

INTERVIEWER: Did you notice any change with 9/11?

PROFESSOR HASSAN: Yeah, I did. Many changes actually . . . Some changes were positive, and some changes were negative. People questioned why Muslims do such acts . . . Some staff would say hurtful things . . . but they'll make you feel that you're different. You have other people who were more sympathizing, or more feeling with you . . . And I think what hurt me the most is how my kids were treated at school. So the kids were picked on, they were bullied, they were told, "You're a terrorist," or "You're Saddam's cousins," for example. Even now my kids sometimes . . . say, "Well, you did not do anything about it." And I said, "Well, I cannot. What can I do about that?" I think that . . . was bringing a lot of tension too, family-wise, work-wise. People start . . . double guessing you or—are you good or are you bad? Are you with us or are you with them?

Or are you going to hurt someone? People start being not sure about you as a person … That was very tough. Very tough. It was very tough also for another reason, because I had a family member whose plane was diverted and he stayed there for ten days. He had a heart attack. So for me, it was a very stressful time, but yet I know that the American people suffered, but I was suffering too. My family were suffering too. But of course this was not about you. Your suffering, nobody cares about. [nursing faculty]

Professor Said described feelings of alienation post-9/11:

I remember driving to work that day and I heard the news on the radio. The first thing in the morning there was a program faculty meeting, and people couldn't function. They were crying. Throughout the day everyone had on a TV or radio. No one was working. They were all immobilized by grief. So many people distraught and crying. Of course I felt sympathy for the victims and their families and for the faculty in pain. But I can tell you what stood out for me that day is what little value my friends and colleagues placed on the lives of innocent Arabs, babies, who have been dying for a very long time. They [faculty] basically could not function because of these deaths in New York. The number of deaths from 9/11 was very small compared to the number of deaths that have happened in Palestine, in Iraq, and other places and no one bats an eye when those events happen even though they are tied to US policies. It struck me. I kind of knew it all along. But seeing the difference in their response, I really felt how different I was. I saw value in lives they didn't. Lives like mine. If I was distraught and became immobile every time 3,000 people in the Middle East died, I'd be fired. But the truth is these tragedies do affect me. It is hard to take. One positive aspect is that I understand what it is to struggle, what it means to be dehumanized, and this allows me to provide support to students of color regardless of their racial or ethnic background, in ways that most white faculty don't seem to be able to do. [nursing faculty]

Participants were not asked to reveal their religious identity or spiritual beliefs during interviews. Therefore, findings about this aspect of identity are not based on systematic collection of data. However, a few participants did disclose their religious affiliation as part of their stories. Christian participants described their faith as a source of strength rather than as a social marker. In contrast, Muslim participants described their religion as a source of discrimination. Professor

Hamid described how stereotypes of Muslim men as oppressive influenced his relationships with colleagues:

> My wife is wearing the headscarf, which is called hijab, . . . and she's actually a faculty [member] also at my institution. And one time another faculty [member] who is a close friend to me, she told me, "Okay, I want to tell you something, and I won't argue because I know you are a great guy and I really trust you, but I have a question that everyone is talking about, and I feel [I] need to talk with you about it." I said, "What about?" and she said, "Your wife is wearing a headscarf and long clothes, and this is very hard where it's almost 100 degrees, and the other faculty in the department are saying that you are forcing her to do that because it's the culture of the Middle East to force their women to wear the clothes that the men want." And I told her, "No, why did you assume that? She has her own ideas, and she took that decision to wear these clothes. I know they are heavy, and it's very hot outside, but this is her decision and it's not mine." . . . I believe that happens a lot . . . people talk [even when they] speak with me frankly about their concerns about why my wife is wearing headscarf especially in the very hot weather, they can't understand although I explain to them . . . and that is a problem for me. [pharmacy faculty]

Middle Eastern and North African faculty are an understudied group. To my knowledge, with the exception of a single narrative with findings similar to this study (415), this study is the first to explore the experiences of Middle Eastern faculty in health professions education. Greater attention to the experiences of this group in the United States is warranted, given its increasing size and the widespread xenophobia targeting Middle Easterners and Northern Africans and Muslims, suggesting these groups are particularly vulnerable to negative stereotyping and discrimination.

NATIVE AMERICAN FACULTY

Demographics. In 2010 Native Americans and Alaska Natives (0.9 percent) and Native Americans and Alaska Natives in combination with one or more other races (0.7 percent) made up 1.7 percent of the US population, a 9.7 percent increase over the previous decade (416). The small numbers of Native Americans and Alaska Natives are a consequence of the holocaust inflicted on them following white colonization of North America (417). Currently, 22 percent of American Indians and Alaska Natives live on reservations or other trust lands, and 60 percent live in metropolitan areas (418). Poverty rates for Native Americans and Alaska Natives are similar to those of blacks and Latino/as, with one in four living in poverty (419).

Three Native Americans participated in the study. Although these three participants were highly satisfied with their positions, this satisfaction was contingent on institutional support and respect for their work in Native American health. The higher education literature supports the importance of institutional support for Native American cultural values and tribal connections (150, 298, 309). Reports from Native American faculty in the literature whose commitments to their tribes have not been honored by their institutions have described this as an invalidating and oppressive experience (315, 420).

The experiences of Native American faculty. Some Native American participants reported being perceived by others as ethnically indistinct, resulting in experiences similar to those described by some Latino/a and Middle Eastern participants. Participants also described encountering disrespectful comments about Native cultures and expectations that were antithetical to their values in academe. Finally, institutional support for work with tribal communities was critical to participants' satisfaction and success.

Professor Smith endured disrespectful comments related to Native American cultures:

> It's not glaringly evident that I'm American Indian. People will look at me and say, "Is he African American? Is he Hispanic? Is he Italian?" I mean because of my skin color and some of my physical features, they know that I'm not from eastern or northern Europe, but they wouldn't necessarily connect me with being American Indian, and so there's been times when people have made off-color comments, some related to American Indians. Sometimes they're unintentional, and sometimes you kind of wonder if it's completely intentional. I mean, people make comments about, "Let's have a pow-wow" ... and they don't have a cultural reference; they're just using our phrase. "We have too many chiefs, not enough Indians involved in this project." Stuff like that, where it just rubs you the wrong way and you recognize that. Why are we still using these old references, ... even in a place where you think people would know better? [medical faculty]

Invalidation of Native values at Professor Yazzie's first institution contributed to her decision to leave her position:

I was put on a tenure track, and one of the things you're supposed to do is tell everybody about all your accomplishments, write up this yearly event, saying, "I did this, I did that," and that's kind of not Native . . . However, that's part of the tenure track. You're supposed to write out your portfolio. You're supposed to do all that. However, it's very counterintuitive to Native culture. Passive forbearance or Native noninterference [holds that] you don't interfere with somebody else's right to be who and what they are . . . It was like a daily occurrence . . . It was just like how the world was; it was culture shock for me . . . I was a new mother . . . I remember one time going to graduation, and one of the faculty said, "People need to hire sitters like we did when we had our kids, and leave their kids at home instead of bringing them to graduation." And I thought, well, not all the people are like you. I didn't say anything. But in Native American culture, we bring our children to everything. That's just how it is. I understand not all the mainstream is like that. And I had a young daughter who was sick all the time, so I was really trying to balance being a professor, taking care of her, and trying to get my research going and all of these kinds of things. And I knew they didn't make allowances. I had read, like two or three times, that if you were going to have children, don't have them until after you were tenured, because there was no mercy . . . The turning point was [when] they had . . . a forum . . . They took four faculty [members] and had them speak about being on the tenure track and their experience in getting tenure. One was an African American, one was Hispanic, one was Asian, and one was Navajo or Native American. And the first three people talked, and then the fourth person was the Navajo woman, and she was kind of young, about my age. She got up there and she started talking, and then she started crying, which is sort of unusual for a Navajo. And she couldn't, she didn't bawl, but just got choked up, and it took her several minutes. And then finally she told her story and her path to getting tenure . . . The auditorium was packed . . . This Navajo woman pretty much said some of the things that I had said, but not directly . . . which is part of being Native, that passive forbearance, not being confrontational. She did it in an indirect way. So afterward, I was walking back to the college and two or three or four of the faculty caught up with me and had a lot of questions for me. And basically, they asked me if it was the same for me. And I said, "Well, yeah. I had some of those same experiences." [nursing faculty]

Professor Yazzie's cultural values, such as welcoming children as part of the community and passive forbearance, were not respected; she left her position and found another one where she was able to translate her cultural values into her faculty role. Support for Native culture and health were integral to her job satisfaction.

Professor Cleary described her contribution to Native American health and the support she received from her institution:

> Being an American Indian helps this research aspect, which was lacking on our campus . . . The college has supported that and encouraged that . . . That is my area, and that's why they're able to develop a research center that crosses the school of medicine and college of pharmacy. We're situated next to the reservations here. Several reservations, and we're very close in proximity to one in particular. It's definitely facilitated my research that way. [pharmacy faculty]

Similarly, Professor Smith described the institutional support he received for his work:

> There's one other faculty member who came on a year ago who is identified as American Indian, but for a long time I was the only faculty member, and so there's been a lot of really good experiences added as a result of that . . . The good experiences are partly the result of having a very supportive . . . division head who always recognized the value of health disparities research, recognized the value of having someone like myself who was connected to the American Indian communities here in the state. I was also at the time well connected to our state health department, and so it was also value there . . . Now being the co-director of our center here . . . has . . . elevated what I do across the institution. In my role as a center director I'm a member of our faculty executive committee, which only opens to department chairs that are directors and institute directors. [medical faculty]

Participants all made critical contributions to Native American health and education. Each was connected to tribes in his or her state and mentored Native American students. Institutional support and recognition of this important work was key to these participants' satisfaction and success.

Historically Black Colleges and Universities

Historically black colleges and universities were established to serve the educational needs of black Americans at a time when they were denied admission to white institutions. The history of historically black colleges and universities is rooted in black communities' commitment to education and empowerment, which has been "particularly meaningful given the sociopolitical policies and practices that deemed black men and women as incapable of succeeding as learners because of the unfounded belief that their race made them inferior and unable to appreciate the benefits of postsecondary education" (421) p.312. Prior to the *Brown v. Board of Education* decision in 1954, 90 percent of black students attended a historically black college or university. As a result, historically black colleges and universities have a long history of providing access to education for blacks as well as other first-generation, low-income, and historically underrepresented populations (422). Given increasing enrollment of black students in predominantly white institutions, some have raised questions about the continued need for historically black colleges and universities. Such questions are predicated on the assumption that predominantly white institutions, benchmarks, and standards are the norm against which all other higher education institutions should be judged (423). Yet there is evidence to suggest that despite significant inequities in political and financial resources between historically black colleges and universities and predominantly white institutions, historically black colleges and universities serve greater numbers of socioeconomically disadvantaged and URM students while better preparing them for future employment (424, 425).

Although black students now have access to predominantly white institutions, and historically black colleges and universities make up only 2 percent of postsecondary institutions (426), historically black colleges and universities continue to graduate 50 percent of black professionals (422). In 2011, 24 percent of black doctoral degree holders in science and engineering received their baccalaureate degrees from a historically black college or university (427). In addition, the social mission of historically black colleges and universities for health-care students makes significant contributions to primary care and care of the underserved. A study of US medical schools found that three historically black colleges and universities ranked highest in the social mission of medical education. Interestingly, social mission ranking was inversely related to NIH funding, suggesting that some institutions prioritize getting research funding over graduating a health-care workforce that will directly affect health inequities (428). Historically black colleges and universities also outperform predominantly white institutions in the racial and ethnic diversity of their faculty and leadership opportunities for women and faculty of color. As an example, 60 percent of medical school faculty at historically black colleges and universities are black, compared to 2.6 percent at non-historically black colleges and universities. Similarly, 73 percent of chairs in medical schools at historically black colleges and universities are black, compared with 2.2 percent at non-historically black colleges and universities (429). Clearly, historically black colleges and universities are a critical resource for diversifying the faculty of health professions academe and the health-care workforce and for providing leadership 90opportunities for faculty of color. Despite their important contributions, historically black colleges and universities continue to be inequitably funded relative to predominantly white institutions, resulting in chronic financial challenges (423).

DEMOGRAPHICS

In 2008 the percentages of blacks in nursing, medicine, pharmacy, dentistry, and public health who received their health professions degrees from historically black colleges and universities were 9.1, 14.6, 46.2, 38.4, and 8.2 respectively (107). In 2009 historically black colleges and universities accounted for 17 percent of all health professions degrees earned by blacks (430). An impressive 65 percent and 70 percent of black physicians and dentists respectively graduated from historically black colleges and universities (422). Participants from historically black colleges and universities in the study included one dental and four nursing school faculty members.

THE EXPERIENCES OF FACULTY FROM HISTORICALLY
BLACK COLLEGES AND UNIVERSITIES

Unlike participants at predominantly white institutions, participants at historically black colleges and universities spoke of a racially diverse environment that was inclusive of faculty of color. Professors Yates, Ross, and Finch, all faculty at historically black colleges and universities, described the large proportion of URMs that made up the faculty and student bodies at their institutions:

PROFESSOR YATES: The full-time faculty, I really couldn't give you a number right now, but estimating . . . I would say 98 percent are faculty of color. And the dean is a person of color. [nursing faculty]

Professor Ross: I would say that maybe 50 percent or less of our students are African American, and maybe forty, forty-five-plus students are West African, followed by West Indians, and then we're getting other minorities as well . . . There [is] a mix of people . . . The mix is predominantly black. [nursing faculty]

PROFESSOR FINCH: When people speak of diversity at professional schools, I can tell you this dental school is as diverse as you can ever get just in origin, where people come from, be it from Africa, Iran, Caribbean, Africa again. It's just a very diverse population . . . I would invite anyone if they want to see diversity at their professional schools. [dental faculty]

The large number of faculty and students of color at historically black colleges and universities created an environment of comfort for participants, as described by Professors Finch and Wakefield:

PROFESSOR FINCH: It feels like you're home in an African American setting. It gives you a certain comfort level. You deal with your people. That's the best way I can put it. So there's a certain comfort level. You can say certain things without having to worry too much . . . what the reaction will be of the person you are speaking to. You pretty much are all, to a large extent, on the same wavelength and even when you're not, you can agree or disagree agreeably. It's a different comfort level. [dental faculty]

PROFESSOR WAKEFIELD: There's always somebody you can talk to if you need to talk to somebody. Whereas when I was at my two previous institutions that were predominantly white, there might be a couple of people you could talk to, but they weren't really interested. They weren't supportive. I just feel a greater sense of trust, and I feel like people have a vested interest in my success. [nursing faculty]

Professor Finch went on to speak of a strong commitment to the education of black students at historically black colleges and universities:

If you're an African American person, person of color, if you will, you're with your people. You don't want to do them wrong; you want to do the best for them. Now this is not to say if you were in a predominantly white setting you would want to do the white students wrong. You want to see them succeed absolutely. You want to see them succeed. Not that you wouldn't want a Caucasian student to succeed, because we have those at the school, also, but you just want to give it the best you can give it. Maybe I'm being idealistic, but that's my approach to it. [dental faculty]

In turn, students treated faculty with respect, an experience that was not always the case in predominantly white settings, as described by Professor Wakefield:

Here I would say that there is almost implicit respect from students . . . and I think that's part of being a student in a relationship with a faculty of color. [nursing faculty]

Professor Ross, who had a white supervisor, was the only participant from a historically black college who did not describe comfortable race relations:

The dean and I are of different ethnic backgrounds. The dean is a European, and she tends to recommend I follow other disciplines within this college . . . that have nothing to do with nursing . . . For her to recommend [that] I follow an allied health model is demeaning . . . So I'm not sure exactly the reasoning, but it feels like racism because everything I do, her response is that I need to follow someone else. In the city, all of the city, and in health-related initiatives I'm viewed as a leader. But the person I work for believes that I need to follow someone else. [nursing faculty]

Other challenges described by participants included lack of mentorship for faculty, as described by professors Yates and Wakefield:

PROFESSOR YATES: I think for me the biggest concern from [a] faculty standpoint is the lack of mentorship for new faculty. I am not an educator . . . I'm a clinician who is teaching a clinical master's program, so I'm really coming from that standpoint. I'm not understanding the learning theories and the curriculum developments, etc., I see at school. Even if I did come from an experienced background, just to understand the system as a whole, [there] was little mentorship offered . . . If I consider teaching after my contract ends . . . [I will] see if there are mentorships. And I asked that on my interview. I did ask that, and they told me that "there's nothing formal but I am here," that was the dean at the time, as your mentor. I'm not so sure she is available for that . . . My question about mentoring new faculty would be my number one question if looking for a new position, and if there is not something formal in place, it would not interest me. [nursing faculty]

PROFESSOR WAKEFIELD: The new faculty are not getting as much mentoring as they need. I don't think there's anyone that they can't go to if they need help, but I think it should have been built in. [nursing faculty]

Professors Finch and Ross described lack of resources at historically black colleges and universities as a serious problem affecting faculty recruitment and retention and program quality:

PROFESSOR FINCH: The simple fact is they don't pay enough money. They don't pay enough money. You need to be doing this out of [the] goodness of your heart, except if you don't really need that salary to live on. I guess maybe just like most historically black universities, they just don't, at least the dental schools, just don't pay that well. The predominantly white universities have the endowed chairs and endowments and stuff like that; they can offer these salaries. We just cannot do it. To be quite frank with you, I don't know if you've kept up with the reports about how they're in dire straits . . . Because of the salary, the young people that I know that have left here go to the VA [Veterans Administration], where they get paid a whole lot more money. If that continues, if that trend continues, I think it's a bad trend and does not portend well for the future, and students lose because they don't get the attention they should be getting. [dental faculty]

PROFESSOR ROSS: That's one issue here is salary, number one. And it's, to me, I need to be tipped for staying so long with the salary as it is. And I say to myself, I think, I hope, I keep hoping that it will get better. Is that ridiculous? [nursing faculty]

Professor Ross went on to describe the lack of resources at her nursing program:

As I sit in this office and look around, it does not speak to the level expected for the section of nursing. I had two people that I interviewed. They were European. They came in, both of them looked around this office and said, "Where's the program office?" I said "This is it." Needless to say, the next day they declined the offer, because even though this is a clean room and it doesn't have a lot of clutter, it doesn't speak to what people think a program office or a dean's office should look like . . . The programs actually added a secretarial position, a typist, and two adjuncts in order to become successful for their accreditation . . . Even the accreditors recognized that we were a low-resource program. And then they were surprised that we were able to do the things we were able to do. [nursing faculty]

Despite the fact that historically black colleges and universities are underresourced, they serve a large number of students who speak English as a second language. Professor Wakefield explained:

A challenge for a lot of historically black universities and colleges, especially if they are located in diverse cities, is they are faced with individuals [for whom] English is their second language. So they're struggling with not only concepts of nursing and skill, but language. Language. I mean you talk about English with them . . . And I understand it's okay, but it's hard enough for students for whom English is their primary language, American born and raised, to even think of what is this English person asking me, much less somebody [for whom] English is their second language. [nursing faculty]

Although historically black colleges and universities serve large student populations with additional learning needs while being underresourced, participants expressed a commitment to working at these institutions. Professor Ross described her commitment:

INTERVIEWER: What influenced your decision to work at a historically black university?

PROFESSOR ROSS: I attended one as an undergrad, and as a graduate student my doctoral program was in a majority school, but in the doctoral program as well . . . the faculty was very diverse. So of course when you have had [a] positive experience, you feel you want to share that experience with those who may not have [had] that experience. I felt confident and positive, plus my doctoral thrust was in speaking for those who don't have a voice. So my service has always been in the public sector, trying to uplift those who have had challenges. Whether it was in accessing health care or accessing a quality education or gaining the confidence you need in order for individuals to do whatever they needed to do in the profession. And after all, I am the one that can help others. [nursing faculty]

Although lack of mentoring was a problem mentioned by participants at all institution types, only participants from historically black colleges and universities described the challenges of educating large numbers of students with English as a second language and significant institutional financial challenges. These findings reflect the diverse populations traditionally served by historically black colleges and universities as well as chronic inequities in funding experienced by these institutions relative to predominantly white institutions (423). In contrast, satisfaction with the institutional social mission and the diversity and equity climate was higher in participants at historically black colleges and universities than among those working at predominantly white institutions.

Summary and Recommendations

The mosaic and hybridization of cultures in the United States create experiences that include areas of commonality and difference among faculty of color. Social hierarchies that pervade US society are also reproduced in health professions academe, with marginalization across gender, class, country of origin, language, and the color line. All groups have something to contribute to education and patient care because they reflect a segment of the US population, and through their diversity, strengthen the excellence of health professions academe. In addition, although most participants were concerned about providing care to minorities and the medically underserved and supporting students of color, each racial and ethnic group in the sample had something unique to offer, with greater awareness of the challenges faced by people of like background. Examples included Latino/a participant concerns about undocumented youth and Native American participants' connections with tribal nations.

Women faced disadvantages in male-dominated fields, particularly in medicine. In addition, the negative experiences of black men in nursing were notable. Fear of black boys and men, grounded in stereotypes, results in disproportionate disciplinary action in the K–12 system against black boys (431) and incarceration of black men at unconscionably high rates relative to all other groups (432). These inequities place this group at a disadvantage, sending negative messages that must be overcome if we are to see growth in the numbers of black men in health professions faculty. Disparities between undergraduate enrollment and graduation rates for black men and black women at predominantly white institutions and historically black colleges and universities further reflect the importance of attending to recruitment and graduation of black men in health professions education and mentoring members of this group for an academic career (433). The AAMC has raised concerns about declining enrollment of black men in medical schools, highlighting the need to attend to this group (434).

Underrepresented minority physicians serve a disproportionately large share of racial and ethnic minorities, uninsured, and people on Medicaid. Furthermore, URM physicians from all class backgrounds serve greater numbers of uninsured and people on Medicaid than white physicians, including those from working-class backgrounds (364). However, findings from this study suggest that clinicians' class background influences their ability to understand and connect to people of color from working-class backgrounds. Hence greater representation of faculty of color from disadvantaged economic backgrounds is a critical priority. This does not mean that students of color from middle- and upper-middle-class backgrounds who apply to health professions schools do not need to be admitted in greater numbers. It means additional efforts to ensure representation of people of color from disadvantaged economic backgrounds in the health professions are vital to ensure quality care for all people.

Foreign-born faculty make vital contributions to health professions education and care, especially in light of the rapid influx of immigrants into the United States and increasing numbers of international students. Despite the importance of foreign-born faculty, greater attention to the numbers of US-born URMs is needed. Collection of data to track representation of US-born URMs has been neglected by health professions schools and educational organizations. This recommendation should not be interpreted as meaning that the number of foreign-born URMs, whose contributions are vital, should be decreased. Rather, it raises the possibility that attention to factors inhibiting representation of US-born URMs in health professions faculty may be needed in order to increase their numbers.

Results from the small sample of Middle Eastern participants provide preliminary evidence that this group is also worthy of greater attention. The negative stereotypes and low job satisfaction reported by most participants, combined with the virtual absence of information about their experiences, is striking. The possibility of a continued influx of refugees and skilled workers into the United States from the Middle East and North Africa in the future and the increasingly negative attitudes toward this group highlight the need for further investigation.

Finally, study findings highlight the important role of historically black colleges and universities in the education of black and economically and educationally disadvantaged students. The positive racial climate present at these institutions, compared to that at predominantly white institutions, provides evidence for the effectiveness of a large mass of faculty of color to improve institutional climate. The diverse student body, including a large number of English-as-a-second-language students served by historically black colleges and universities, warrants greater funding, not less, as has chronically been the case for these institutions. Historically black colleges and universities play a critical role in advancing health professions education, providing a model of service to the community and graduating large numbers of URMs while providing a climate of respect for faculty of color. Predominantly white Institutions should look to historically black colleges and universities, not only as sites to recruit diverse graduate students and faculty, as has often been the case, but as institutions with missions, cultures, and traditions from which much can be learned to promote racial and ethnic diversity in health professions education.

Voices of Change

LESSONS LEARNED FROM THE

EXPERIENCES OF FACULTY OF COLOR

IN THE HEALTH PROFESSIONS

If access to health care is considered a human right,
who is considered human enough to have that right?

Paul Farmer (435) p.206

The determination of who is worthy to be admitted to a profession
in many ways defines that profession.

Geneviève Moineau (436) p.9

Health professions education has a moral obligation to serve the nation's health based on the assumption that all human lives, regardless of social background, are of equal value. Most health professions' ethical codes, although largely focused on the care of individuals, also recognize the importance of working to ensure just health outcomes (437–444). As described in the preceding chapters, the hegemonic norms of whiteness give birth to policies and practices that perpetuate educational and health inequities and detrimentally affect the satisfaction and success of faculty of color. White racial domination was reflected in participants' reports of exclusion and control; the common occurrence of exclusionary institutional climates; and narrow understandings of what it means to be a good scholar, clinician, or student in the health professions. The problem of underrepresentation and isolation of faculty of color at predominantly white institutions is not a new finding but is important nonetheless. The negative effect of isolation on participants' opportunities for collaboration, mentorship, and promotion and on their personal well-being was often severe.

Leaders' commitment to nurture, protect, mentor, and hire faculty of color for leadership roles is vital to achieving equity. Underrepresentation of faculty of color in leadership negatively affected the satisfaction and success of participants. Although several participants were themselves in leadership roles, many also reported barriers to leadership opportunities. Participants described leaders of color as sensitive to the needs of faculty and students of color and committed to educational and health equity more often than they described white leaders as being so. History has shown that the racially homogeneous leadership of health professions education has not engaged in the kind of decision making needed to achieve educational and health equity since passage of the 1964 Civil Rights Act (445, 446). The responsibility of leadership in health professions education for human suffering over this sustained period of time is real.

Connecting Social Justice with Racial and Ethnic Diversity in the Health Professions

The United States contains inequalities that are morally alarming, and the gap between racial and ethnic minorities and whites, rich and poor, is widening. The chance of being born one race or ethnicity rather than another determines the life chances of every child who is born. If you are a black child born in America, you are four times more likely than a white child to be born into poverty; the future of a black boy is six times more likely to include a prison term prison than that of a white boy (447, 448). Regardless of poverty level, schools serving mostly racial and ethnic minority children are underfunded compared to districts that are 90 percent or more white (449, 450). Societal inequities create gaps affecting the odds of becoming a health-care professional as early as third grade (451). Any attempt to address the state of diversity in the health professions, and along with it the satisfaction and success of faculty of color, must confront these inequalities and the challenges they pose.

For health professions education to help make a better world, "we must acknowledge right now that we are citizens of one interdependent world, held together by mutual fellowship as well as the pursuit of mutual advantage, by compassion as well as self-interest, by a love of human dignity in all people, even when there is nothing we have to gain from co-operating with them. Or rather, even when what we have to gain is the biggest thing of all: participation in a just and morally decent world" (452) p.18. Many health professionals who are embedded in the current system of inequity experience moral distress, reflecting their connection with the human beings they care for (453, 454). It is this inner voice that health professions educators must attune themselves to for change to occur. Working to make social justice the overarching paradigm of health professions education promotes human fulfillment while providing a blueprint to achieve equity.

Making a Personal Commitment to Social Justice

My father introduced me to social justice struggle. In 1948 he was driven from his home in Lydda, Palestine, at gunpoint, part of a mass exodus that would later be referred to as a death march (455). A Palestinian historian quoted my uncle Haj As'ad Hassouneh, who described the miles-long march on foot in the summer heat: "There was no water. People began to die of thirst. Some women died and their babies nursed from their dead bodies. Many of the elderly died on the way . . . Many buried their dead in the leaves of corn" (455) p.71. This trauma haunts our family and shaped my upbringing in the diaspora. At the same time, as an Arab Muslim girl I also experienced gender oppression in my community. Violence and abuse was tolerated, and I was married to an abusive man at the age of fifteen. When I left the marriage at age twenty-three my soon to be ex-husband tried to murder me. People I had known since I was a child put up money to bail my abuser out of jail; a series of judgments and rationalizations had rendered my life worthless in their eyes. Soon after that I married an American black man. When we met, some of his family resided in the public housing he had grown up in, and I became familiar with the challenges people living in that community faced. Later I met Lizzi, a woman with quadriplegia, who became my closest friend. Although Lizzi was a leader in the disability community, an activist, and a scholar, she faced social barriers to personal freedom, respect, and health care. Through these relationships and my own experiences, I have seen and experienced oppression through multiple lenses. My resistance to interlocking systems of oppression such as racism, sexism, heterosexism, disablism, and the violence of colonialism, all hierarchies governing unequal resource distribution, is an affirmation of my own human life. Every health professions faculty member can also choose to make this commitment; those who remain silent are also making a choice. There is no neutral ground.

Human Agency and Implicit Bias

Implicit biases, which are pervasive and robust, have a number of negative effects on education, health, housing, employment, and the criminal justice system (456). Some participants attributed their experiences of exclusion and control to implicit bias, while others were suspicious of this explanation. Perhaps this is because both implicit and conscious biases are malleable. Human agency is made possible by the interplay of automatic and conscious mental processes. Because "conscious mental causation is at play in matters we really care about," implicit bias can be overcome (457) p.458. Any assertion that whites cannot conquer racial bias is a refusal to privilege the history of whites who have given their lives in the struggle for racial justice over those who have chosen to maintain racist thinking (368). Hence, implicit biases can be changed with conscious intention and time should people choose to do this work.

The Fallacy of Race-Neutral Policies

Race-conscious strategies to achieve educational and health equity, which are intended to repair the damage done by discrimination, serve a compelling societal interest. The advent of color-blind racism and attacks on distributive justice in the post–civil rights era have decreased the use of race-conscious strategies, supporting use of race-neutral approaches to student admissions and hiring. In a survey on race in America conducted in 2015, the Kaiser Family Foundation found that 78 percent of Americans believe hiring, promotion, and college admission should be based strictly on merit and qualifications other than race or ethnicity, yet the qualities and achievements that constitute merit have evolved in the context of a white supremacist society (458). Race-neutral policies do not allow for procedural differences in the treatment of individuals by race or ethnicity, but the population outcomes of such policies belie claims of neutrality. Participants reported pervasive racial biases in admissions, hiring, and promotion under the guise of policies that were purportedly race neutral. As long as policies are enacted by people who fail to challenge white racial dominance and possess implicit and conscious biases, and occur in exclusionary institutional climates, race-neutral policies serve the purpose of perpetuating the status quo. The perception of race-neutral policies as just is predicated on the assumption that racial inequities in the post–civil rights era are not caused by racism but rather by cultural deficiencies and individual failure (445). The narratives provided by participants in this book reject and refute these beliefs and offer a testament to the dedication of scholars, teachers, and clinicians with a passion to serve.

The Need for Race-Conscious Strategies to Effect Change

Recognizing the role white supremacy has played and continues to play in shaping the current state of health professions education is necessary to effect change. Implementation of race-conscious strategies in teaching, practice, and research reflect a commitment to diversity and equity and a rejection of the status quo that perpetuates disparate outcomes for faculty, students, and communities of color.

VALUING THE CONTRIBUTIONS OF HISTORICALLY BLACK COLLEGES AND UNIVERSITIES

The *Merriam-Webster's Learner's Dictionary* defines *elite* as "people who have the most wealth and status in a society: the most successful or powerful group of people" (459). This describes the majority of students served by elite academic institutions, which largely exclude people from disadvantaged economic and educational backgrounds while privileging the wealthy. Despite their exclusion of working-class people and people of color, elite institutions enjoy tremendous prestige in health professions education. In contrast, historically black colleges and universities, although underresourced, have a distinguished tradition of accepting students from economically deprived K–12 systems to improve access to higher education while providing a strong education and graduating successful clinicians (422). Participants' stories reflect the commitment of faculty of color at historically black colleges and universities to the success of all students, particularly students of color. Reflecting the sway of whiteness in higher education, some historically black colleges and universities have been stigmatized for enacting policies that challenge academic elitism instead of being recognized for their contributions. Moreover, since historically white institutions have opened their doors to students of color (460), questions have been raised about the relevance of historically black colleges and universities (422, 423, 461). Such attitudes reflect a disturbing assumption that predominantly white institutions are the bar against which historically black colleges and universities should be measured. In truth, predominantly white institutions have much to learn from historically black colleges and universities' longstanding commitment to educational and health equity.

Whether they are beneficiaries of affirmative action or not, faculty of color may be seen as undeserving of their positions and find that the merit of their work often goes unrecognized (225). Such perceptions and the consequences that ensue arise from color-blind racist assumptions. Addressing this racist behavior is important for the successful implementation of race-conscious strategies to increase racial and ethnic diversity in the health professions.

This study suggests that faculty of color are concerned about the effects of racial bias on student admissions. Qualitative research is needed to shed light on these concerns. In addition, because race-neutral policies are commonly seen as fair, and because racial inequities are endemic to the K–12 system and the distribution of wealth, many URM applicants to health professions programs are turned away. These applicants may have slightly lower GPAs and test scores than whites, even though such criteria are not the sole determinants of success. Hence there is a talent pool waiting to be developed that health professions education has passed by. As historically black colleges and universities have shown, good talent can be developed even if students arrive in need of additional supports and preparation. Waiting for a supply of URM applicants proportional to their representation in the US population with access to educational and economic advantages equal to whites is a futile strategy, given the profound societal inequities affecting children and youth in the pipeline. Working with the K–12 system and providing adequate supports for educationally disadvantaged students when they enter health professions education to ensure graduation are remedies that can be used if the will is there; some leaders have successfully used these strategies (462). Yet admission of URMs with slightly lower grade point averages or test scores is seen by some as a path to the production of substandard clinicians. A comment posted by Charles in response to "How Hard Is It to Get into Medical School? Depends on Your Ethnicity" provides an example of this thinking:

> Affirmative action needs to go away. Applications should not have the race, religion, or gender. When I want a doctor I want the best people possible. I do not want someone who got in because the standards were lower for them.

I don't care if this means there are a disproportionate number of Asians and whites. Diversity for diversity sake is bad. Let the best candidate for the job get the job. (463)

Charles's view reflects common, unsubstantiated assumptions that (1) grade point averages and test scores are the most important qualities we should be looking for to produce health professionals who are best qualified to serve and protect the nation's health, (2) race-conscious admissions decrease the quality of the health-care workforce, and (3) racial and ethnic diversity in the health professions does not offer any benefits to health care. Those who view applicants of color with slightly lower test scores or grades as weak are choosing to see them through a deficit lens instead of recognizing the critical strengths they bring to educational excellence and health equity. In contrast, whites with good test scores and grades who are often ill equipped to address health inequities are typically seen as strong applicants. In the face of persistent and embarrassing health inequities, health professions education has recognized the need to develop cultural and social competencies in its primarily white student body. Hence, development of competencies in white talent is an accepted practice. In contrast, the idea of providing additional academic supports to develop talent in people of color from disadvantaged educational backgrounds is commonly disparaged. These assumptions, and the color-blind racism from which they arise, must be combated as part of the struggle to achieve educational and health equity.

In the recent opinion in *Fisher v. University of Texas* (2016), the US Supreme Court stated that race and ethnicity may be considered a positive feature of a minority student's application even it if is just "a 'factor of a factor of a factor' in the holistic-review calculus" (464) p.5. In light of the continued constitutional precedent allowing for race-conscious admissions and the urgent need to increase racial and ethnic diversity in health professions education and the health-care workforce, accreditation standards requiring use of holistic admissions, which typically consider race as a factor, are needed. Additional criteria focused on the potential to improve health equity, which is directly relevant to national goals, may offer added weight to a person of color's application for admission. In states where race-conscious admissions have been banned, a focus on the potential of candidates to improve health equity offers a non-race-based admissions standard that may indirectly improve racial and ethnic student diversity.

Hiring faculty of color requires engaging in action to counteract the status quo of white racial dominance that disadvantages racially and ethnically diverse candidates. Growing your own faculty while providing candidates with the necessary supports for success is a critical and viable strategy to creating a critical mass of racially and ethnically diverse faculty in a department or unit. Further, as Turner and Myer's analysis of the effects of market supply on racial and ethnic minority faculty representation revealed, health professions education will need to make an academic career more welcoming and lucrative to attract more faculty of color (83). To introduce more diverse perspectives and reduce the hegemonic influence of whiteness on admissions and hiring, panels made up of persons from communities of color should be given authority to contribute to decision-making processes, especially at institutions where the underrepresentation of blacks, Latino/as, and Native Americans is significant.

RACE-CONSCIOUS EDUCATION AND PRACTICE

Participants identified dialogue as an essential strategy to improve institutional climate while also reporting an absence of critical conversations about racism. Institutional silence about racism and avoidance of race talk is a powerful socializing force that retards future health professionals' ability to serve patients who face racism in everyday life and combat structural racism affecting health. Hence, institutional silence on racism flies in the face of the educational needs of students in what are often overwhelmingly white institutions. Although in part a function of being a demographic majority, whites are more isolated from people of other races, while blacks and Latino/as are members of more diverse communities. The Kaiser Family Foundation survey found only 37 percent of whites reported that people in their neighborhood or the people they socialize with are mostly of a different race, compared to 72 percent of Hispanics and 70 percent of blacks. Higher income blacks and lower income whites were more likely than their counterparts to live in or socialize with racially and ethnically diverse communities (458). The commonplace nature of whites' social segregation suggests many applicants to health professions programs are ill equipped to provide care to people of other races and ethnicities. Participants' reports of white colleagues' stereotyping of racial and ethnic minority faculty and students support this concern. Curricular changes that promote racial literacy are needed to address this weakness. According to Guinier,

[r]acial literacy is an interactive process in which race functions as a tool of diagnosis, feedback, and assessment ... [It] emphasizes the relationship between
race and power. Racial literacy reads race in its psychological, interpersonal,
and structural dimensions. It acknowledges the importance of individual
agency but refuses to lose sight of institutional and environmental forces
that both shape and reflect that agency. It sees little to celebrate when formal
equality is claimed within a racialized hierarchy ... [W]hile racial literacy
never loses sight of race, it does not focus exclusivity on race. It constantly
interrogates the dynamic relationship among race, class, geography, gender,
and other explanatory variables. It sees the danger of basing a strategy for
monumental social change on assumptions about individual prejudice and
individual victims. (124) p.115

Addressing implicit bias is integral to the development of racial literacy.
Counterstereotype training, collaborative intergroup contact, deliberative
self-monitoring, and learning to take the perspective of others are promising
strategies (456). Finally, the development of critical consciousness facilitated
through classroom discussion, service learning, and longitudinal clinical experiences in racially and ethnically diverse communities is essential to the
production of a racially literate health professions workforce.

CRITICAL RACE SCHOLARSHIP

Eliminating racism is required to achieve health equity. Hence, scholarship in
the health sciences must be responsive to structural racism's contemporary
influence on health, health inequities, and science itself. The work of critical
scholars exposes how racism produces disparate rates of morbidity, mortality, and overall well-being based on socially constructed identities. Scholars
engaged in this kind of knowledge production attend to equity while carrying
out research, scholarship, and practice that seek to transform the hierarchies
they identify in their work (465).

Faculty whose scholarly work uses critical theoretical approaches and meth-
odologies are typically a minority voice within their department or area of
study in the health sciences. Scholarly work that challenges the status quo may
encounter significant resistance. Such biases affect the availability of mentorship, acceptance of diverse philosophical and methodological approaches to

research, quality of evaluation, and funding priorities (466). Currently the NIH is conducting studies to determine if reviewer bias explains racially disparate patterns in R01 awards (467). My own experience on an NIH study section supports this concern. The extent to which my experience is generalizable remains to be seen, but it highlights the need for far greater numbers of racial and ethnic minority reviewers on NIH panels. Having only a few scholars of color on panels is insufficient to protect them from the consequences of challenging a racist hierarchy should the need arise during review processes. Greater attention to racial and ethnic diversity in the leadership of funding agencies and review panels is needed to help address this inequity. Prioritizing and rewarding health equity research, challenging the hegemonic influence of whiteness in funding agencies, weeding out reviewer bias, and promoting philosophical and methodological pluralism are essential steps to creating a national research agenda that values the lives of people of color.

Summary

The stories of participants challenge the invisibility of whiteness and provide evidence to support use of race-conscious strategies in health professions education. Participants were constrained by exclusion and control processes and exclusionary climates in health professions education at the same time that they strategically advanced their careers and worked to achieve educational and health equity. Yet even thriving participants often paid a price as they struggled to resist the oppressive contexts, policies, and practices that pervade health professions education. I invite readers to read the narratives in this book closely. Through the stories of others, faculty of color may find both validation and useful strategies for thriving in health professions education. Moreover, I call on white faculty to consider the effect of whiteness on participants' stories and the role of white leaders and colleagues in shaping participants' experiences. Responsibility for changing an unjust educational and health system does not lie with a fraction of faculty, whether they be racial and ethnic minorities or white, but instead belongs to everyone. Racial and ethnic diversity is central to equity and excellence in health professions education and for that reason is foundational to the nation's health. Achieving equity and openness to different ways of doing health professions education is within our grasp. Listening to and valuing the voices of faculty of color is vital to achieving these goals.

REFERENCES

1. Powers B, White A, Oriol N, Jain S. Race-conscious professionalism and African American representation in academic medicine. Academic Medicine. 2016;91(7):913–5.

2. Lorde A. Sister outsider: essays and speeches by Audre Lorde. Berkeley, CA: The Crossing Press; 1984.

3. Sullivan Commission on Diversity in the Health Care Workforce. Missing persons: minorities in the health professions. Washington, DC: Sullivan Commission; 2004.

4. Smith D. Diversity's promise for higher education: making it work. 2nd ed. Baltimore: Johns Hopkins University Press; 2015.

5. Garrison-Wade D, Diggs G, Estrada D, Galindo R. Lift every voice and sing: faculty of color face the challenges of the tenure track. Urban Review: Issues and Ideas in Public Education. 2012;44:90–112.

6. Ahmed S. On being included: racism and diversity in institutional life. London: Duke University Press; 2012.

7. Dowd A, Bensimon E. Engaging the "race question": accountability and equity in U.S. higher education. New York: Teacher's College Press; 2015.

8. Smith M. Gender, whiteness, and the "other Others" in the academy. In: Razack S, Smith M, Thobani S, editors. States of race: critical feminism for the 21st century. Toronto: Between the Lines; 2010. p.37–58.

9. Ahmed S. The language of diversity. Ethnic & Racial Studies. 2007;30(2):235–56.

10. Mirchandani K, Butler, A. Beyond inclusion and equity: contributions from transnational anti-racist feminism. In: Konrad A, Prasad P, Pringle J, editors. Handbook of workplace diversity. Thousand Oaks, CA: Sage; 2006. p.475–88.

11. US Department of Health and Human Services, Health Resources and Services Administration, National Center for Health Workforce Analysis. Sex, race, and ethnic diversity of U.S. health occupations (2010–2012). Rockville, MD: U.S. Department of Health and Human Services; 2014. Available from https://bhw.hrsa.gov/sites/default/files/bhw/nchwa/diversityushealthoccupations.pdf.

12. Gasman M, Travers C, Abioloa U. Diversity and senior leadership at elite institutions of higher education. Journal of Diversity in Higher Education. 2015;18(1):1–14.

13. Lin S, Frances H, Minor L, Eisele D. Faculty diversity and inclusion program outcomes at an academic otolaryngology department. The Laryngoscope. 2016;126(2):352–60.

14. Mendoza F, Walker L, Stoll B, Fuentes-Afflick E, Geme J, Cheng T, et al. Diversity and inclusion training in pediatric departments. Pediatrics. 2015;135(4):707–13.

15. Shaw G. Where more can be done to promote diverse leadership in neurology. Neurology Today. 2016;16(9):19–21.

16. Yu P, Hassanein O, Rogers S, Chang D. Minorities struggle to advance in academic medicine—a 12-year review of diversity at the highest levels of America's teaching institutions. Journal of Surgical Residence. 2013;182(2):212–8.

17. Grumbach K, Mendoza R. Disparities in human resources: addressing the lack of diversity in the health professions. Health Affairs. 2008;27(2):413–22.

18. Fang D, Li Y, Stauffer D, Trautman D. 2015–2016 salaries of instructional and administrative nursing faculty in baccalaureate and graduate programs in nursing. Washington, DC: American Association of Colleges of Nursing; 2016. Contract No.: 15-16-02.

19. American Association of Medical Colleges. AAMC faculty roster. Table 3: Distribution of U.S. medical school faculty by rank and race/ethnicity. 2015. Available from: https://www.aamc.org/download/453416/data/15table3.pdf.

20. Taylor D, Taylor J, Nguyen N. 2015–2016 profile of pharmacy faculty. Alexandria, VA: American Association of Colleges of Pharmacy; 2016.

21. Moody J. Faculty diversity: removing the barriers. 2nd ed. New York: Routledge; 2012.

22. Cokley K, Obaseki V, Moran-Jackson K, Jones L, Vohra-Gupta S. College access improves for black students but for which ones? are selective colleges as selective as they could be in choosing among black students for admission? Phi Delta Kappan. 2016;97(5):43–8.

23. Nivet M. Minorities in academic medicine: review of the literature. Journal of Vascular Surgery. 2010;51:53S–58S.

24. American Association of Medical Colleges. Striving toward excellence: faculty diversity in medical education. Washington, DC: American Association of Medical Colleges; 2009.

25. National League for Nursing. Achieving diversity and meaningful inclusion in nursing education: a living document from the National League for Nursing 2016. Available from: http://www.nln.org/docs/default-source/about/vision-statement-achieving-diversity.pdf?sfvrsn=2.

26. Johnson & Johnson. The campaign for nursing's future: choose your school 2011. Available from: https://www.discovernursing.com/schools#no-filters.

27. American Association of Medical Colleges. AAMC 2015 annual report. American Association of Medical Colleges; 2011 Available from: https://www. aamc.org/about/451624/annual-report-2015.html#highlights.

28. American Association of Colleges of Osteopathic Medicine. Osteopathic medical college information book: entering class 2017. Chevy Chase, MD: American Association of Colleges of Osteopathic Medicine; 2016 [cited May 16, 2016]. Available from: http://www.aacom.org/docs/default-source/cib/2017_com-map.pdf?sfvrsn=10.

29. American Association of Colleges of Pharmacy. Academic pharmacy's vital statistics. American Association of Colleges of Pharmacy; 2015 Available from: http://www.aacp.org/about/pages/vitalstats.aspx.

30. American Dental Education Association. ADEA snapshot of dental education 2016–2017. Washington, DC: American Dental Education Association; 2016.

31. Bureau of Labor Statistics, US Department of Labor. Occupational employment and wages, May 2015: 25-1072 nursing instructors and teachers, postsecondary. Bureau of Labor Statistics U.S. Department of Labor; 2016 [cited March 30, 2016]. Available from: http://www.bls.gov/oes/current/oes251072.htm.

32. American Association of Colleges of Osteopathic Medicine. 2015–16 Osteopathic medical college faculty by race/ethnicity. Chevy Chase, MD: American Association of Colleges of Osteopathic Medicine; 2016. Available from: https://www. aacom.org/docs/default-source/data-and-trends/2015-16-COM-FacbyRE.pdf?sfvrsn=4.

33. American Association of Colleges of Osteopathic Medicine. 2015–16 Osteopathic medical college basic science faculty by rank. Chevy Chase, MD: American Association of Colleges of Osteopathic Medicine; 2016. Available from: http://www.aacp.org/about/pages/vitalstats.aspx.

34. Nunez-Smith M, Ciarleglio M, Sandoval-Schaefer T, Elumn J, Castillo-Page L, Peduzzi P, et al. Institutional variation in promotion of racial/ethnic minority faculty at US medical schools. American Journal of Public Health. 2012;102(5):852–8.

35. Fang D, Moy E, Colburn L, Hurley J. Racial and ethnic disparities in faculty promotion in academic medicine. JAMA. 2000;284(9):1085–92.

36. Castro C. Women of color navigating the academy: the discursive power of professionalism [Dissertation]. Philadelphia: Temple University; 2012.

37. Heckler M. Report of the Secretary's Task Force on black & minority health. Washington DC: U.S. Department of Health and Human Services; 1985. Contract No.: MH10D9924.

38. Smedley B, Stith A, Nelson A, editors. Unequal treatment: confronting racial and ethnic disparities in health care. Committee on Understanding and Eliminating Racial and Ethnic Disparities in Health Care, Board on Health Sciences Policy, Institute of Medicine. Washington, DC: National Academies Press; 2003.

39. Smedley A, Butler A, Bristow L, editors. In the nation's compelling interest: ensuring diversity in the health care workforce. Committee on Institutional and Policy-Level Strategies for Increasing the Diversity of the U.S. Healthcare Workforce, Board on Health Sciences Policy, Institute of Medicine. Washington, DC: National Academies Press; 2004.

40. Pew Research Center. King's dream remains an elusive goal; many Americans see racial disparities 2013. Available from: http://www.pewsocialtrends.org/2013/08/22/kings-dream-remains-an-elusive-goal-many-americans-see-racial-disparities/.

41. Sandhu G. When I say . . . social accountability in medical education. Medical Education. 2015;49(1):23–4.

42. Chisholm M. Diversity: a missing link to professionalism. American Journal of Pharmaceutical Education. 2004;68(5):1–3.

43. Johnson A. Minority recruitment at school psychology graduate programs. [Dissertation]. Indiana: Indiana University of Pennsylvania; 2008. Available from: http://knowledge.library.iup.edu/cgi/viewcontent.cgi?article=1821&context=etd.

44. Jacob S, Sánchez Z. The challenge of closing the diversity gap: development of Hispanic nursing faculty through a Health Resources and Services Administration Minority Faculty Fellowship Program grant. Journal of Professional Nursing. 2011;27(2):108–13.

45. Richert A, Campbell K, Rodriguez J, Borowsky I, Parikh R. ACU workforce column: expanding and supporting the healthcare workforce. Journal of Health Care for the Poor and Underserved. 2013;24(4):1423–31.

46. Fitzpatrick L, Sutton M, Greenberg A. Toward eliminating health disparities in HIV/AIDS: the importance of the minority investigator in addressing scientific gaps in black and Latino communities. Journal of the National Medical Association. 2006;98(12):1906–11.

47. Cargill V. Recruiting, retaining, and maintaining racial and ethnic minority investigators: why we should bother, why we should care. American Journal of Public Health. 2009;99(S1):S5–S7.

48. Turner C, González J, Wood J. Faculty of color in academe: what 20 years of literature tells us. Journal of Diversity in Higher Education. 2008;1(3):139–68.

49. Coleman M. Racism in academia: the white superiority supposition in the "unbiased search" for knowledge. European Journal of Political Economy. 2005;21:762–74.

50. Arnold N. Psychological heuristics: mental/emotional designs of racial battle fatigue and the tenure/promotion terrain for faculty of color. In: Fasching-Varner K, Albert K, Mitchell R, Allen C, editors. Racial battle fatigue in higher education: exposing the myth of post-racial America. London: Rowman & Littlefield; 2015. p.77–89.

51. Locher H, Ropers-Huilman R. Wearing you down: the influence of racial battle fatigue on academic freedom for faculty of color. In: Fasching-Varner K, Albert K, Mitchell R, Allen C, editors. Racial battle fatigue in higher education: exposing the myth of post-racial America. London: Rowman & Littlefield Publishing; 2015. p.103–14.

52. Anderson-Thompkins S. Race scholars on the politics of race, research, and risk in the academy: a narrative inquiry. [Dissertation]. Atlanta: Georgia State University; 2010. Available from: http://scholarworks.gsu.edu/cgi/viewcontent.cgi?article=1043&context=eps_diss.

53. Bernal, D, Villalpando O. An apartheid of knowledge in academia: the struggle for "legitimate" knowledge for faculty of color. Equity & Excellence in Education. 2002;35(2):169–80.

54. Healy G. The politics of equality and diversity: history, society, and biography. In: Bendl R, Bleijenbergh I, Henttonen E, Mills A, editors. The Oxford handbook of diversity in organizations. Oxford: Oxford University Press; 2015. p.15–38.

55. Villalpando O, Bernal D. A critical race theory analysis of barriers that impede the success of faculty of color. In: Smith W, Altbach P, Lomotey K, editors. The racial crisis in American education: continuing challenges for the twenty-first century. rev. ed. Albany: State University of New York Press; 2002. p.243–69.

56. Gates P, Ganey J, Brown M. Building the minority faculty development pipeline. Journal of Dental Education. 2003;67(9):1034–8.

57. Johnson J, Jayadevappa R, Taylor L, Askew A, Williams B, Johnson B. Extending the pipeline for minority physicians: a comprehensive program for minority faculty development. Academic Medicine. 1998;73(3):237–44.

58. Gates P, Ubu N, Smithey L, Rogers J, Haden N, Rodriguez T, et al. Faculty development for underrepresented minority dental faculty and residents. Journal of Dental Education. 2013;77(3):276–91.

59. Stanley J, Capers C, Berlin L. Changing the face of nursing faculty: minority faculty recruitment and retention. Journal of Professional Nursing. 2007;23(5):253–61.

60. Beech B, Calles-Escandon J, Hairston K, Langdon S, Latham-Sadler B, Bell R. Mentoring programs for underrepresented minority faculty in academic medical centers: a systematic review of the literature. Academic Medicine. 2013;88(4):541–9.

61. Daley S, Palermo A, Nivet M, Soto-Greene M, Taylor V, Butts G, et al. No 6—Successful programs in minority faculty development: ingredients of success. Diversity in academic medicine, special issue of Mount Sinai Journal of Medicine. 2008;75(6):533–51.

62. Buchwald D, Dick R. Weaving the Native Web: using social network analysis to demonstrate the value of a minority career development program. Academic Medicine. 2011;86(6):778–86.

63. Equality Challenge Unit. Unconscious bias in higher education London; 2013. Available from: http://www.ecu.ac.uk/wp-content/uploads/2014/07/unconscious-bias-and-higher-education.pdf.

64. Pachter L, Kodjo C. New century scholars: a mentorship program to increase workforce diversity in academic pediatrics. Academic Medicine. 2015;90(7):881–7.

65. Viets V, Baca C, Verney S, Venner K, Parker T, Wallerstein N. Reducing health disparities through a culturally centered mentorship program for minority faculty: the Southwest Addictions Research Group (SARG) experience. Academic Medicine. 2009;84(8):1118–26.

66. Goldstein Hode M, Meisenbach R. Reproducing whiteness through diversity: a critical discourse analysis of the pro-affirmative action amicus briefs in the *Fisher* case. Journal of Diversity in Higher Education. 2017; 10(2): 162–80. Available from: http://dx.doi.org/10.1037/dhe0000014.

67. Center for the Study of Social Policy. Race equity—glossary of terms. Available from: http://www.cssp.org/about/race-equity/GLOSSARY-OF-TERMS.pdf.

68. American Dental Education Association. Statement of the American Dental Education Association: the voice of dental education. Senate Committee on Health, Ed-

ucation, Labor, and Pensions Hearing: "Addressing health care workforce issues"; 2008 Available from: http://www.allhealth.org/briefingmaterials/adea-helptestimony-1268 .pdf.

69. National League for Nursing. NLN nurse educator fact sheet 2013. Available from: http://www.nln.org/docs/default-source/advocacy-public-policy/nurse-faculty-shortage -fact-sheet-pdf.pdf?sfvrsn=0.

70. Yanchick V, Baldwin J, Bootman J, Carter R, Crabtree B, Maine L. Report of the 2013–2014 Argus Commission: diversity and inclusion in pharmacy education. American Journal of Pharmaceutical Education. 2014;78(10):S21.

71. Fang D, Li Y, Stauffer D, Trautman D. 2015–2016 enrollment and graduations in baccalaureate and graduate programs in nursing. Washington DC; American Association of Colleges of Nursing; 2016.

72. American Association of Medical Colleges. Table B-5: total enrollment by U.S. medical school and race/ethnicity, 2015–2016. American Association of Medical Colleges; 2016 Available from: https://www.aamc.org/download/321540/data/factstableb5.pdf.

73. American Association of Colleges of Pharmacy. Profile of pharmacy students: fall 2015. Alexandria, VA: American Association of Colleges of Pharmacy; 2015. Available from: http://www.aacp.org/resources/research/institutionalresearch/Documents /Introduction.pdf.

74. National Center for Education Statistics. Table 306.30: fall enrollment of U.S. residents in degree-granting postsecondary institutions, by race/ethnicity: selected years, 1976 through 2025. U.S. Department of Education; 2015. Available from: https://nces .ed.gov/programs/digest/d15/tables/dt15_306.30.asp.

75. US Bureau of The Census. Quick facts; 2015. Available from: https://www.census .gov/quickfacts/table/RHI825215/00.

76. American Dental Education Association. Full-time dental school faculty by gender, and race, and ethnicity, 2013–2014 academic year. American Dental Education Association; 2014. Available from: http://www.adea.org/publications-and-data/data-analysis -and-research/faculty.aspx.

77. National Center for Education Statistics. Table 315.20: Full-time faculty in degree-granting postsecondary institutions, by race/ethnicity, sex, and academic rank: fall 2009, fall 2011, and fall 2013. US Department of Education; 2014. Available from: https:// nces.ed.gov/programs/digest/d14/tables/dt14_315.20.asp.

78. Krogstad J, Lopez M. Hispanic population reaches record 55 million, but growth has cooled: Pew Research Center; 2015 [updated June 25, 2015]. Available from: http:// www.pewresearch.org/fact-tank/2015/06/25/u-s-hispanic-population-growth-surge -cools/ft_15-06-25_hispanic_percent/.

79. Castillo-Page L. Diversity in medical education: facts and figures 2012. Washington, DC: American Association of Medical Colleges; 2012.

80. Beardsley R, Matzke G, Rospond R, Williams J, Knapp K, Kradjan W, et al. Fac-

tors influencing the pharmacy faculty workforce. American Journal of Pharmaceutical Education. 2008;72(2):1–11.

81. American Dental Education Association. Dental school faculty by gender, race and ethnicity, and employment status, 2009–2010. 2010. Available from: http://www .adea.org/uploadedFiles/ADEA/Content_Conversion/publications/TrendsinDental Education2009/TDEFaculty/Documents/Faculty_VacanciesSeparations_files/SeeAll FacultySlides.pdf.

82. Smith D. How to diversify the faculty. Academe. 2000;86(5):48–52.

83. Turner C, Myers S. Faculty of color in academe: bittersweet success. Needham Heights, MA: Allyn & Bacon; 2000.

84. Corrice A. Unconscious bias in faculty and leadership recruitment: a literature review. Analysis in brief. Washington, DC: American Association of Medical Colleges; 2009. Available from: https://www.aamc.org/download/102364/data/aibvol9no2.pdf.

85. Rutledge D. Social Darwinism, scientific racism, and the metaphysics of race. Journal of Negro Education. 1995;64(3):243–52.

86. Bynum B. Discarded diagnoses. Lancet. 2000;356(9241):1615.

87. Weisberg M. Remeasuring man. Evolution & Development. 2014;16(3):166–78.

88. Balter M. Geneticists decry book on race and evolution. American Association for the Advancement of Science; 2014 [updated August 8, 2014]. Available from: http:// www.sciencemag.org/news/2014/08/geneticists-decry-book-race-and-evolution.

89. Beaver K, Nedelec J, Barnes J, Boutwell B, Boccio C. The association between intelligence and personal victimization in adolescence and adulthood. Personality and Individual Differences. 2016;98:355–60.

90. Lynn R, Cheng H. Recent data for majority and racial minority differences in intelligence of 5 year olds in the United Kingdom. Intelligence. 2013;41(5):452–5.

91. Flynn J. The spectacles through which I see the race and IQ debate. Intelligence. 2010;38(4):363–6.

92. Wicherts J, Dolan C, van der Maas H. A systematic literature review of the average IQ of sub-Saharan Africans. Intelligence. 2010;38(1):1–20.

93. Richards G. "Race," racism and psychology: towards a reflexive history. 2nd ed. New York: Routledge; 2016.

94. Braun L. Breathing race into the machine: the surprising career of the spirometer from plantation to genetics. Minneapolis: University of Minnesota Press; 2014.

95. Fryberg S. Constructing junior faculty of color as strugglers: the implications for tenure and promotion. In: Little D, Mohanty S, editors. The future of diversity: academic leaders reflect on American higher education. New York: Palgrave Macmillan; 2010. p.181–217.

96. Plaut V, Fryberg S, Martinez E. Officially advocated, but institutionally undermined: diversity rhetoric subjective realities of junior faculty of color. International Journal of Diversity in Organizations, Communities and Nations. 2012;11(2):101–16.

97. Gasman M, Conrad C. Minority serving institutions: educating all students. Philadelphia: University of Pennsylvania Center for Minority Serving Institutions; 2013. Available from: http://www.gse.upenn.edu/pdf/cmsi/msis_educating_all_students.pdf.

98. Gasman M. The changing face of historically black colleges and universities. Philadelphia: University of Pennsylvania Center for Minority Serving Institutions; 2013. Available from: http://www.gse.upenn.edu/pdf/cmsi/Changing_Face_HBCUs.pdf.

99. Excelencia in Education. Hispanic Serving Institutions 2013–2014. Washington, DC; 2015. Available from: http://www.edexcelencia.org/gateway/download/23767/1472418085.

100. Gasman M, Nguyen T, Conrad C,. Lives intertwined: a primer on the history and emergence of minority serving institutions. Journal of Diversity in Higher Education. 2015;8(2):120–38.

101. The Penn Center for Minority Serving Institutions. Redefining success: how tribal colleges and universities build nations, strengthen sovereignty, and persevere through challenges. Philadelphia: University of Pennsylvania Center for Minority Serving Institutions; 2015 Available from: https://www2.gse.upenn.edu/cmsi/sites/gse.upenn.edu.cmsi/files/MSI_TBLCLLGreport_Final.pdf.

102. National Commission on Asian American and Pacific Islander Research in Education. Partnership in equity through research in education (PEER): findings from the first year of research on AANAPISIs. 2013. Available from: http://www.apiasf.org/pdfs/2013_peer_report/APIASF_and_CARE_PEER_Report_June_2013.pdf.

103. U.S. Department of Education. List of FY 2016 eligible Asian American and Native American Pacific Islander-serving institutions. 2016. Available from: https://www2.ed.gov/programs/aanapi/aanapi-eligibles-2016.pdf.

104. Fiegener M, Proudfoot S. Baccaulaureate origins of U.S.-trained S&E doctorate recipients. National Science Foundation; 2013. Available from: https://www.nsf.gov/statistics/infbrief/nsf13323/nsf13323.pdf.

105. Hispanic Association of Colleges & Universities. HSI STEM degree production. Hispanic Association of Colleges & Universities; 2013. Available from: http://www.hacu.net/hacu/HSIs_and_STEM.asp.

106. The Penn Center for Minority Serving Institutions. On their own terms: two-year minority serving institutions. Philadelphia: University of Pennsylvania, Center for Minority Serving Institutions; 2015. Available from: http://www2.gse.upenn.edu/cmsi/sites/gse.upenn.edu.cmsi/files/MSI_CCreport_FINAL.pdf.

107. Noonan A, Lindong I, Jaitley V. The role of historically black colleges and universities in training the health care workforce. American Journal of Public Health. 2013;103(3):412–5.

108. Santiago D; Galdeano E, Taylor M. Excelencia in Education. Finding your workforce: Latinos in health. Washington, DC: Excelencia in Education; 2015.

109. Hispanic-Serving Health Professions Schools. About us. [Internet] 2012. Available from: http://www.hshps.org/about.

110. Hispanic-Serving Health Professions Schools. Hispanic Serving Health Professions Schools member institutions. 2015. Available from: http://www.hshps.org/about/member-institutions/2015.

111. Carter R. Genes, genomes, and genealogies: the return of scientific racism? Ethnic and Racial Studies. 2007;30(4):546–56.

112. Azoulay K. Reflections on race and the biologization of difference. Patterns of Prejudice. 2006;40(4–5):353–79.

113. Phillips D, Drevdahl D. Race and the difficulties of language. Advances in Nursing Science. 2003;26(1):17–29.

114. Glaser B. Theoretical sensitivity. Mill Valley, CA: The Sociology Press; 1978.

115. Charmaz K. Grounded theory in the 21st century: applications for advancing social justice studies. In: Denzin N, Lincoln Y, editors. The handbook of qualitative research. 3rd ed. Thousand Oaks, CA: Sage; 2005. p.507–35.

116. Charmaz K. Grounded theory methods in social justice research. In: Denzin N, Lincoln Y, editors. The Sage handbook of qualitative research. 4th ed. Thousand Oaks, CA: Sage; 2011. p.359–80.

117. Desmond-Harris J. Black doc sues UCLA, cites racist treatment. 2012 [posted May 31, 2012]. Available from: http://www.theroot.com/articles/politics/2012/05/dr_christian_head_ucla_medical_center_racism_case_interview.html.

118. Said E. Orientalism. New York: Vintage; 1979.

119. Lensmire T. White men's racial others. Teachers College Record. 2014;116(3):1–32.

120. Myser C. Differences from somewhere: the normativity of whiteness in bioethics in the United States. American Journal of Bioethics. 2003;3(2):1–11.

121. Zinn H. A people's history of the United States: 1492–present. New York: HarperCollins; 1999.

122. Drakeford L. The pathology of color blindness: a historical account. In: Drakeford L, editor. The race controversy in American education. Santa Barbara, CA: Praeger; 2015. p.33–68.

123. Bonilla-Silva E. Down the rabbit hole: color-blind racism in Obamerica. In: Neville H, Gallardo M, Sue D, editors. The myth of racial color blindness: manifestations, dynamics, and impact. Washington, DC: American Psychological Association; 2016. p.25–38.

124. Guinier L. From racial liberalism to racial literacy: Brown v. Board of Education and the interest-divergence dilemma. Journal of American History. 2004;91(1):92–118.

125. Bonilla-Silva E. The structure of racism in color-blind, "post-racial" America. American Behavioral Scientist. 2015;59(11):1358–76.

126. Norton M, Sommers S. Whites see racism as a zero-sum game that they are now losing. Perspectives on Psychological Science. 2011;6(3):215–8.

127. Tuitt F, Bonner F. Introduction. In: Bonner F, marbley a, Tuitt F, Robinson P, Banda R, Hughes R, editors. Black faculty in the academy: narratives for negotiating identity and achieving career success. New York: Routledge; 2015. p.1–9.

128. Bell L. Telling on racism: developing a race-conscious agenda. In: Neville H, Gallardo M, Sue D, editors. The myth of racial color blindness: manifestations, dynamics, and impact. Washington, DC: American Psychological Association; 2016. p.105–22.

129. Fryberg S, Martínez E. Constructed strugglers: the impact of diversity narratives on junior faculty of color. In: Fryberg S, Martínez E, editors. The truly diverse faculty: new dialogues in American higher education. New York: Palgrave Macmillan; 2014. p.3–34.

130. Goff P. Saying "no" to whiteness: negotiating the unstated requests of the academy. In: Fryberg S, Martínez E, editors. The truly diverse faculty: new dialogues in American higher education. New York: Palgrave Macmillan; 2014. p.125–55.

131. Harris F, Lieberman R. Introduction—Beyond discrimination: racial inequality in the age of Obama. In: Beyond discrimination: racial inequality in a postracist era. New York: Russell Sage Foundation; 2013. p.1–36.

132. Hall W, Chapman M, Lee K, Merino Y, Thomas T, Payne B, et al. Implicit racial/ethnic bias among health care professionals and its influence on health care outcomes: a systematic review. American Journal of Public Health. 2015;105(12):e60–e76.

133. White A. Seeing patients: unconscious bias in health care. Cambridge, MA: Harvard University Press; 2011.

134. Greenwald A, Krieger L. Implicit bias: scientific foundations. California Law Review. 2006;94(4):945–68.

135. Mathew D. Just medicine: a cure for racial inequality in American health care. New York: New York University Press; 2015.

136. Gaertner S, Dovidio J. Reducing intergroup bias. The common ingroup identity model. New York: Routledge; 2012.

137. Robbins C, Quaye S. Racial privilege, gender oppression, and intersectionality. In: Mitchell D, Simmons C, Greyerbiehl L, editors. Intersectionality & higher education: theory, research, & praxis. New York: Peter Lang; 2014. p.20–30.

138. Wjeyesinghe C, Jones S. Intersectionality, identity, and systems of power and inequality. In: Mitchell D, Simmons C, Greyerbiehl L, editors. Intersectionality & higher education: theory, research, & praxis. New York: Peter Lang; 2014. p.9–19.

139. Anders A, DeVita J. Intersectionality: a legacy from critical legal studies and critical race theory. In: Mitchell D, Simmons C, Greyerbiehl L, editors. Intersectionality & higher education: theory, research, & praxis. New York: Peter Lang; 2014. p.31–44.

140. Crenshaw K. Mapping the margins: intersectionality, identity politics, and violence against women of color. In: Crenshaw K, Gotanda N, Peller G, Kendall, T, editors, Critical race theory—the key writings that formed the movement. New York: New Press; 1995. p.357–83.

141. Turner J, González J, Wong K. Faculty women of color: the critical nexus of race and gender. Journal of Diversity in Higher Education. 2011;4(4):199–211.

142. Monrouxe L. When I say . . . intersectionality in medical education research. Medical Education. 2015;49(1):21–2.

143. Hassouneh D, Lutz K, Beckett A, Junkins E, Horton L. The experiences of underrepresented minority faculty in medicine. Medical Education Online. 2014;19. Available from: http://med-ed-online.net/index.php/meo/article/view/24768.

144. Hassouneh D, Akeroyd J, Lutz K, Beckett A. Exclusion and control: patterns aimed at limiting the influence of faculty of color. Journal of Nursing Education. 2012;51(6):314–25.

145. Goff P, Steele C, Davies P. The space between us: stereotype threat and distance in interracial contexts. Journal of Personality and Social Psychology. 2008;94(1):91–107.

146. Quinn D, Kallen R, Spencer S. Stereotype threat. In: Dovidio J, Hewstone M, Glick P, Esses V, editors. The Sage handbook of prejudice, stereotyping, and discrimination. Thousand Oaks, CA: Sage; 2010. p.379–94.

147. Niemann Y. The making of a token: a case study of stereotype threat, stigma, racism, and tokenism in academe. In: Muhs G, Niemann Y, Gonzáles C, Harris A, editors. Presumed incompetent: the intersections of race and class for women in academia. Boulder: University Press of Colorado; 2012. p.336–55.

148. Eagan M, Garvey J. Stressing out: connecting race, gender, and stress with faculty productivity. Journal of Higher Education. 2015;86(6):923–54.

149. Curtis-Boles H. An African American woman's experience in the academy: negotiating cultures. In: Curtis-Boles H, Adams D, Jenkins-Monroe V, editors. Making our voices heard: women of color in academia. New York: Nova Science; 2012. p.9–19.

150. Elliot B, Dorscher J, Wirta A, Hill D. Staying connected: Native American women faculty members on experiencing success. Academic Medicine. 2010;85(4):675–9.

151. Karabel J. The chosen: the hidden history of admission and exclusion at Harvard, Yale, and Princeton. New York: Houghton Mifflin Harcourt; 2006.

152. Wilder C. Ebony & ivy: race, slavery, and the troubled history of America's universities. New York: Bloomsbury Press; 2013.

153. Harris A, Gonzáles C. Introduction. In: Muhs G, Niemann Y, Gonzáles C, Harris A, editors. Presumed incompetent: the intersections of race and class for women in academia. Boulder: University Press of Colorado; 2012. p.1–14.

154. Ford K. Race, gender, and bodily (mis)recognitions: women of color faculty experiences with white students in the college classroom. Journal of Higher Education. 2011;82(4):444–78.

155. Mahoney M, Wilson E, Odom K, Flowers L, Adler S. Minority faculty voices on diversity in academic medicine. Academic Medicine. 2008;83(8):781–6.

156. Davis S, Davis M. Experiences of ethnic minority faculty employed in predominantly white schools of nursing. Journal of Cultural Diversity. 1998;5(2):68–76.

157. Kolade F. The lived experience of minority nursing faculty: a phenomenological study. Journal of Professional Nursing. 2016;32(2):107–14.

158. Carr P, Paplepu A, Szalacha L, Caswell C, Inui T. "Flying below the radar": a qualitative study of minority experience and management of discrimination in academic medicine. Medical Education. 2007;4(6):601–9.

159. Pololi L, Cooper L, Carr P. Race, disadvantage and faculty experiences in academic medicine. Journal of General Internal Medicine. 2010;25(12):1363–9.

160. Wingard D, Reznik V, Daley S. Career experiences and perceptions of underrepresented minority medical school faculty. Journal of the National Medical Association. 2008;100(9):1084–7.

161. Rodriguez J, Campbell K, Fogarty J, Williams R. Underrepresented minority faculty in academic medicine: a systematic review. Family Medicine. 2014;46(2):100–4.

162. Price E, Powe N, Kern D, Golden S, Wand G, Cooper L. Improving the diversity climate in academic medicine: faculty perceptions as a catalyst for institutional change. Academic Medicine. 2009;84(1):95–105.

163. Peterson N, Friedman R, Ash A, Franco S, Carr P. Faculty self-reported experience with racial and ethnic discrimination in academic medicine. Journal of General Internal Medicine. 2004;19(3):259–65.

164. Kim E, Hogge I, Mok G, Nishida H. Work experiences of foreign-born Asian women counseling and psychology faculty. Journal of Multicultural Counseling and Development. 2014;42(3):147–60.

165. Jayakumar U, Howard T, Allen W, Han J. Racial privilege in the professoriate: an exploration of campus climate, retention, and satisfaction. Journal of Higher Education. 2009;80(5):538–63.

166. Kelly B, McCann K. Women faculty of color: stories behind the statistics. Urban Review: Issues and Ideas in Public Education. 2014;46(4):681–702.

167. Hartlep N. An adopted Korean speaks out about his racialized experiences as a faculty member at a predominantly white institution. In: Fasching-Varner K, Albert K, Mitchell R, Allen C, editors. Racial battle fatigue in higher education: exposing the myth of post-racial America. London: Rowman & Littlefield; 2015. p.115–22.

168. Bower B. Campus life for faculty of color: still strangers after all these years? New Directions for Community Colleges. 2002;118:79–88.

169. Garcia A. Latina faculty narratives and the challenges of tenure: identifying strategies, institutionalizing accountability. In: Mack D, Watson E, Camacho M, editors. Mentoring faculty of color: essays on professional development and advancement in colleges and universities. Jefferson, NC: McFarland & Company; 2013. p.69–87.

170. Essien V. Visible and invisible barriers to the incorporation of faculty of color in predominantly white law schools. Journal of Black Studies. 2003;34(1):63–71.

171. Mohamed T. Surviving the academy: the continuing struggle of minority faculty on mainstream campuses. International Journal of Diversity in Organizations, Communities and Nations. 2010;10(4):41–52.

172. Giles M. Behind enemy lines: critical race theory, racial battle fatigue and higher education. In: Fasching-Varner K, Albert K, Mitchell R, Allen C, editors. Racial battle fatigue in higher education: exposing the myth of post-racial America. London: Rowman & Littlefield; 2015. p.169–78.

173. Jenkins T. Black. Woman. Nontraditional other: creating hybrid spaces in higher education. In: Fasching-Varner K, Albert K, Mitchell R, Allen C, editors. Racial battle fatigue in higher education: exposing the myth of post-racial America. London: Rowman & Littlefield; 2015. p.37–44.

174. Pérez D. A hyphenated life: power and liberation within the research academy. In: Fasching-Varner K, Albert K, Mitchell R, Allen C, editors. Racial battle fatigue in higher education: exposing the myth of post-racial America. London: Rowman & Littlefield; 2015. p.179–88.

175. Mitchell R, Fasching-Varner K, Albert K, Allen C. Introduction. In: Fasching-Varner K, Albert K, Mitchell R, Allen C, editors. Racial battle fatigue in higher education: exposing the myth of post-racial America. London: Rowman & Littlefield; 2015. p.xv–xxiii.

176. Altbach P, Lomotey K, Rivers S. Race in higher education: the continuing crisis. In: Smith A, Altbach P, Lomotey K, editors. The racial crisis in American higher education: continuing challenges for the twenty-first century. rev. ed. Albany: State University of New York Press; 2002. p.23–41.

177. Monzó L, SooHoo S. Translating the academy: learning the racialized languages of academia. Journal of Diversity in Higher Education. 2014;7(3):147–65.

178. Mitchell D. Introduction. In: Mitchell D, Simmons C, Greyerbiehl L, editors. Intersectionality & higher education: theory, research, & praxis. New York: Peter Lang; 2014. p.1–6.

179. Maydun N, Williams S, McGee E, Milner H. On the importance of African-American faculty in higher education: implications and recommendations. Educational Foundations. 2013:65–84.

180. Lopez M, Johnson K. Presumed incompetent: important lessons for university leaders on the professional lives of women faculty of color. Berkeley Journal of Gender, Law, & Justice. 2014;29(2):388–405.

181. Diggs G, Garrison-Wade D, Estrada D, Galindo R. Smiling faces and colored spaces: the experiences of faculty of color pursing tenure in the academy. Urban Review: Issues and Ideas in Public Education. 2009;41:312–33.

182. Leyens J, Demoulin S. Ethnocentrism and group realities. In: Dovidio J, Hewstone M, Glick P, Esses V, editors. The Sage handbook of prejudice, stereotyping, and discrimination. Thousand Oaks, CA: Sage; 2010. p.194–208.

183. Hammond W, Gillen M, Yen I. Workplace discrimination and depressive symptoms: a study of multi-ethnic hospital employees. Race and Social Problems. 2010;2(1):19–30.

184. Cartwright B, Washington R, McConnell R. Examining racial microaggressions in rehabilitation counselor education. Rehabilitation Education. 2009;23(2):171–82.

185. Hodge S, Wiggins D. The African American experience in physical education and kinesiology: plight, pitfalls, and possibilities. Quest. 2010;62(1):35–60.

186. Razack S, Hodges B, Steinert Y, Maguire M. Seeking inclusion in an exclusive process: discourses of medical school student selection. Medical Education. 2015;49(1):36–47.

187. Jenkins T. The myth of meritocracy in the American medical profession. XVIII ISA World Congress of Sociology, facing an unequal world: challenges for global sociology. July 15, 2014. Available from: https://isaconf.confex.com/isaconf/wc2014/webprogram/Paper59218.html.

188. McNamee S, Miller R. The meritocracy myth. 3rd ed. Plymouth, UK: Rowman & Littlefield; 2013.

189. Guinier L. The tyranny of the meritocracy: democratizing higher education in America. Boston: Beacon Press; 2015.

190. Knowles E, Lowery B. Meritocracy, self-concerns, and whites' denial of racial inequity. Self and Identity. 2012;11:202–22.

191. Shavers M, Butler Y, Moore J. Cultural taxation and the over-commitment of service at predominantly white institutions. In: Bonner F, marbley a, Tuitt F, Robinson P, Banda R, Hughes R, editors. Black faculty in the academy: narratives for negotiating identity and achieving career success. New York: Routledge; 2015. p.41–51.

192. Gonzales L. Faculty inside a changing university: constructing roles, making spaces [Dissertation]. El Paso: University of Texas; 2010.

193. Allen W, Epps E, Guillory E, Suh S, Bonous-Hammarth M, Stassen M. Outsiders within: race, gender, and faculty status in U.S. higher education. In: Smith W, Altbach P, Lomotey K, editors. The racial crisis in American higher education: continuing challenges for the twenty-first century. rev. ed. Albany: State University of New York Press; 2002. p.189–220.

194. Borges N, Navarro A, Grover A, Hoban J. How, when, and why do physicians choose careers in academic medicine? a literature review. Academic Medicine. 2010;85(4):680–6.

195. Minnich E. Transforming knowledge. Philadelphia: Temple University Press; 1990.

196. Bonner F. The critical need for faculty mentoring. Say brother, can you spare the time? In: Bonner F, marbley a, Tuitt F, Robinson P, Banda R, Hughes R, editors. Black faculty in the academy: narratives for negotiating identity and achieving career success. New York: Routledge; 2015. p.123–36.

197. Rockquemore K, Laszloffy T. The black academic's guide to winning tenure— without losing your soul. Boulder: Lynne Rienner Publishers; 2008.

198. Andrews D. Navigating race-gendered microaggressions: The experiences of a tenure-track black female scholar. In: Bonner F, marbley a, Tuitt F, Robinson P, Banda R, Hughes R, editors. Black faculty in the academy: narratives for negotiating identity and achieving career success. New York: Routledge; 2015. p.79–88.

199. Chesler M, Lewis A, Crowfoot J. Challenging racism in higher education: promoting justice. Lanham, MD: Rowman & Littlefield; 2005.

200. Young E. Legal and educational foundations in critical race theory. In: Brooks J, Witherspoon-Arnold N, editors. Confronting racism in higher education: problems and

possibilities for fighting ignorance, bigotry and isolation. Charlotte, NC: Information Age; 2013. p.111–38.

201. Benschop Y, Holgersson C, Van den Brink M, Wahl A. Future challenges for practices of diversity management in organizations. In: Bendl R, Bleijenbergh I, Henttonen E, Mills A, editors. The Oxford handbook of diversity in organizations. New York: Oxford University Press; 2015. p.553–74.

202. Bezrukova K, Jehn K, Spell C. Reviewing diversity training: where we have been and where we should go. Academy of Management Learning & Education. 2012;11(2):207–27.

203. DiAngelo R. Nothing to add: a challenge to white silence in racial discussions. Understanding & Dismantling Privilege. 2012;2(1):1–17.

204. Johnson A. Privilege, power, and difference. 2nd ed. New York: McGraw-Hill; 2006.

205. Project Implicit. Implicit association test. Available from: https://implicit.harvard .edu/implicit/takeatest.html.

206. Pederson A, Walker I, Rapley M, Wise M. Anti-racism—what works? an evaluation of the effectiveness of anti-racism strategies. 2nd ed. Perth, Western Australia: Centre for Social Change & Social Equity Murdoch University; 2003. Available from: http://www .omi.wa.gov.au/resources/clearinghouse/antiracism_what_works.pdf.

207. Singleton G, Linton C. Courageous conversations about race: a field guide for achieving equity in schools. 2nd ed. Thousand Oaks, CA: Corwin Press; 2015.

208. Acosta D, Ackerman-Barger K. Breaking the silence: time to talk about race and racism. Academic Medicine. 2017; 92(3): 285–8. Available from: http://journals.lww.com/academic medicine/Abstract/publishahead/Breaking_the_Silence___Time_to_Talk_About_Race _and.98396.aspx.

209. Gates E. My daddy, the jailbird. The Daily Beast. July 21, 2009 [cited July 15, 2016]. Available from: http://www.thedailybeast.com/articles/2009/07/22/my-daddy -the-jailbird.html.

210. Davis A. Lecture on slavery and the prison industrial complex, delivered at Southern Illinois University, Carbondale. YouTube video; 2014. Available from: https://www .youtube.com/watch?v=6s8QCucFADc.

211. Kennedy Group Executive. Culture versus climate. n.d. Available from: http:// thekennedygroup. com/_pdfs/culture_vs_climate.pdf.

212. Victorino C, Nylund-Gibson K, Conley S. Campus racial climate: a litmus test for faculty satisfaction at four-year colleges and universities. Journal of Higher Education. 2013;84(6):769–805.

213. Litvin D. Diversity: making space for a better case. In: Konrad A, Prasad P, Pringle J, editors. Handbook of workplace diversity. Thousand Oaks, CA: Sage; 2006. p.75–94.

214. Salazar C. Strategies to survive and thrive in academia: the collective voices of counseling faculty of color. International Journal of Advanced Counseling. 2009;31:181–91.

215. Harvey W, Scott-Jones D. We can't find any: the elusiveness of black faculty members in American higher education. Issues in Education. 1985;3(1):68–76.

216. American Association of Medical Colleges. Table B6: total graduates by U.S. medical school and race / ethnicity, 2014–2015; 2015. Available from: https://www.aamc .org/download/321538/data/factstableb6.pdf.

217. Taylor D, Taylor J. The pharmacy student population: applications received 2010–2011, degrees conferred 2010–2011, fall enrollments. AACP Reports. American Journal of Pharmaceutical Education. 2012;76(6): S2. Available from: http://www.ajpe.org/doi /pdf/10.5688/ajpe766S2.

218. Gibbs K, Griffin K. What do I want to be with my PhD? the roles of personal values and structural dynamics in shaping the career interests of recent biomedical science PhD graduates. CBE-Life Sciences Education. 2013;12(4):711–23.

219. Hershel A, Lang J. The long-term retention and attrition of U.S. medical school faculty. Analysis in brief, 8(4). Washington, DC. American Association of Medical Colleges; 2008. Available from: https://www.aamc.org/download/67968/data/aibvol8no4.pdf.

220. Pololi L, Krupat E, Civian J, Ash A, Brennan R. Why are a quarter of faculty considering leaving academic medicine? a study of their perceptions of institutional culture and intentions to leave at 26 representative U.S. medical schools. Academic Medicine. 2012;87(7):859–69.

221. Fang D, Bednash. Attrition of full-time faculty from schools of nursing with baccalaureate and graduate programs, 2010 to 2011. Nursing Outlook. 2014;62(3):164–73.

222. Liu C, Morrison E. U.S. medical school full-time faculty attrition. Analysis in Brief. 2014;14(2):2. Washington, DC: American Association of Medical Colleges.

223. Moreno J, Smith D, Clayton-Pederson A, Parker S, Teraguchi D. The revolving door for underrepresented minority faculty in higher education: an analysis from the campus diversity initiative: The James Irvine Foundation; 2006. Available from: https:// folio.iupui.edu/bitstream/handle/10244/50/insight_Revolving_Door.pdf?sequence=1.

224. Ahmed S. "You end up doing the document rather than doing the doing": diversity, race equality and the politics of documentation. Ethnic & Racial Studies. 2007;30(4):590–609.

225. Zambrana R, Rashawn R, Espino M, Cohen B, Eliason J. "Don't leave us behind": the importance of mentoring for underrepresented minority faculty. American Educational Research Journal. 2015;52(1):40–72.

226. Osei-Kofi N. Junior faculty of color in the corporate university: implications of neoliberalism and neoconservativism on research, teaching, and service. In: Fryberg S, Martínez E, editors. The truly diverse faculty: new dialogues in American higher education. New York: Palgrave Macmillan; 2012. p.69–96.

227. Liaison Committee on Medical Education. Functions and structure of a medical school: standards for accreditation of medical education programs leading to the MD degree. Standards effective July 1, 2017. Liaison Committee on Medical Education;

2016. Available from: https://med.virginia.edu/ume-curriculum/wp-content/uploads/sites/216/2016/07/2017-18_Functions-and-Structure_2016-03-24.pdf/.

228. Commission on Osteopathic Colleges Accreditation. Accreditation of colleges of osteopathic medicine: COM accreditation standards and procedures. Chicago: American Osteopathic Association; 2016. Available from: https://www.osteopathic.org/inside-aoa/accreditation/COM-accreditation/Documents/com-accreditation-standards-7-1-16.pdf.

229. Commission on Dental Accreditation. Accreditation standards for dental education programs. Chicago: Commission on Dental Accreditation; 2016. Available from: http://www.ada.org/~/media/CODA/Files/predoc.ashx.

230. Commission on Dental Accreditation. Accreditation standards for dental therapy education programs. Chicago: Commission on Dental Accreditation; 2015. Available from: http://www.ada.org/~/media/CODA/Files/dt.pdf?la=en.

231. Accreditation Council for Pharmacy Education. Accreditation standards and key elements for the professional program in pharmacy leading to the doctor of pharmacy degree ("standards 2016"). Chicago: Accreditation Council for Pharmacy Education; 2015.

232. Commission for Nursing Education Accreditation: Accrediting standards for nursing education programs. Washington, DC: National League for Nursing; 2016.

233. Commission on Collegiate Nursing Education. Standards for accreditation of baccalaureate and graduate nursing programs, amended 2013. Washington, DC: Commission on Collegiate Nursing Education; 2013.

234. Accreditation Commission for Midwifery Education. Criteria for programmatic accreditation of midwifery education programs, with instructions for elaboration and documentation: Accreditation Commission for Midwifery Education; 2015. Available from: http://www.midwife.org/ACNM/files/ccLibraryFiles/Filename/000000006173/CriteriaforProgrammaticAccreditationofMidwiferyEducationPrograms(June2013April2015)updatedpassrateinstructionsforclarityJune2016.pdf.

235. Council on Accreditation of Nurse Anesthesia Educational Programs. Park Ridge, IL: Council on Accreditation of Nurse Anesthesia Educational Programs; 2016. Available from: http://home.coa.us.com/accreditation/Documents/Standards%20for%20Accreditation%20of%20Nurse%20Anesthesia%20Programs%20-%20Practice%20Doctorate,%20rev%20June%202016.pdf.

236. Accreditation Commission for Education in Nursing. Accreditation manual. Accreditation Commission for Education in Nursing; 2016. Available from: http://www.acenursing.org/accreditation-manual/.

237. Bureau of Labor Statistics, US Department of Labor. Registered nurses have highest employment in healthcare occupations; anesthesiologists earn the most. Bureau of Labor Statistics, US Department of Labor; July 13, 2015. Available from: http://www.bls.gov/opub/ted/2015/registered-nurses-have-highest-employment-in-healthcare-occupations-anesthesiologists-earn-the-most.htm.

238. Giles M. Acclimating to the institutional climate: there's a "chill" in the air. In:

Bonner F, marbley a, Tuitt F, Robinson P, Banda R, Hughes R, editors. Black faculty in the academy: narratives for negotiating identity and achieving career success. New York: Routledge; 2015. p.13–22.

239. Smith D. The diversity imperative: moving to the next generation. In: Bastedo M, Altbach P, Gumport P, editors. American higher education in the twenty-first century: political, social, and economic challenges 4th ed. Baltimore: Johns Hopkins University Press; 2016. p.375–400.

240. Whittaker J, Montgomery B, Acosta V. Retention of underrepresented minority faculty: strategic initiatives for institutional value proposition based on perspectives from a range of academic institutions. Journal of Undergraduate Neuroscience Education. 2015;13(3):A136–A45.

241. Stewart P. The uphill climb: scholars see little progress in efforts to diversify faculty ranks. Diverse Issues in Higher Education. 2012;29(11):16–7.

242. Relf M. Advancing diversity in academic nursing. Journal of Professional Nursing. 2016;32(5S):S42–S47.

243. Angelou M. A conversation with Dr. Maya Angelou. In: LaNae T, editor. Beautifully Said Magazine. 2012. Available from: http://beautifullysmagazine.com/201207feature -of-the-month-3/.

244. Law A, Bottenberg M, Brozick A, Currie J, DiVall M, Haines S, et al. A checklist for the development of faculty mentorship programs. American Journal of Pharmaceutical Education. 2014;78(5):98.

245. Eiland L, Marlowe K, Sacks G. Development of faculty mentor teams in a pharmacy practice department. Currents in Pharmacy Teaching and Learning. 2014;6(6):759–66.

246. Palepu A, Friedman R, Barnett R, Carr P, Ash A, Szalacha L, et al. Junior faculty members' mentoring relationships and their professional development in U.S. medical schools. Academic Medicine. 1998;73(3):318–23.

247. Sambunjak D, Straus S, Marušić A. Mentoring in academic medicine: a systematic review. JAMA. 2006;296(9):1103–15.

248. Byington C, Keenan H, Phillips J, Childs R, Wachs E, Berzins M, et al. A matrix mentoring model that effectively supports clinical and translational scientists and increases inclusion in biomedical research: lessons from the University of Utah. Academic Medicine. 2016;91(4):497–502.

249. Fuller K, Maniscalco-Feichtl M, Droege M. The role of the mentor in retaining junior pharmacy faculty members. American Journal of Pharmaceutical Education. 2008;72(2):41.

250. Kohn H. A mentoring program to help junior faculty members achieve scholarship success. American Journal of Pharmaceutical Education. 2014;78(2):29.

251. Mkandawire-Valhmu L, Kako P, Stevens P. Mentoring women faculty of color in nursing academia: creating an environment that supports scholarly growth and retention. Nursing Outlook. 2010;58(3):135–41.

252. Shollen S, Bland C, Center B, Finstad D, Taylor A. Relating mentor type and

mentoring behaviors to academic medicine faculty satisfaction and productivity at one medical school. Academic Medicine. 2014;89(9):1267–75.

253. Gwyn P. The quality of mentoring relationships' impact on the occupational commitment of nursing faculty. Journal of Professional Nursing. 2011;27(5):292–8.

254. Dunham-Taylor J, Lynn C, Moore P, McDaniel S, Walker J. What goes around comes around: improving faculty retention through more effective mentoring. Journal of Professional Nursing. 2008;24(6):337–46.

255. Chung C, Kowalski S. Job stress, mentoring, psychological empowerment, and job satisfaction among nursing faculty. Journal of Nursing Education. 2012;51(7):381–8.

256. Reid M, Misky G, Harrison R, Sharpe B, Auerbach A, Glasheen J. Mentorship, productivity, and promotion among academic hospitalists. Journal of General Internal Medicine. 2012;27(1):23–7.

257. Wasserstein A, Quistberg A, Shea J. Mentoring at the University of Pennsylvania: results of a faculty survey. Journal of General Internal Medicine. 2007;22:210–4.

258. Franko D. From nothing to something: the nuts and bolts of building a mentoring program in a health sciences college. Mentoring & Tutoring: Partnership in Learning. 2016;24(2):109–23.

259. Straus S, Johnson M, Marquez C, Feldman M. Characteristics of successful and failed mentoring relationships: a qualitative study across two academic health centers. Academic Medicine. 2013;88(1):82–9.

260. Cora-Bramble D, Zhang K, Castillo-Page L. Minority faculty members' resilience and academic productivity: are they related? Academic Medicine. 2010;85(9):1492–8.

261. Burden J, Harrison L, Hodge S. Perceptions of African American faculty in kinesiology-based programs at predominantly white American institutions of higher education. Research Quarterly for Exercise & Sport. 2005;76(2):224–37.

262. Zambrana R. Inequality in higher education: diversity or transformation? In: Palmer S., Gyllensten, K, editors. Psychological stress, v. 1. The history and development of theories: stress. London: SAGE Ltd.; 2015:109–15. Available from: http://www.crge.umd.edu/pdf/rez/2015%20Zambrana%20Inequality%20in%20Higher%20Ed.pdf.

263. Hill J, Del Favero M, Ropers-Huilman B. The role of mentoring in developing African American nurse leaders. Research and Theory in Nursing Practice: An International Journal. 2005;19(4):341–56.

264. Ramanan R, Phillips R, Davis R, Silen W, Reede J. Mentoring in medicine: keys to satisfaction. American Journal of Medicine. 2002;112(4):336–41.

265. Pololi L, Evans A, Civian J, Vasiliou V, Coplit L, Gillum L, et al. Mentoring faculty: a US national survey of its adequacy and linkage to culture in academic health centers. Journal of Continuing Education in the Health Professions. 2015;35(3):176–84.

266. Pololi L, Evans A, Gibbs B, Krupat E, Brennan R, Civian J. The experience of minority faculty who are underrepresented in medicine, at 26 representative U.S. medical schools. Academic Medicine. 2013;88(9):1308–14.

267. Byrne D. The attraction paradigm. New York: Academic Press; 1971.

268. Hu C, Thomas K, Lance C. Intentions to initiate mentoring relationships: understanding the impact of race, proactivity, feelings of deprivation, and relationship roles. Journal of Social Psychology. 2008;148(6):727–44.

269. Ginther D, Schaffer W, Schnell J, Masimore B, Liu F, Haak L, et al. Race, ethnicity, and NIH research awards. Science. 2011;333(6045):1015–9.

270. Warner E, Carapinha R, Weber G, Hill E, Reede J. Faculty promotion and attrition: the importance of coauthor network reach at an academic medical center. Journal of General Internal Medicine. 2016;31(1):60–7.

271. Victorino C. Examining faculty satisfaction, productivity, and collegiality in higher education: contemporary contexts and modern methods. Dissertation Abstracts International Section A: Humanities and Social Sciences. 2013;74(2-A(E)).

272. Payton T, Howe L, Timmons S, Richardson M. African American nursing students' perceptions about mentoring. Nursing Education Perspectives. 2013;34(3):173–87.

273. Thomas K, Willis, L, Davis, J. Mentoring minority graduate students: issues and strategies for institutions, faculty, and students. Educational Opportunities International. 2007;26(3):178–92.

274. Wong R, Sullivan M, Yeo H, Roman S, Bell R, Sosa J. Race and surgical residency: results from a national survey of 4339 U.S. general surgery residents. Annals of Surgery. 2013;257(4):782–7.

275. McCoy D, Winkle-Wagner R, Luedke C. Colorblind mentoring? exploring white faculty mentoring of students of color. Journal of Diversity in Higher Education. 2015;8(4):225–42.

276. Bond M, Cason C, Baxley S. Institutional support for diverse populations: perceptions of Hispanic and African American students and program faculty. Nurse Educator. 2015;40(3):134–48.

277. Dickerson S, Neary M, Hyche-Johnson M. Native American graduate nursing students' learning experiences. Journal of Nursing Scholarship. 2000;32(2):189–96.

278. Mainah F, Perkins V. Challenges facing female leaders of color in U.S. higher education. International Journal of African Development. 2015;2(2):5–13.

279. US Department of Labor. A solid investment: making full use of the nation's human capital. Recommendations of the Federal Glass Ceiling Commission. Washington, DC: US Government Printing Office; 1995. Available from: http://digitalcommons.ilr.cornell.edu/cgi/viewcontent.cgi?article=1117&context=key_workplace.

280. Fang D, Li Y, Stauffer DC, Trautman DE. 2015–2016 salaries of deans in baccalaureate and graduate programs in nursing. Washington, DC: American Association of Colleges of Nursing; 2016.

281. Chmar J, Weaver R, Ranney R, Haden N, Valochovic R. A profile of dental school deans, 2002. Journal of Dental Education. 2004;68(4):475–87.

282. Haden N, Ditmyer M, Rodriguez T, Mobley C, Beck L, Valachovic R. A profile of dental school deans, 2014. Journal of Dental Education. 2015;79(10):1243–50.

283. Rodriguez T, Zhang M, Tucker-Lively F, Ditmyer M, Brallier L, Haden N, et al. Profile of department chairs in U.S. and Canadian dental schools: demographics, requirements for success, and professional development needs. Journal of Dental Education. 2016;80(3):365–73.

284. Rayburn W, Alexander H, Lang J, Scott J. First-time department chairs at U.S. medical schools: a 29 year perspective on recruitment and retention. Academic Medicine. 2009;84(10):1336–41.

285. Kosoko-Lasaki O, Sonnino R, Voytko M. Mentoring for women and underrepresented minority faculty and students: experience at two institutions of higher education. Journal of the National Medical Association. 2006;98(9):1449–59.

286. Palermo A, Soto-Greene M, Taylor V, Cornbill R, Johnson J, Mindt M, et al. No. 5—Successful programs in minority faculty development: overview. Diversity in academic medicine, special issue of Mount Sinai Journal of Medicine. 2008;75(6):523–32.

287. Lewellen-Williams C, Johnson V, Deloney L, Thomas B, Goyol A, Henry-Tillman R. The POD: a new model for mentoring underrepresented minority faculty. Academic Medicine. 2006;81(3):275–9.

288. Adanga E, Avakame E, Carthon M, Guevara J. An environmental scan of faculty diversity programs at U.S. medical schools. Academic Medicine. 2012;87(11):1540–7.

289. Johnson W. On being a mentor: a guide for higher education faculty. 2nd ed. New York: Routledge; 2016.

290. Sambunjak D, Straus S, Marusic A. A systematic review of qualitative research on the meaning and characteristics of mentoring in academic medicine. Journal of General Internal Medicine. 2010;25(1):72–8.

291. Tran N. The role of mentoring in the success of women leaders of color in higher education. Mentoring and Tutoring: Partnership in Learning. 2014;22(4):302–15.

292. Mainah F. The rising of black women in academic leadership positions in USA: lived experiences of black female faculty [Dissertation]. Chicago: Chicago School of Professional Psychology; 2016.

293. Munden S. Starting at the top: increasing African American female representation at higher education administration in the United States [Dissertation]. Boston: Northeastern University; 2015.

294. Savala L. The experiences of Latina/o executives in higher education [Dissertation]. Kalamazoo: Western Michigan University; 2014.

295. Peek M, Kim K, Johnson J, Vela M. "URM candidates are encouraged to apply": a national study to identify effective strategies to enhance racial and ethnic faculty diversity in academic departments of medicine. Academic Medicine. 2013;88(3):405–12.

296. Gray J, Carter P. Growing our own: building a Native research team. Journal of Psychoactive Drugs. 2012;44(2):160–5.

297. Sinkford J, Valachovic R, Weaver R, West J. Minority dental faculty development: responsibility and challenge. Journal of Dental Education. 2010;74(12):1388–93.

298. Smalling S. American Indians in social work education: addressing issues of recruitment, retention and inclusion [Dissertation]. Cleveland: Case Western Reserve University; 2012. Available from: https://etd.ohiolink.edu/pg_10?0::NO:10:P10_ACCESSION_NUM:case1333400579#abstract-files.

299. Padilla R. Barriers to accessing the professoriate. In: Castellanos J, Jones L, editors. The majority in the minority: expanding the representation of Latino/a faculty, administrators and students in higher education. Sterling, VA: Stylus; 2003. p.179–204.

300. Guevera J, Adanga E, Avakame E, Carthorn M. Minority faculty development programs and underrepresented minority faculty representation at US medical schools. JAMA. 2013;310(21):2297–304.

301. Zachery L. The mentor's guide: facilitating effective learning relationships. 2nd ed. San Francisco: Jossey-Bass; 2011.

302. Johnson-Bailey J, Cervero R. Mentoring in black and white: the intricacies of cross-cultural mentoring. Mentoring and Tutoring. 2004;12(1):7–21.

303. Stanley C, Lincoln Y. Cross-race faculty mentoring. Change: The Magazine of Higher Learning. 2005;37(2):44–50.

304. Rabionet S, Santiago L, Zorilla C. A multifaceted mentoring model for minority researchers to address HIV health disparities. American Journal of Public Health. 2009;99(S1):S65–S70.

305. Sinkford J, West J, Weaver R, Valochovic R. Modeling mentoring: early lessons from the W. K. Kellogg ADEA Minority Dental Faculty Development Program. Journal of Dental Education. 2009;73(6):753–63.

306. Wilson D, Spitzer C. Wilson's way: win, don't whine; a minority medical leader's relentless rise to the top. San Bernardino, CA: BookSurge Publisher; 2009.

307. marbley a, Rouson L, Li J, Huang S, Taylor C. Black faculty negotiating the microaggressions in scholarship. In: Bonner F, marbley a, Tuitt F, Robinson O, Banda R, Hughes R, editors. Black faculty in the academy: narratives for negotiating identity and achieving career success. New York: Routledge; 2015. p.55–66.

308. Lutz K, Hassouneh D, Akeroyd J, Beckett A. Balancing survival and resistance: experiences of faculty of color in predominantly Euro-American schools of nursing. Journal of Diversity in Higher Education. 2013;6(2):127–46.

309. Boyd-Ball A. Who am I (swit I? skwist) as an American Indian woman in academia: traversing two worlds. In: Curtis-Boles H, Adams D, Jenkins-Monroe, V, editors. Making our voices heard: women of color in academia. New York: Nova Science Publishers; 2012. p.63–76.

310. Miranda A. Tenure on my terms. In: Stanley C, editor. Faculty of color: teaching in predominantly white colleges and universities. Bolton, MA: Anker Publishing; 2006. p.225–33.

311. Stanley C. An overview of the literature. In: Stanley C, editor. Faculty of color: teaching in predominantly white colleges and universities. Bolton, MA: Anker Publishing; 2006. p.1–29.

312. Alexander R, Moore S. The benefits, challenges, and strategies of African American faculty teaching in predominantly white institutions. Journal of African American Studies. 2008;12(1):4–18.

313. Jarmon B. Unwritten rules of the game. In: Mabokela R, Green A, editors. Sisters of the academy: emergent black women scholars in higher education. Sterling, VA: Stylus; 2001. p.175–82.

314. Ross A. Learning to play the game. In: Stanley C, editor. Faculty of color: teaching in predominantly white colleges and universities. Bolton, MA: Anker Publishing; 2006. p.263–82.

315. Monture P. Race, gender, and the university: strategies for survival. In: Razack S, Smith M, Thobani S, editors. States of race: critical feminism for the 21st century. Toronto: Between the Lines; 2010. p.23–35.

316. Alfred M. Success in the ivory tower: lessons learned from black tenured female faculty at a major research university. In: Mabokela R, Green A, editors. Sisters of the academy: emergent black women scholars in higher education. Sterling, VA: Stylus; 2001. p.57–79.

317. Adams S. Succeeding in the face of doubt. In: Stanley C, editor. Faculty of color: teaching in predominantly white colleges and universities. Bolton, MA: Anker Publishing; 2006. p.30–40.

318. Temple J, Thao Y, Henry S. Multiple voices: same song. In: Mack D, Watson E, Camacho M, editors. Mentoring faculty of color: essays on professional development and advancement in colleges and universities. Jefferson, NC: McFarland & Company; 2013. p.140–52.

319. Holmes D, Murray S, Perron A, Rail G. Deconstructing the evidence-based discourse in health sciences: truth, power, and fascism. International Journal of Evidence Based Health Care. 2006;4(3):180–6.

320. Jenkins-Monroe V. How I got over: supports and lifelines in my journey to the academy. In: Curtis-Boles H, Adams D, Jenkins-Monroe V, editors. Making our voices heard: women of color in academia. New York: Nova Science Publishers; 2012. p.89–98.

321. Buettner-Schmidt K, Lobo M. Social justice: a concept analysis. Journal of Advanced Nursing. 2012;68(4):948–58.

322. Joseph T, Hirshfield L. "Why don't you get somebody new to do it?" Race and cultural taxation in the academy. Journal of Racial and Ethnic Studies. 2010;34(1):121–41.

323. Turner, C. Defining success: promotion and tenure—planning for each stage and beyond. In: García M, editor. Succeeding in an academic career: a guide for faculty of color. Westport, CT: Greenwood Press; 2000. p.111–40.

324. Edwards J, Bryant S, Clark T. African American female social work educators in predominantly white schools of social work: strategies for thriving. Journal of African American Studies. 2008;12(1):37–49.

325. Robinson O. Characteristics of racism and the health consequences experienced by black nursing faculty. ABNF Journal. 2014;25(4):110–5.

326. Watson L. The politics of tenure and promotion of African-American faculty. In: Jones L, editor. Retaining African Americans in higher education: challenging paradigms for retaining students, faculty & administrators. Sterling, VA: Stylus; 2001. p.235–45.

327. Hu-DeHart E. Office politics and departmental culture. In: García M, editor. Succeeding in an academic career: a guide for faculty of color. Westport, CT: Greenwood Publishing; 2000. p.27–38.

328. Adams D. Racism, trauma, and being the Other in the classroom. In: Curtis-Boles H, Adams D, , Jenkins-Monroe, V, editors. Making our voices heard: women of color in academia. New York: Nova Science; 2012. p.35–46.

329. Moore A. The life of a black male scholar: contesting racial microaggressions in academe. In: Bonner F, marbley a, Tuitt F, Robinson P, Banda R, Hughes R, editors. Black faculty in the academy: narratives for negotiating identity and achieving career success. New York: Routledge; 2015. p.23–32.

330. Allen B. Resisting power to survive and thrive in academia. In: Curtis-Boles H, Adams D, Jenkins-Monroe V, editors. Making our voices heard: women of color in academia. New York: Nova Science; 2012. p.99–105.

331. Liu J. An open letter on how to succeed in academic life. In: Mack D, Watson E, Camacho M, editors. Mentoring faculty of color: essays on professional development and advancement in colleges and universities. Jefferson, NC: McFarland & Company; 2013. p.103–15.

332. Morrison T. The truest eye of the greater good. O Magazine. 2003;(November). Available from: http://www.oprah.com/omagazine/toni-morrison-talks-love.

333. Rodriguez J, Campbell K, Pololi L. Addressing disparities in academic medicine: what of the minority tax? BMC Medical Education. 2015;15(6):1–5.

334. Zirkel S. Is there a place for me? Role models and academic identity among white students and students of color. Teachers College Record. 2002;104(2):357–76.

335. Sue D. Microaggressions in everyday life. Race, gender, and sexual orientation. Hoboken, NJ: John Wiley & Sons; 2010.

336. Coleman S, Stevenson H. The racial stress of membership: development of the faculty inventory of racialized experiences in schools. Psychology in the Schools. 2013;50(6):548–66.

337. Thomas F. Experiences of black women who persist to graduation at predominantly white schools of nursing. [Dissertation]. New Orleans, LA: University of New Orleans; 2009. Available from: http://scholarworks.uno.edu/cgi/viewcontent.cgi?article=2007&context=td.

338. Hassouneh D, Beckett A. An education in racism. Journal of Nursing Education. 2003;42(6):258–65.

339. White B, Fulton J. Common experiences of African American nursing students: an integrative review. Nursing Education Perspectives. 2015;36(3):167–75.

340. Dyrbye L, Thomas M, Eacker A, et al. Race, ethnicity, and medical student well-being in the United States. Archives of Internal Medicine. 2007;167(19):2103–9.

341. Odom K, Roberts L, Johnson R, Cooper L. Exploring obstacles to and opportunities for professional success among ethnic minority medical students. Academic Medicine. 2007;82(2):146–53.

342. Hassouneh D, Lutz K. Having influence: faculty of color having influence. Nursing Outlook. 2013;61(3):153–63.

343. Umbach P. The contribution of faculty of color to undergraduate education. Research in Higher Education. 2006;47(3):317–45.

344. Bowman N. How much diversity is enough? The curvilinear relationship between college diversity interactions and first-year student outcomes. Research in Higher Education. 2013;54(8):874–94.

345. Baker C. Social support and success in higher education: the influence of on-campus support on African American and Latino college students. Urban Review: Issues and Ideas in Public Education. 2013;45(5):632–50.

346. Smith C, Ester T, Inglehart M. Dental education and care for underserved patients: an analysis of students' intentions and alumni behavior. Journal of Dental Education. 2006;70(4):398–408.

347. Crandall S, Davis S, Broeseker A, Hildebrandt C. A longitudinal comparison of pharmacy and medical students' attitudes toward the medically underserved. American Journal of Pharmaceutical Education. 2008;72(6):148.

348. Major N, McQuistan M, Qian F. Changes in dental students' attitudes about treating underserved populations: a longitudinal study. Journal of Dental Education. 2016;80(5):517–25.

349. Habibian M, Seirawan H, Mulligan R. Dental students' attitudes toward underserved populations across four years of dental school. Journal of Dental Education. 2011;75(8):1020–29.

350. Stephens M, Landers G, Davis S, Durning S, Crandall S. Medical student attitudes toward the medically underserved: the USU perspective. Military Medicine. 2015;180(4):61.

351. Baez B. Race-related service and faculty of color: conceptualizing critical agency in academe. Higher Education. 2000;39(3):363–91.

352. Ross L. Blackballed: the black and white politics of race on America's campuses. New York: St. Martin's Press; 2015.

353. Potter H. What can we learn from states that ban affirmative action? The Century Foundation; June 26, 2014. Available from: https://tcf.org/content/commentary/what-can-we-learn-from-states-that-ban-affirmative-action/.

354. DeSantis N. Supreme Court upholds use of race-conscious admissions at U. of Texas. Chronicle of Higher Education. June 23, 2016. Available from: http://www.chronicle.com/blogs/ticker/supreme-court-upholds-use-of-race-conscious-admissions-at-u-of-texas-3/112357.

355. Wall A, Aljets A, Ellis S, Hansen D, Moore M, Petrelli H, et al. White paper on pharmacy admissions: developing a diverse work force to meet the health-care needs of an increasingly diverse society—recommendations of the American Association of

Colleges of Pharmacy Special Committee on Admissions. American Journal of Pharmaceutical Education. 2015;79(7):S7.

356. Adams A, Bletzinger R, Sondheimer H, White S, Johnson L. Roadmap to diversity: integrating holistic review practices into medical school admission processes. Association of American Medical Colleges; 2010. Available from: https://members.aamc.org /eweb/upload/Roadmap%20to%20Diversity%20Integrating%20Holistic%20Review.pdf.

357. American Dental Education Association. Incorporating holistic review in admissions practices: resources. Washington, DC: American Dental Education Association; n.d. Available from: http://www.adea.org/HolisticReview/Incorporating-Holistic-Review .aspx.

358. American Association of Colleges of Nursing. Holistic admissions review in nursing. Washington, DC: American Association of Colleges of Nursing; 2016. Available from: http://www.aacn. nche.edu/education-resources/holistic-review.

359. Price S, Grant-Mills D. Effective admissions practices to achieve greater student diversity in dental schools. Journal of Dental Education. 2010;74(10):S87–S97.

360. Urban Universities for Health. Holistic admissions in the health professions: findings from a national survey [cited September 2014]. Available from: http:// urbanuniversitiesforhealth.org/media/documents/Holistic_Admissions_in_the_Health _Professions.pdf.

361. Felix H, Laird J, Ennulat C, Donkers K, Garrubba C, Hawkins S, et al. Holistic admissions process: an initiative to support diversity in medical education. Journal of Physician Assistant Education. 2012;23(3):21–7.

362. Terregino C, McConnell M, Reiter H. The effect of differential weighting of academics, experiences, and competencies measured by the multiple mini interview (MMI) on race and ethnicity of cohorts accepted to one medical school. Academic Medicine. 2015;90(12):1651–7.

363. Brotherton S, Stoddard J, Tang S. Minority and nonminority pediatricians' care of minority and poor children. Archives of Pediatrics & Adolescent Medicine. 2000;154(9):912–7.

364. Saha S, Shipman S. Race-neutral versus race-conscious workforce policy to improve access to care. Health Affairs. 2008;27(1):234–45.

365. US Department of Health & Human Services. 20 million people have gained health insurance coverage because of the Affordable Care Act, new estimates show [updated March 3, 2016]. Available from: https://www.hhs.gov/about/news/2016/03/03 /20-million-people-have-gained-health-insurance-coverage-because-affordable-care -act-new-estimates.

366. Nivet M. Commentary: diversity 3.0: a necessary systems upgrade. Academic Medicine. 2011;86(12):1487–9.

367. Albino J, Inglehart M, Tedesco L. Dental education and changing oral health care needs: disparities and demands. Journal of Dental Education. 2012;76(1):75–88.

368. hooks b. Killing rage: ending racism. New York: Henry Holt; 1995.

369. Flagg B. Whiteness: some critical perspectives. Foreword: whiteness as metaprivilege. Washington University Journal of Law and Policy. 2005;18(1–2):1–11.

370. Sinkford J, Harrison S, Brunson W, Valachovic R. Advancement of women in dental education: expanding opportunities, enriching the pool. Journal of Dental Education. 2011;75(5):707–11.

371. Zhuge Y, Kaufman J, Simeone D, Chen H, Velazquez O. Is there still a glass ceiling for women in academic surgery? Annals of Surgery. 2011;253(4):637–43.

372. Kleinman C. Understanding and capitalizing on men's advantages in nursing. Journal of Nursing Administration. 2004;34(2):78–82.

373. Kouta C, Kaite C. Gender discrimination and nursing: a literature review. Journal of Professional Nursing. 2011;27(1):59–63.

374. Williams C. The glass escalator: hidden advantages for men in the "female" professions. Social Problems. 1992;39(3):253–67.

375. Muench U, Sindelar J, Busch S, Buerhaus P. Salary differences between male and female registered nurses in the United States. JAMA. 2015;313(12):1265–7.

376. Westphal J. Characteristics of nurse leaders in hospitals in the USA from 1992 to 2008. Journal of Nursing Management. 2012;20(7):928–37.

377. Williams C. Hidden advantages for men in nursing. Nursing Administration Quarterly. 1995;19(2):63–70.

378. Buhr K. Is there a glass escalator for male nurses in Canada? Nursing Leadership. 2011;24(3):86–100.

379. Maume D. Glass ceilings and glass escalators: occupational segregation and race and sex differences in managerial positions. Work and Occupations. 1999;26(4):483–509.

380. Landivar C. Men in nursing occupations: American community surveys highlight report. US Census Bureau; February 2013. Available from: https://www.census.gov/people/io/files/Men_in_Nursing_Occupations.pdf.

381. Wingfield A. Racializing the glass escalator: reconsidering men's experiences with women's work. Gender & Society. 2009;23(1):5–26.

382. Dodani, S, LaPorte, R. Brain drain from developing countries: how can brain drain be converted into wisdom gain? Journal of the Royal Society of Medicine. 2005;98(11):487–91.

383. Pew Research Center. Modern immigration wave brings 59 million to U.S., driving population growth and change through 2065: views of immigrations' impact on U.S. society mixed. Chapter 5, U.S. foreign born population trends. 2015. Available from: http://www.pewhispanic.org/2015/09/28/chapter-5-u-s-foreign-born-population-trends/.

384. Gahungu A. Integration of foreign-born faculty in academia: foreignness as an asset. International Journal of Educational Leadership Preparation. 2011;6(1):1–22.

385. Zeng L, Yan-he G. A comparative study of refereed journal articles published by native and foreign born faculty in the United States. US-China Education Review. 2010;7(8):78–86.

386. National Science Foundation. Science and engineering indicators 2014. Chapter 5,

academic research and development: doctoral scientists and engineers in academia. 2014. Available from: http://www.nsf.gov/statistics/seind14/index.cfm/chapter-5/c5s3.htm.

387. McCabe K. Foreign-born health care workers in the United States. Migration Policy Institute; 2012 [updated June 27, 2012]. Available from: http://www.migrationpolicy.org /article/foreign-born-health-care-workers-united-states.

388. Opoku S. Assessing geographic variation and migration behaviors of foreign-born medical graduates in the United States. [Dissertation]. Omaha: University of Nebraska Medical Center; 2015.

389. Mick S, Lee S, Wodchis W. Variations in geographical distribution of foreign and domestically trained physicians in the United States: "safety nets" or "surplus exacerbation"? Social Science & Medicine. 2000;50(2):185–202.

390. Pew Research Center. Social and demographic trends: the rise of Asians. 2012. Available from: http://www.pewsocialtrends.org/2012/06/19/the-rise-of-asian-americans/.

391. Hoeffel E, Rastogi S, Kim M, Shahid H. The Asian population: 2010. 2012. Available from: https://www.census.gov/prod/cen2010/briefs/c2010br-11.pdf.

392. Kim J. Asian American racial identity development theory. In: Wijeyesinghe C, Jackson B, editors. New perspectives on racial identify development: integrating emerging frameworks. 2nd ed. New York: New York University Press; 2012. p.138–60.

393. Suh S. The significance of race for Asian Americans: access, rewards, and workplace experiences of academics [Dissertation]. Los Angeles: University of California Los Angeles; 2008.

394. Rastogi S, Johnson T, Hoeffel E, Drewery M. The black population: 2010. 2011. Report No.: C2010BR-06.

395. Kochhar R, Fry R. Wealth inequality has widened along racial, ethnic lines since end of Great Recession. Pew Research Center; 2014 [updated December, 12, 2014]. Available from: http://www.pewresearch.org/fact-tank/2014/12/12/racial-wealth-gaps-great -recession/.

396. Benson J. Exploring the racial identity of black immigrants in the United States. Sociological Forum. 2006;21(2):219–47.

397. Guenther K, Pendaz S, Makene F. The impact of intersecting dimensions of inequality and identity on the racial status of Eastern African immigrants. Sociological Forum. 2011;26(1):98–120.

398. American Association of Medical Colleges. Table A12: applicants, first-time applicants, acceptees, and matriculants to U.S. medical schools by race/ethnicity, 2013–2014 through 2016–2017. American Association of Medical Colleges; 2013. Available from: https://www.aamc.org/download/321480/data/factstablea12.pdf.

399. American Dental Education Association. ADEA survey of U.S. dental school applicants and enrollees, 2010 entering class. American Dental Education Association; 2012. Available from: http://www.adea.org/publications/library/ADEAsurveysreports /Pages/ADEASurveyofUSDentalSchoolApplicantsandEnrollees20102011.aspx.

400. Brown A. U.S. Hispanic and Asian populations growing, but for different reasons. Pew Research Center; June 26, 2014. Available from: http://www.pewresearch.org/fact-tank/2014/06/26/u-s-hispanic-and-asian-populations-growing-but-for-different-reasons/.

401. Ennis R, Rios-Vargas M, Albert N. The Hispanic population: 2010. 2011. Available from: http://www.nsf.gov/statistics/infbrief/nsf13323/nsf13323.pdf.

402. Gonzalez-Barrera B, Lopez M. Is being Hispanic a matter of race, ethnicity or both? Pew Research Center; 2015. Available from: http://www.pewresearch.org/fact-tank/2015/06/15/is-being-hispanic-a-matter-of-race-ethnicity-or-both/.

403. Humes K, Ramirez R, Jones N, Rios M, Buchanan A, Marks R. Meeting summary, Forum on Ethnic Groups from the Middle East and North Africa. May 29, 2015. Suitland, MD: US Census Bureau; 2015. Available from: http://www.census.gov/library/working-papers/2015/demo/2015-MENA-Experts.html.

404. Dudar H. Arabs, others feel overlooked, undercounted. The Blade; 2014 [updated January 20, 2014]. Available from: http://www.toledoblade. com/Culture/2014/01/19/Arabs-others-feel-overlooked-undercounted.html.

405. Pavlovskaya M, Bier J. Mapping census data for difference: towards the heterogeneous geographies of Arab American communities in the New York metropolitan area. Geoforum. 2012;43(3):483–96.

406. Krogstad J. Census Bureau explores new Middle East/North Africa ethnic category. 2014. Available from: http://www.pewresearch.org/fact-tank/2014/03/24/census-bureau-explores-new-middle-eastnorth-africa-ethnic-category/.

407. Arab American Institute. Quick facts about Arab Americans. 2011. Available from: http://b. 3cdn. net/aai/fcc68db3efdd45f613_vim6ii3a7.pdf.

408. Ajrouch K, Jamal A. Assimilating to a white identity: the case of Arab Americans. International Migration Review. 2007;41(4):860–79.

409. Lipton E. Panel says census move on Arab-Americans recalls World War II internments. New York Times. November 10, 2004. Available from: http://query.nytimes.com/gst/fullpage.html?res=9802E1DA113CF933A25752C1A9629C8B63.

410. Zong J, Batalova J. Middle Eastern and Northern African immigrants in the United States. 2015 [updated June 3, 2015]. Available from: http://www.migrationpolicy.org/article/middle-eastern-and-north-african-immigrants-united-states.

411. Arab American Institute. Demographics. 2014. Available from: https://d3n8a8pro7vhmx.cloudfront.net/aai/pages/9843/attachments/original/1460668240/National_Demographic_Profile_2014.pdf?1460668240.

412. Arab American Institute. Attitudes toward Arabs and Muslims. December 21, 2015. Available from: https://d3n8a8pro7vhmx.cloudfront.net/aai/pages/11126/attachments/original/1450651184/2015_American_Attitudes_Toward_Arabs_and_Muslims.pdf?1450651184.

413. Pew Research Center. Views of government's handling of terrorism fall to post-

9/11 low: little change in views of relationship between Islam and violence. Pew Research Center; December 15, 2015. Available from: http://www.people-press.org/2015/12/15/views-of-governments-handling-of-terrorism-fall-to-post-911-low/.

414. Mir A, Toor S, Mir R. Of race and religion: understanding the roots of anti-Muslim prejudice in the United States. In: Bendl R, Bleijenbergh I, Henttonen E, Mills A, editors. The Oxford handbook of diversity in organizations. New York: Oxford University Press. 2015; p.499–517.

415. Haj-Ali R. Just because I choose to be me. In: Stanley C, editor. Faculty of color: teaching in predominantly white colleges and universities. Bolton, MA: Anker Publishing; 2006. p.175–81.

416. Norris T, Vines P, Hoeffel E. The American Indian and Alaska Native population 2010. 2012. Report No.: C2010BR-10.

417. Stannard D. American holocaust: the conquest of the new world. New York: Oxford University Press; 1992.

418. Artiga S, Arguello R, Duckett P. Health coverage and care for American Indians and Alaska Natives: executive summary. Menlo Park, CA: Henry Kaiser Family Foundation; October 7, 2013.

419. Krogstad J. One-in-four Native American and Alaska Natives are living in poverty. Pew Research Center; 2014. Available from: http://www.pewresearch.org/fact-tank/2014/06/13/1-in-4-native-americans-and-alaska-natives-are-living-in-poverty/.

420. Jacobson M. Breaking silence, building solutions: the role of social justice group work in the retention of faculty of color. Social Work with Groups. 2012;35(3):267–86.

421. Albritton T. Educating our own: the historical legacy of HBCUs and their relevance for educating a new generation of leaders. Urban Review: Issues and Ideas in Public Education. 2012;44:311–31.

422. Bettez S, Suggs V. Centering the educational and social significance of HBCUs: a focus on the journeys and thoughts of African American scholars. Urban Review: Issues and Ideas in Public Education. 2012;44:303–10.

423. Wooten M. In the face of inequality: how black colleges adapt. Albany: State University of New York Press; 2015.

424. Lee J. Moving beyond racial and ethnic diversity at HBCUs. In: Palmer R, Shorette R, Gasman M, editors. Exploring diversity at historically black colleges and universities: implications for policy and practice. San Francisco: Jossey-Bass; 2015. p.17–35.

425. Seymour S, Ray J. Grads of historically black colleges have well-being edge. Gallup; 2015 [updated October 17, 2015]. Available from: http://www.gallup. com/poll/186362/grads-historically-black-colleges-edge.aspx.

426. National Center for Education Statistics. Integrated post-secondary education data system. Institute for Education Sciences; 2014. Available from: http://nces.ed.gov/ipeds/Home/UseTheData.

427. National Science Foundation. Science and engineering indicators in 2014. 2013. Available from: http://www.nsf.gov/statistics/seind14/index. cfm/chapter-5/c5s3. htm.

428. Mullan F, Chen C, Petterson S, Kolsky G, Spagnola M. The social mission of medical education: ranking the schools. Annals of Internal Medicine. 2010;152:804–11.

429. Mader E, Rodriguez J, Campbell K, Smilnak T, Bazemore A, Petterson S, et al. Status of underrepresented minority and female faculty at medical schools located within historically black colleges and in Puerto Rico. Medical Education Online. 2016;21. Available from: http://med-ed-online.net/index.php/meo/article/view/29535.

430. Post Secondary National Policy Institute. Historically black colleges and universities (HBCUs): a background primer. New America; January 1, 2015. Available from: https://www.newamerica.org/post-secondary-national-policy-institute/our-blog /historically-black-colleges-and-universities-hbcus/.

431. Rudd T. Racial disproportionality in school discipline: implicit bias is heavily implicated. Columbus: Kirwan Institute for the Study of Race and Ethnicity, Ohio State University; 2014.

432. Weaver V. Unhappy harmony: accounting for black mass incarceration in a "postracial" America. In: Harris F, Lieberman R, editors. Beyond discrimination: racial inequality in a postracist era. New York: Russell Sage Foundation; 2013. p.215-256.

433. Lundy-Wagner V, Gasman M. When gender issues are not just about women: reconsidering male students at historically black colleges and universities. Teachers College Record. 2011;113(5):934–68.

434. American Association of Medical Colleges. Altering the course: black males in medicine. Washington, DC; 2015. Available from: https://members.aamc.org/eweb /upload/Black_Males_in_Medicine_Report_WEB.pdf.

435. Farmer P. Pathologies of power: health, human rights, and the new war on the poor. London: University of California Press; 2005.

436. Moineau G. Our social accountability: when will we walk the talk? Medical Education. 2015;49(1):9–11.

437. American College of Nurse-Midwives Ethics Committee. Code of ethics. Silver Springs, MD: American Colleges of Nurse-Midwives; 2013. Available from: http://www. midwife.org/ACNM/files/ACNMLibraryData/UPLOADFILENAME/000000000048 /Code-of-Ethics.pdf.

438. American Nurses Association. Code of ethics for nurses with interpretive statements. Silver Spring, MD: American Nurses Association; 2015.

439. American Medical Association. AMA code of medical ethics. American Medical Association; 2016. Available from: http://www.ama-assn.org/ama/pub/physician -resources/medical-ethics/code-medical-ethics.page.

440. Thomas J, Sage M, Dillenberg J, Guillory V. A code of ethics for public health. American Journal of Public Health. 2002;92(7):1057–60.

441. National Association of Social Workers. Code of ethics of the National Association of Social Workers: approved by the 1996 NASW Delegate Assembly and revised by the 2008 NASW Delegate Assembly. 2008. Available from: https://www.socialworkers .org/pubs/code/code.asp.

442. American Dental Association. Principles of ethics and code of professional conduct, with official advisory opinions, revised to April 2012. Chicago: American Dental Association; 2012. Available from: http://www.ada.org/~/media/ADA/About%20the%20 ADA/Files/code_of_ethics_2012.pdf?la=en.

443. American Pharmaceutical Association and American Society of Health Systems Pharmacists. Code of ethics for pharmacists. 1994. Available from: https://www.ashp .org/DocLibrary/BestPractices/EthicsEndCode.aspx.

444. American Academy of Physician Assistants. Guidelines for ethical conduct for the physician assistant profession. American Academy of Physician Assistants; 2013. Available from: https://www.aapa.org/workarea/downloadasset.aspx?id=815.

445. Valdez Z. The abandoned promise of civil rights. Sociological Forum. 2015;30(S1):612–26.

446. Myers S, Fealing K. Changes in the representation of women and minorities in biomedical careers. Academic Medicine. 2012;87(11):1525–9.

447. Patten E, Krogstad J. Black child poverty rate holds steady, even as other groups see declines. Pew Research Center; 2015 [updated July 14, 2015]. Available from: http:// www.pewresearch.org/fact-tank/2015/07/14/black-child-poverty-rate-holds-steady-even -as-other-groups-see-declines/.

448. The Sentencing Project. The United States is the world's leader in incarceration. Washington, DC: The Sentencing Project; 2016. Available from: http://www.sentencing project.org/criminal-justice-facts/.

449. White G. The data are damning: how race influences school funding. 2015 [updated September 30, 2015]. Available from: http://www.theatlantic.com/business /archive/2015/09/public-school-funding-and-the-role-of-race/408085/.

450. Spatig-Amerikaner A. Unequal education: federal loophole enables lower spending on students of color. Center for American Progress; 2012. Available from: https:// www.americanprogress.org/wp-content/uploads/2012/08/UnequalEduation.pdf.

451. Lupkin S. Why America's minority doctor problem begins in the third grade. 2016 [updated March 16, 2016]. Available from: https://news. vice. com/article/why-are -there-so-few-minority-doctors-united-states.

452. Nussbaum M. Beyond the social contract: capabilities and global justice. An Olaf Palme Lecture, delivered in Oxford on June 19, 2003. Oxford Development Studies. 2004;32(1):3–18.

453. Fried A. Moral stress in mental health practice and research. Center for Ethics Education, Fordham University; 2016 [updated April 22, 2016]. Available from: http://www .socialjusticesolutions.org/2016/04/22/moral-stress-mental-health-practice-research/.

454. Musto L, Rodney P, Vanderheide R. Toward interventions to address moral distress: navigating structure and agency. Nursing Ethics. 2015;22(1):91–102.

455. Saleh A. Zionist massacres: the creation of the Palestinian refugee problem in the 1948 war. In: Benvenisti E, Gans C, Hanafi S, editors. Israel and the Palestinian refugees. New York: Springer; 2007. p.59–128.

456. Staats C, Capatosto K, Wright R, Jackson V. State of the science: implicit bias review, 2016. Kirwan Institute for the Study of Race and Ethnicity, Ohio State University; 2016. Available from: http://kirwaninstitute.osu.edu/wp-content/uploads/2016/07/implicit-bias-2016.pdf.

457. Pacherie E. Self agency. In: Gallaher S, editor. The Oxford handbook of the self. Oxford: Oxford University Press; 2011. p.440–62.

458. DiJulio B, Norton M, Jackson S, Brodie M. Kaiser Family Foundation/CNN survey of Americans on race. Henry J. Kaiser Family Foundation; November 2015. Report No.: 8805.

459. Merriam-Webster's learner's dictionary. 2017. Available from: http://www.learnersdictionary.com/definition/elite.

460. Bonilla-Silva E. The invisible weight of whiteness: the racial grammar of everyday life in contemporary America. Ethnic & Racial Studies. 2012;35(2):173–94.

461. Palmer R, Walker L. Defending the relevance, importance of HBCUs in a white privileged society. Diverse Issues in Higher Education. December 2, 2015. Available from: http://diverseeducation. com/article/79271/.

462. Lathrop B. Nursing leadership in addressing the social determinants of health. Policy, Politics, & Nursing Practice. 2013;14(1):41–7.

463. How hard is it to get into medical school? Depends on your ethnicity. 2016. Available from: http://www.medicalschoolsuccess.com/how-hard-is-it-to-get-into-medical-school/.

464. Supreme Court of the United States. Slip opinion, Fisher v. University of Texas at Austin et al. Certiorari to the United States Court of Appeals for the Fifth Circuit. No. 14-981. Argued December 9, 2015; decided June 23, 2016. 2016. Available from: https://www.supremecourt.gov/opinions/15pdf/14-981_4g15.pdf.

465. Ford C, Airhihenbuwa C. Critical race theory, race equity, and public health: toward antiracism praxis. American Journal of Public Health. 2010;100(Supp. 1):S30–S35.

466. Stanley C. Summary and key recommendations for the recruitment and retention of faculty of color. In: Stanley C, editor. Faculty of color: teaching in predominantly white colleges and universities. Bolton, MA: Anker Publishing; 2006. p.361–73.

467. Mervis, J. In an effort to understand continuing racial disparities, NIH to test for bias in study sections. Science Magazine. June 9, 2016. Available from: http://www.sciencemag.org/news/2016/06/effort-understand-continuing-racial-disparities-nih-test-bias-study-sections.

INDEX

Page numbers in italics indicate tables.

Castro, Connie, 195
Charmaz, Kathy, 16
civil rights movement, 9, 21, 244
Clark, Trenette T., 165
class: differences in color experiences, 18–19; health insurance and access to care, 241; in health professions institutions, 202–5; Native American poverty, 230–31; US racial disparities in wealth, 214
climate: of exclusion, 31; defined, 56; dialogue and, 59–60, 92–96; diversity programs, 79, 80–84; for equity, 1–2; faculty and student diversity, 72; at historically black colleges and universities, 42; institutional components of, 17–18, 111–12; leadership and, 98–99; participant satisfaction and, 110–11; recruitment and retention, 57–60, 58–59; reports of racism and, 88–89; sensitivity to, 54; thriving strategies and, 172; wealth inequality for blacks, 214
color blindness, 21, 46, 53, 61, 115–16, 126, 246, 248–49
coping strategies, 1–2, 50–51, 166–71
criminal justice system, 4–5, 23–24
Cuban Americans, 6, 220, 224
culture: academic, 27–28, 38, 46, 210; climate and, 56; of diversity, 109; dominant and nondominant, 18, 47, 212, 231–33; hybridization of, 240; mentoring and, 143, 217; organizational, racism in, 166; real inclusion and, 78, 88, 98; recruitment and, 184–85; role models and, 175–77; subcultures in health professions, 3

dentistry: complaints of discrimination, 91–92; diversity standards for accreditation, 108–9; education, diversity in, 6–9, 73; holistic admissions, 191; reports of racism and, 91–92; in study design, 15; URM faculty hiring statistics, 63, 198
dialogue(s): beginning inclusion and, 96–97; climate and, 59–60, 92–93, 111, 250; covert exclusion and, 93–94; "difficult," 111; indifference and, 94–96; real inclusion and, 97–98, 106; social change and, 100
DiAngelo, Robin, 94
difference: as inclusion goal, 3, 78, 88; ornamental diversity and, 111; patients of color and, 187, 192–93; in perspectives and experiences, 4–5, 18–19, 236–38; racial, framework of, 10, 23; recognition of, 53
diversity: beginning inclusion and, 75–76, 85–87; "caring for," 76; climate stages of, 57–60, 58–59; covert exclusion and, 72–75, 80–84; defined, 2; excellence and, 195; "grow your own" recruitment and, 122–26; in health professions education, 6–9, 7, 8; indifference and, 72–75, 84–85, 101; institutional, tools for, 17; in leadership roles, 129–33; privilege and, 2; programs, 79, 80–84; race-conscious strategies for, 245–52; real inclusion, 78–79, 87–88, 97–98; teaching/service relating to, 186–89; tokenism, 39–40, 195–96
Dorsey, Archie, 152–53

education. See health professions education
Edwards, Janice Berry, 165
Ellison, Ralph, 22–23
equity: absent from workplace treatment,

32–37; climates fostering, 1–2; climate stages of, 57; defined, 2; and ethical codes in health profession, 243–44; excellence and, 195; in health professions, 6; implicit bias and, 21–22, 246, 251; institutional, tools for, 17; investment in research time, 3–4; participant satisfaction and, 110–11; practice/research and, 192–96; privilege and, 2; race-conscious strategies for, 245–52; research on, 116–17, 251–52; teaching/service relating to, 186–89; as trigger for racism, 168

ethnicity: differences in experience of color, 18–19; discrimination in health professions, 211–14, 216; exclusion and control and, 50–51; type of institution as factor in exclusion, 42–44; US government categories, 220, 225–26

exclusion and control: in admissions interviews, 190; consequences, 44; covert, 60–64, 72–75, 93–94, 99–101; dialogue and, 93–94; diversity programs and, 80–84; experiences of black faculty, 215–16; indifference, 64–67, 72–75, 84–85, 89–92; intersectionality and, 22; leadership and, 91–92, 99–101; mentoring and, 138–39, 179–83; overview, 29–31; prevalence in health education, 28; reports of racism and, 88–89; seeking supports and, 165; strategies of, 22; type of institution as factor, 42–44. See also inclusion; isolation

faculty members of color: benefits, 1; black, 214; contributions in health education, 5, 18; foreign-born, 206–11; hiring statistics for, 62–63, 66–67, 198; mentoring needs, 17–18; overview of

experiences, 215–16, 240–42; racial perceptions of, 10; salaries, 9; students of color and, 4; study methodology for, 14. See also recruitment and retention

Fisher v. University of Texas, 191, 249–50

Ford Foundation, 111

foreign-born status: of blacks, 214; demographics, 205–6; differences in experience of color, 18–19, 205; immigrant versus domestic nonimmigrant groups, 217–19; out-group status and, 29; URM experiences and, 206–11. See also immigration

Garrison-Wade, Dorothy F., 1

Gasman, Marybeth, 13

gender: angry black woman stereotype, 199–200, 203; differences in experience of color, 18–19; exclusion and control and, 50–51; experience by race and, 22; in health professions institutions, 198–202; leadership stresses on black women, 130; nursing as gendered profession, 200–202; personal values for success and, 153; retention of female faculty, 96; type of institution as factor in exclusion, 42–44

Ginther, Donna, 116–17

Glaser, Barney, 16

Guevara, James P., 142–43

Guinier, Lani, 189, 250–51

Harvard Medical School, 119

Harvey, William B., 62–63

Head, Christian, 20

health professions education: black faculty, 214; career trajectory and, 120–22; commitment to social justice in, 245; contributions by faculty of color, 5, 18; diversity in, 3; employment of foreign born in, 205–11; ethical codes and obligations, 243–44; faculty collegiality, 119–20; historically black colleges and universities, 234–40; institutions serving minorities, 10–11; promotion and tenure, 45–47; race-conscious education and practice, 250; racist processes in, 16–17; social hierarchies in higher education, 38–39, 51; tradition of exclusion in, 28; type of institution as factor in exclusion, 42–44; URM faculty hiring statistics, 63, 66–67, 198

Heckler Report, 4

Hispanic Americans: dialogue and, 95; faculty experiences, 219–25; institutions serving, 10–11, 13; mentoring and, 177, 184–85; representation in health professions, 6. *See also* Latinos/Latinas; Puerto Ricans

historically black colleges and universities: climate at, 31; contributions to social justice, 247–48; foreign- versus US-born students, 216–17; health professions pipeline and, 10–11; importance in health professions education, 241–42; overview, 234–40; recognition of difference at, 197–98; STEM degrees at, 12; study subjects from, 14–15. *See also* black Americans

Hu-DeHart, Evelyn, 170

human agency, 172, 246

humility (cultural), 5, 18, 27, 113, 143, 186–87

immigration: attitudes toward African immigrants, 205; demographics,

205–6; generational experiences, 216, 218; immigrant versus domestic nonimmigrant groups, 217–19; Immigration and Nationality Act of 1965, 205; out-group status and, 29; Puerto Ricans as immigrants, 177; undocumented immigrants in health care, 224–25; US quota system, 226. *See also* foreign-born status; language

implicit bias, 21–22, 52, 246, 251

inclusion: beginning dialogue on, 95–96; comfort with difference and, 3, 78, 88; diversity and, 75–76, 78–79, 85–88, 97–98; leadership and, 70–72, 79, 96–98, 102–6; overview, 57–60, 58–59, 67–70; real, and participant satisfaction, 110–11. *See also* exclusion and control

indifference: climate stages for inclusion, 57–60, 58–59, 64–67, 72–75, 84–85; color blindness and, 21; dialogue and, 94–95; leadership and, 91–92, 95, 101; as most prevalent climate, 111; reports of racism and, 89–92

individuality, 16–17, 22–23, 28

Institute of Medicine, 6

institutions serving minorities: demographics, 10–11; opportunities in, 13–14; STEM degrees and, 12

intersectionality: Asian American intersectional experiences, 211–14, 216; class in health professions institutions, 202–5; differences in color experiences, 18–19; exclusion and control and, 22, 50–51; foreign-born experiences of, 206–11; gender in health professions institutions, 198–202; interview format and, 15–16; prejudice and, 118; recognition of difference and, 197–98 invalidation: of cultural norms, 27–28; denial of professional status, 23–24; in job applications, 32; job performance expectations and, 34–35; overview, 22–28; of professional knowledge, 26–27; in promotion and tenure, 46–47; proving and, 47–49; of role authority, 40–42; self-confidence and, 49–50

invisibility, 22–23

Islam, 214, 226–30

isolation: climate and, 59, 73–75, 92–93; dialogue and, 92–93; "grow your own" recruitment and, 70; loneliness, 164–65; mentoring and, 137; outsider treatment, 29–31; overview, 17, 44–45; proactive networking and, 156; tenure review and, 46. *See also* exclusion and control

Johnson, Brad W., 52

Junkins, Edward, 14

Kaite, Charis P., 200

Kouta, Christiana, 200

language (non-English): foreign-born faculty members of color, 206–8, 211; in health professions education, 176–77; at historically black colleges and universities, 239, 242; in patient care, 103, 213, 220, 223–25

Laszloffy, Tracey, 148–49

Latinos/Latinas: climate of indifference and, 66; faculty experiences, 219–25; faculty hiring statistics, 63, 198; racial and national identification of, 220–22; representation in health professions, 3, 6–9; type of institution as factor in exclusion, 43; US attitudes toward, 205. *See also* Hispanic Americans

leadership: beginning inclusion and, 96–97, 102–5; commitment to diversity, 17–18, 51, 52–55, 63–64, 73, 79, 86–88, 142; covert exclusion and, 91–92, 99–101; demographic data for, 131–32; development of URM leaders, 69–70; importance for climate, 58–59, 98–99, 111–12; indifference and, 91–92, 95, 101; mentoring for, 129–33; real inclusion and, 70–72, 79, 97–98, 105–6; white dominance in, 3, 28, 91, 101, 105

Lutz, Kristin, 14, 132

Mainah, Fredah, 130, 153

medicine: diversity in medical education, 74; diversity standards for accreditation, 108–9; mentoring, 124–28; in study design, 15; URM faculty hiring statistics, 63, 66–67, 198

mentoring: accidental, 126–28; best practices for, 143; climate of exclusion and, 138–39, 179–83; climate of indifference and, 66; cross-race competencies, 116–17, 138–39, 143; cultural change and, 147; by faculty supervisor, 128–29; "godfathers" in promotion and tenure, 47; "grow your own" strategy, 122–26; at historically black colleges and universities, 236–40; inadequate, 119–22, 160–61; needs of faculty of color, 17–18, 135–36, 142; nourishing the pipeline, 183–86; at other institutions, 126; proactive engagement of, 155–58, 162–64; programs for, 133–35, 142–43; role models, 175–77; sources of, 122–23; statistics and studies on, 113–16, 119, 129–30; targeted recruitment and, 68–70; validation of personal experience, 136–42, 177–78

and, 207; freedom of speech and, 89–90; in health professions education, 16–17; implicit bias and, 21–22, 52, 246, 251; intervention versus silence and, 51, 52–53, 90–91, 93; medical faculty, racial bias of, 20; microaggression, 164–65; Middle Eastern racial identity, 226–27; minority tax, 174, 196; Native American racial identity, 231; origin of racial hierarchies, 20–21; "race rules" for advancement, 57, 148–53; racial literacy, 250–51; racial prejudice of mentors, 116–17; rejection of difference and, 197–98; silencing of challenges to, 38–39; similarity-attraction theory, 115; strategic engagement/disengagement, 168–71; type of institution as factor in exclusion, 42–44; US government racial categories, 220; as Western contrivance, 14; white accountability and, 89–90; white intellectual superiority, belief in, 10. *See also* black Americans; stereotype(s); structural racism

racial literacy, 250–51

Rayburn, William F., 132

recruitment and retention, 9; benefits of diversity and, 67–68, 122–26; climate elements, overview, 57–60, 58–59; "grow your own" strategy, 69–70, 122–26; health professions, overview, 5–6; institutional reputation and, 74–77; mentoring and, 120–26; race-conscious hiring, 248–49; sense of safety and, 76–77; targeted initiatives, 68–70. *See also* faculty members of color

religion, 27, 214, 226–30

research: on equity, 116–17, 251–52; minority, support for; Native

American approaches to, 27; race-related stress and, 25; racial experiences and, 42–44, 43; as tenure factor, 3–4; URM subjects of, 5, 13, 36–37, 68

Rockquemore, Kerry Ann, 148–49

Scott-Jones, Diane, 62–63

silencing: control strategies and, 22; in faculty-student dialogue, 93–94; intervention versus silence in racial experiences, 51, 52–53, 90–91, 93; overview, 37–39

similarity-attraction theory, 115

Smith, Daryl G., 9, 111, 201

Stanley, Christine A., 165

STEM (science, technology, engineering, and math), 12

stereotype(s): angry black woman, 199–200, 203; assertive versus aggressive behavior, 215; fear of black men, 24–25, 241; presumption of criminality, 23–24; threats, 25–26. *See also* race and racism

structural racism: color blindness and, 21, 46, 53, 61, 115–16, 126, 246, 248–49; individual experiences of, 1–2; investment in research time, 3–4

Student National Medical Association (SNMA), 85

students: exclusionary climates and, 179–83; faculty members of color and, 4, 23; mentoring students, 174–75; minority recruitment, 5; nourishing the pipeline, 183–86

Sullivan Commission, 1

Syrian refugees, 218

tenure and promotion. *See* promotion and tenure

testocratic merit, 189

thriving strategies: being proactive, 155–58; choosing opportunities, 158–62; climate and, 172; coping with everyday racism, 166–71; having a vision, 145–48, 173; knowing the game, 148–53; living your values, 153–55, 161–62, 172–73; overview, 18, 144–45, 171–72; seeking mentorship, 162–64; seeking supports, 164–66

tokenism, 39–40

Trump, Donald, 197

Turner, Caroline S. T., 9, 27, 164, 250

underrepresented minorities (URMs): diverse climate and, 110–11; foreign- versus US-born, 218–19; insurance and access to health care and, 241; overview of health professions, 3, 6–9; promotion and tenure, 45–47; recruitment, 9

using, 39–40

Victorino, Christine A., 56

Westphal, Judith A., 201

whiteness: affirmative action and, 9–10, 248–50; defined, 197–98; diversity versus equity and, 2, 21; dominant in health professions, 3, 10–11, 13, 28; Eurocentric traits and norms, 23, 27; freedom of speech and, 89–90; intervention versus silence in racial experiences, 51, 52–53, 90–91, 93; invalidation and, 22; invisibility in, 252; in leadership roles, 3, 28, 91; patients of color and, 1; perception of racial experience and, 4–5; postraciality and, 21, 246–47; and privilege, 2, 16–17, 20–21, 32, 34–35, 37, 51, 53; racial stereotypes of, 24–25; white antiracism, 52–55

Williams, Christine L., 201

Wilson, Donald E., 145

Wingfield, Adia H., 201

Zirkel, Sabrina, 175